Studies in Systems, Decision and Control

Volume 513

The series "Studies in Systems, Decision and Control" (SSDC) covers both new developments and advances, as well as the state of the art, in the various areas of broadly perceived systems, decision making and control–quickly, up to date and with a high quality. The intent is to cover the theory, applications, and perspectives on the state of the art and future developments relevant to systems, decision making, control, complex processes and related areas, as embedded in the fields of engineering, computer science, physics, economics, social and life sciences, as well as the paradigms and methodologies behind them. The series contains monographs, textbooks, lecture notes and edited volumes in systems, decision making and control spanning the areas of Cyber-Physical Systems, Autonomous Systems, Sensor Networks, Control Systems, Energy Systems, Automotive Systems, Biological Systems, Vehicular Networking and Connected Vehicles, Aerospace Systems, Automation, Manufacturing, Smart Grids, Nonlinear Systems, Power Systems, Robotics, Social Systems, Economic Systems and other. Of particular value to both the contributors and the readership are the short publication timeframe and the world-wide distribution and exposure which enable both a wide and rapid dissemination of research output.

Indexed by SCOPUS, DBLP, WTI Frankfurt eG, zbMATH, SCImago.

All books published in the series are submitted for consideration in Web of Science.

Tofigh Allahviranloo · Farhad Hosseinzadeh Lotfi ·
Zohreh Moghaddas · Mohsen Vaez-Ghasemi
Editors

Decision Making in Healthcare Systems

Springer

Editors
Tofigh Allahviranloo
Faculty of Engineering and Natural Sciences
Istinye University
İstanbul, Türkiye

Farhad Hosseinzadeh Lotfi
Department of Mathematics
Science and Research Branch
Islamic Azad University
Tehran, Iran

Zohreh Moghaddas
School of Information Technology
Deakin University, Waurn Ponds Campus
Geelong, VIC, Australia

Mohsen Vaez-Ghasemi
Department of Mathematics
Islamic Azad University
Rasht, Iran

ISSN 2198-4182 ISSN 2198-4190 (electronic)
Studies in Systems, Decision and Control
ISBN 978-3-031-46734-9 ISBN 978-3-031-46735-6 (eBook)
https://doi.org/10.1007/978-3-031-46735-6

This Springer imprint is published by the registered company Springer Nature Switzerland AG
The registered company address is: Gewerbestrasse 11, 6330 Cham, Switzerland

Paper in this product is recyclable.

Contents

Methodologies for Decision-Making in the Health and Medicine Sector

Kemal Gökhan Nalbant and Sevgi Aydin

Abstract The fields of medicine and healthcare have benefited significantly from technological advances, investments, and software in our ever-evolving and transforming world, as they have from these same developments in every other industry. Because of the tremendous strides that have been made in the realm of specialist software in the health industry, the health system has become significantly more technologically advanced and functional. As a consequence of advances in technology, diagnosis and treatment are now more easily available, and favorable outcomes are being achieved with greater frequency. The growth of Artificial Intelligence (AI) technology has resulted in the establishment of ultra-modern medical facilities, such as hospitals and other health institutions. In these hospitals that are getting more and more advanced, robotic surgery techniques are much better than traditional ones. This means that patients can recover faster and have a lower chance of complications. In this chapter, we take a look at the many approaches to decision-making that are utilized in the field of health and medicine. Machine learning, artificial intelligence, the internet of things, deep learning, and natural language processing are just a few of the major methods that are utilized in this discipline. This chapter also delves into the topics of organizational decision-making in healthcare as well as medical decision-making. In addition, the marketing of healthcare services and some of the benefits of using marketing tactics for health services are both covered in this chapter.

Keywords Decision-making · Artificial intelligence · Healthcare marketing · Machine learning · Health sector

---

K. G. Nalbant (✉)
Istanbul Beykent University, Software Engineering, Istanbul, Turkey
e-mail: kemalnalbant@beykent.edu.tr

S. Aydin
Istanbul Beykent University, Business, Istanbul, Turkey

T. Allahviranloo et al. (eds.), *Decision Making in Healthcare Systems*,
Studies in Systems, Decision and Control 513,
https://doi.org/10.1007/978-3-031-46735-6_1

The Internet of Things (IoT), which has emerged as one of the most innovative technologies in recent years, has been largely responsible for the paradigm shift that has been brought about in conventional methods of providing medical treatment. IoT-based eHealth aims to provide intelligent and individualized medical care services by utilizing the principle of frictionless data sharing across connected devices, which is then followed by effective data analytics [11].

The goal of what is known as "artificial intelligence" (AI) is to simulate human cognitive abilities. It is bringing about a paradigm shift in the healthcare industry, which is being propelled by the expanding availability of healthcare data and the quick advancement of analytical tools. There are many different kinds of medical data that can be processed by AI (structured and unstructured). Popular applications of artificial intelligence include methods of machine learning for structured data, such as the traditional support vector machine and neural network, as well as the more recent deep learning and natural language processing for unstructured data. Both of these methods can be used with structured data. Cancer, neurology, and cardiology are examples of important illness areas that make use of AI capabilities [23].

It is becoming increasingly clear that the application of artificial intelligence (AI) approaches will be critical to the improvement of clinical research and care. Natural Language Processing (NLP) and Deep Learning (DL) techniques have been utilized in order to extract information from a significant number of electronic health records (EHR), the majority of which are locked in clinical narratives. In the context of robotics-assisted operations, computer vision techniques can be used for medical imaging, natural language processing techniques can be used for analyzing unstructured information in electronic health records, and reinforcement learning techniques can be used as well [32]. While analyzing text and determining the grammatical relationships between phrases, NLP algorithms can be used to find clinically relevant phenotypes. This can be done while the algorithms are also analyzing the text. In clinical records, rule-based natural language processing approaches may be utilized to achieve high sensitivity (the identification of a significant proportion of actual cases) as well as high positive predictive value. One of the fields in which computer science is becoming increasingly helpful in a wide variety of activities is the healthcare industry. Language processing is at the heart of many of the most exciting new applications for artificial intelligence, and this trend is sweeping the healthcare industry from the most fundamental level practices all the way up to the most specialized areas. The capabilities of these AI algorithms may enable the detection of distinguishing clinical traits among patients, which aids in clinical treatment and reduces methodological heterogeneity in medical research on a wide range of health conditions [22].

4 Medical Decision Making

The process of making medical decisions encompasses decisions made in medicine, policy, or daily contexts that have an effect on the health of individuals or the general population. When compared to other sorts of judgments, the process of making medical decisions is usually fraught with risk and uncertainty, challenging trade-offs, information overload, decisions regarding future consequences, and interdependent behaviors, in addition to a dependence on data. In the field of medical decision-making, research uses people's psychological processes, especially the systematic ways they deviate from rationality, to better understand and improve the health outcomes of decisions, such as by "nudging" people toward healthy choices [24].

Since over half a century ago, formal research and other relevant applications have focused on the process of decision-making in the medical field. There is a professional and academic society devoted to studying and improving decision practices called the Organization for Medical Decision Making (SMDM). This society hosts yearly meetings and publishes a magazine called Sage Publications: Medical Decision Making (Sage Publications). There is also a paradigm for investigating medical decision-making processes that is founded on the normative comparative method. This paradigm has been around for a while and is pretty well established. The archetype of the person who makes medical decisions is that of a stoic, emotionless, and utterly logical doctor who methodically considers well-defined possibilities (i.e., therapeutic choices or diagnostic alternatives) on the basis of a meticulous weighing of the facts. Equally typical is his or her colleague, who is definitely less skilled: a faulty reasoner who is susceptible to biases and particularly incompetent in applying probability theory to choice difficulties. Because of these inadequacies, erroneous decision-making procedures commonly occur [29].

When it comes to medical matters, there is always an element of unpredictability surrounding the consequences of decisions. Incomplete information can be gleaned from clinical examinations and other diagnostic methods. The indications for the majority of therapeutic approaches, in addition to the risks and benefits associated with those approaches, are ill-defined or unknown. When it comes to the vast majority of clinical issues, information gleaned from randomized clinical trials is either inaccessible or cannot be generalized to the patient in question. Probability theory, the threshold model of decision-making, and expected value decision analysis are all examples of useful tools that can be utilized to assist in navigating this uncertainty [26].

With a few significant exceptions, teenagers do not have the legal ability to offer permission for or refuse medical procedures. These exceptions are rare, though. However, there are some circumstances in which the question arises over whether or not a mature child should be allowed to make a life-altering medical choice that would be contested if the decision were made by the minor's parent [13].

the diseases that individuals have, which is done via gene research, it will be possible to forestall the conditions that would result in the appearance of an infection. As a direct result of this, it is possible to avoid contracting the condition, which in turn enables people to enjoy a long and healthy life. The use of robots in the health and medical fields contributes greatly to the reduction of the amount of time spent on treatment as well as the amount of work done by doctors. In addition to that, the circumstances will provide a new perspective on the practice of medicine. Health and medical technology have come a long way, and both people and robots have helped a lot. The advancement of artificial intelligence gadgets will allow future generations to live lives that are both healthier and longer than their predecessors. The use of artificial intelligence technologies has made it feasible for clinicians to treat patients remotely during the pandemic (COVID-19). Interaction between medical staff and patients should be kept to a minimum. Healthcare experts made an effort to protect the patient's health by utilizing equipment that utilizes artificial intelligence. Clinicians are able to diagnose patients, prescribe medications, and provide treatments without ever having to communicate directly with the patients. Additionally, positive identification of COVID-19 cases is achievable through the utilization of artificial intelligence. When it comes to the education of medical professionals, artificial intelligence, robots, and other forms of technology are used rather frequently. Virtual reality (VR) technology that shows human anatomy has made it simpler for students of medicine and health to learn new information. The use of digital technology in the process of decision-making is of crucial relevance in the field of medicine and health.

References

1. Abbasi, F., Allahviranloo, T.: Conception and implementation of a new data-driven fuzzy method for reliability and safety analysis. New Math. Nat. Comput. **16**(02), 339–361 (2020). https://doi.org/10.1142/s1793005720500210
2. Abbasi, F., Allahviranloo, T.: The fuzzy arithmetic operations of transmission average on Pseudo-Hexagonal fuzzy numbers and its application in fuzzy system reliability analysis. Fuzzy Inf. Eng. **13**(1), 58–78 (2021). https://doi.org/10.1080/16168658.2021.1915449
3. Abbasi, F., Allahviranloo, T.: Realistic solution of fuzzy critical path problems, case study: the airport's cargo ground operation systems. Granul. Comput. **8**(3), 617–632 (2022). https://doi.org/10.1007/s41066-022-00347-w
4. Akram, M., Shahzadi, S., Shah, S.M.U., Allahviranloo, T.: A fully Fermatean fuzzy multi-objective transportation model using an extended DEA technique. Granul. Comput. (2023). https://doi.org/10.1007/s41066-023-00399-6
5. Allahviranloo, T., Abbasi, F.: A new estimation of failure analysis in fuzzy environment, case study: the electrical model failure for the football stadium. New Math. Nat. Comput. **18**(03), 791–817 (2022). https://doi.org/10.1142/s1793005722500387
6. Amirteimoori, A., Allahviranloo, T., Kordrostami, S., Bagheri, S.F.: Improving decision-making units in performance analysis methods: a data envelopment analysis approach. Math. Sci. (2023). https://doi.org/10.1007/s40096-023-00512-5
7. Amirteimoori, A., Allahviranloo, T., Zadmirzaei, M.: Scale elasticity and technical efficiency analysis in the European forest sector: a stochastic value-based approach. Eur. J. Forest Res. (2023). https://doi.org/10.1007/s10342-023-01589-2

8. Amirteimoori, A., Allahviranloo, T., Zadmirzaei, M., Hasanzadeh, F.: On the environmental performance analysis: a combined fuzzy data envelopment analysis and artificial intelligence algorithms. Expert Syst. Appl. **224**, 119953 (2023). https://doi.org/10.1016/j.eswa.2023.119953
9. Baek, J.W., Kim, J.C., Chun, J., Chung, K.: Hybrid clustering based health decision-making for improving dietary habits. Technol. Health Care **27**(5), 459–472 (2019)
10. Cai, C.J., Reif, E., Hegde, N., Hipp, J., Kim, B., Smilkov, D., Terry, M.: Human-centered tools for coping with imperfect algorithms during medical decision-making. In: Proceedings of the 2019 Chi Conference on Human Factors in Computing Systems, pp. 1–14 (2019)
11. Chatterjee, P., Cymberknop, L.J., Armentano, R.L.: IoT-based decision support system for intelligent healthcare—applied to cardiovascular diseases. In: 2017 7th International Conference on Communication Systems and Network Technologies (CSNT), pp. 362–366. IEEE (2017)
12. Chowdhury, N.K., Kabir, M.A., Rahman, M.M.: An ensemble-based multi-criteria decision making method for COVID-19 cough classification. arXiv:2110.00508 (2021)
13. Diekema, D.S.: Adolescent brain development and medical decision-making. Pediatrics **146**(Supplement_1), S18–S24 (2020)
14. Domínguez, S., Carnero, M.C.: Fuzzy multicriteria modelling of decision making in the renewal of healthcare technologies. Mathematics **8**(6), 944 (2020)
15. Drake, J.I., de Hart, J.C.T., Monleón, C., Toro, W., Valentim, J.: Utilization of multiple-criteria decision analysis (MCDA) to support healthcare decision-making FIFARMA, 2016. J. Mark. Access Health Policy **5**(1), 1360545 (2017)
16. Glaize, A., Duenas, A., Di Martinelly, C., Fagnot, I.: Healthcare decision-making applications using multicriteria decision analysis: a scoping review. J. Multi-Criteria Decis. Anal. **26**(1–2), 62–83 (2019)
17. Grote, T., Berens, P.: On the ethics of algorithmic decision-making in healthcare. J. Med. Ethics **46**(3), 205–211 (2020)
18. Guo, K.L.: DECIDE: a decision-making model for more effective decision making by health care managers. Health News **39**(3), 133–141 (2020)
19. Hansson, S.O.: Decision theory. A Brief Introduction. Department of Philosophy and the History of technology. Royal Institute of Technology, Stockholm (1994)
20. Harputlugil, T.I.M.U.C.I.N., Prins, M.A.T.T.H.I.J.S., Gültekin, A.T., Topçu, Y.I.: Conceptual framework for potential implementations of multi criteria decision making (MCDM) methods for design quality assessment. In: Management and Innovation for a Sustainable Built Environment MISBE 2011, Amsterdam, The Netherlands, June 20–23. CIB, Working Commissions W55, W65, W89, W112; ENHR and AESP (2011)
21. Henig, M.I., Buchanan, J.T.: Solving MCDM problems: process concepts. J.Multi-Criteria Decis. Anal. **5**(1), 3–21 (1996)
22. Jain, K., Prajapati, V.: NLP/Deep learning techniques in healthcare for decision making. Prim. Health Care Open Access **11**(3), 1–4 (2021)
23. Jiang, F., Jiang, Y., Zhi, H., Dong, Y., Li, H., Ma, S., Wang, Y.: Artificial intelligence in healthcare: past, present and future. Stroke Vasc. Neurol. **2**(4) (2017)
24. Li, M., Chapman, G.B.: Medical decision making. The Wiley Encyclopedia of Health Psychology, pp. 347–353 (2020)
25. Loftus, T.J., Tighe, P.J., Filiberto, A.C., Efron, P.A., Brakenridge, S.C., Mohr, A.M., Bihorac, A.: Artificial intelligence and surgical decision-making. JAMA Surg. **155**(2), 148–158 (2020)
26. Lurie, J.D., Sox, H.C.: Principles of medical decision making. Spine **24**(5), 493–498 (1999)
27. Majumder, M.: Impact of urbanization on uater shortage in face of climatic aberrations. Springer (2015)
28. Mehta, S.: Healthcare marketing. In: Healthcare System Management: Methods and Techniques, pp. 239–260. Springer Nature Singapore, Singapore (2022)
29. Patel, V.L., Kaufman, D.R., Arocha, J.F.: Emerging paradigms of cognition in medical decision-making. J. Biomed. Inform. **35**(1), 52–75 (2002)
30. Pohekar, S.D., Ramachandran, M.: Application of multi-criteria decision making to sustainable energy planning—a review. Renew. Sustain. Energy Rev. **8**(4), 365–381 (2004)

31. Purcarea, E.V.L.: The impact of marketing strategies in healthcare systems. J. Med. Life **12**(2), 93 (2019)
32. Seyyedabbasi, A.: A reinforcement learning-based metaheuristic algorithm for solving global optimization problems. Adv. Eng. Softw. **178**, 103411 (2023). https://doi.org/10.1016/j.advengsoft.2023.10341
33. Shahid, N., Rappon, T., Berta, W.: Applications of artificial neural networks in health care organizational decision-making: a scoping review. PLoS ONE **14**(2), e0212356 (2019)

The Application of System Simulation in the Health Sector: A Rapid Review

Mohammadreza Mobinizadeh, Marita Mohammadshahi, Parisa Aboee, Zeinab Fakoorfard, Alireza Olyaeemanesh, and Efat Mohamadi

Abstract Introduction: Implementation of applied mathematics aligned with evidence informed decision-making methods can be used for improving of health system performance. This research intends to help the policymakers decide on the use of simulation methods (with operations research techniques) in the health care by reviewing the available evidence. Methods: By such rapid-review, Cochrane, PubMed and Google Scholar databases have been searched by April 2023. The inclusion criteria were studies that investigated on the use of various kind of simulation (with operations research techniques) on the health policy context. Results: On the base of retrieved data, system dynamics (SD), discrete event simulation (DES), and agent-based modeling (ABM) were the most commonly used methods. SD is a way of creating computer models that show how complex systems work and change over time. DES refers to how things happen to one person, and what they experience in those situations. The ABM model looks at separate things and shows how they behave by following simple rules. Conclusion: These models (DS) can help combine feedback information with real-time data to create useful tools for managing health care and making health system policies. This new way of collecting information can help decision makers make better decisions.

M. Mobinizadeh · M. Mohammadshahi · P. Aboee · Z. Fakoorfard · A. Olyaeemanesh (✉)
National Institute for Health Research, Tehran University of Medical Sciences, Tehran, Iran
e-mail: arolyaee@gmail.com

M. Mobinizadeh
e-mail: mr.mobini1986@gmail.com

M. Mohammadshahi
e-mail: m.mohamadshahi@gmail.com

P. Aboee
e-mail: abooep65@gmail.com

Z. Fakoorfard
e-mail: zfakoor929@gmail.com

A. Olyaeemanesh · E. Mohamadi
Health Equity research center (HERC), Tehran University of Medical Sciences, Tehran, Iran
e-mail: efat.mohamadi@gmail.com

T. Allahviranloo et al. (eds.), *Decision Making in Healthcare Systems*,
Studies in Systems, Decision and Control 513,
https://doi.org/10.1007/978-3-031-46735-6_2

Data Science in the Field of Health

Handan Kulan and Ezgi Özer

Abstract Data science in healthcare has made great progress using data analysis and machine learning methods that have the potential to detect and help solve healthcare problems. After mortality and during morbidity, relevant data about a health problem have been gathered. This massive amount of data in various forms needs to be handled for any healthcare issues are significant. With the growth of big data in healthcare communities, accurate analysis of medical data has the benefits of early disease detection, improved patient care, and effective community services. Because of its significance, there is a need to develop efficient and better-performing data analytics techniques and tools to analyze medical big data from the gene level to the clinical level. The purpose of data analytics in healthcare is to find new insights in data, at least partially automate tasks such as diagnosing, and to facilitate clinical decision-making. Also, healthcare analytics has the potential to reduce costs of treatment, predict outbreaks of disease, avoid preventable diseases, and improve the quality of life in general. The average human lifespan is increasing across the world population and the application of big data analytics in healthcare are increasing day by day. Different format of health data are used for different types of analyses. For example, IoT gadgets are used by certain patients and clinicians as wearable monitors to track heartbeat and temperature. This signal generated data should be carefully analyzed over time. Also, scans such as X-rays, magnetic resonance images (MRIs), and computed tomography (CAT) scans can be studied with different data analysis techniques and machine learning algorithms to visualize the insides of the body in depth. In addition, data on individual cases of disease are analyzed; data received as text must be sorted, categorized, and coded for statistical analysis; and data from surveys might need to be weighted to produce valid estimates for sampled populations. The number of resources healthcare professionals can obtain from their patients continues to increase. Since these data are normally in different formats and sizes, it can be difficult for analysis. However, the current focus is no longer on how big the data is,

H. Kulan (✉) · E. Özer
Istinye University, Computer Engineering, Istanbul, Turkey
e-mail: handan.kulan@istinye.edu.tr

E. Özer
e-mail: ezgi.ozer@istinye.edu.tr

T. Allahviranloo et al. (eds.), *Decision Making in Healthcare Systems*,
Studies in Systems, Decision and Control 513,
https://doi.org/10.1007/978-3-031-46735-6_3

but how intelligently it is managed by data analysis techniques and machine learning algorithms. This study examines analytical techniques for different forms of health-related data to generate comprehensive healthcare reports and transform them into relevant critical insights that can then be used to provide better care.

Keywords Healthcare · Data analytics · Signal processing · Image processing · Machine learning

1 Introduction and Motivation

Today, the increasing volume of digital data has created new problem areas. The main difficulties are developing methods or systems to handle large amounts of multidimensional and complex data, new types of data and distributed data, and to use and security of data. The enormous amount of health-related data has made it difficult to process these data by traditional data processing methods and has led to the introduction of the concept of big data into health services. They can be analyzed completely and quickly using data science to transform high-volume, fast, and diverse data sets that cannot be stored, managed, and analyzed into meaningful and value-creating results.

Data Science in healthcare collects data and analyzes it with the help of data analytic techniques. The purpose of healthcare data analysis is to predict and solve problem using data-driven findings in a quick way. From the genet level, molecular level, to the clinical level in major healthcare areas such as electronic health record maintenance, disease diagnosis, and prediction of emergency conditions of patients, data are accumulated. This big-style health data refers to the vast quantities of information created by the digitization of everything, that gets consolidated and analyzed by specific analytic techniques. Collected data can be any format; text document, image file or time-stamped data. Doctors can monitor a patient's blood pressure, circadian cycle, and calorie intake using laboratory equipment or analytical tools. If the disease will be tested on animals, an experiment will be conducted in the laboratory and then the data will be evaluated. Documentation output from laboratory tests or analytic tools can be evaluated to identify critical factors in disease. In the preprocessing processes of the document, the missing values must be filled and then normalized. Also, text values need to be converted to numeric values in order to process them with analytical techniques or machine learning algorithms.

Early diagnosis and disease classification are the most important elements of disease management. Investigating disease findings and further examination not only reduces the risk of death of patients but also increases the quality of life of the patients. Depending on the nature of the disease to be diagnosed, both the syndromes seen in the patients and the imaging and/or by analyzing activities recorded as time or frequency series, diseases can be diagnosed. The stage or severity of the disease can be classified, with the help of the findings obtained. Statistical and visual data is obtained from past patients in order to make diagnoses and predictions. In addition, in order to make these diagnoses and inferences, in general terms decision support-based software programs based on statistical and mathematical methods are used.

In recent years, parallel to the development of technology, computers, and computer-aided systems have had an important place in human life. The studies carried out in order to summarize the data, establish a relationship between the data, and interpret the results as a result of these relationships has developed the concept of artificial intelligence. A computer system created using artificial intelligence techniques establishes relationships between events using the available data and has the ability to predict new events to come.

There are different methods for all processes in preprocessing steps. After preprocessing steps, the feature selection methods can be applied to determine critical factors in disease. By evaluating accuracy result of machine learning algorithms, the reliability of text data evaluation is determined. In addition to numeric data evaluation, to characterize trends and detect changes in disease incidence, data must be evaluated either over time span or across image area. Evaluation of numeric data alone pinpoints key factors and provides an overview of the disease process. Time span data show functional change during the incidence and image analysis highlights structural abnormality. Therefore, health data in different formats should be evaluated together in order to evaluate the disease process comprehensively. Thus, a systematic evaluation of the disease process can be made and the underlying factors can be understood.

2 Literature Review

2.1 Numeric Data Evaluation

Healthcare data analytics refers to the collection and analysis of patient data to improve medical care and patient experience. Patients go through a continuum of caregiving from diagnosis to recovery. The data can be obtained from laboratory output, customer service calls, online forms and other digital methods. If the data is in text form, natural language processing (NLP) techniques can be applied for conducting proper text mining. The text data is converted into numeric form by applying different filter methods and algorithms so that it can be understood by computers. The type of analysis is divided into semantic search, sentiment analysis, and named entity recognition (NER). Artificial intelligence, in the form of machine learning, can be applied to this type of analytics to make data analysis faster and more accurate. Combining AI and NLP in healthcare, the semantic insights are gained.

If the output is in the formatted type like excel, csv, sql file format, the missing values must be filled in and the datasets must be normalized at the preprocessing step. Datasets which contain missing values result to misleading predictions for the unknowns. Thus, the missing values must be replaced with different values such as median value, mean value and most frequent term. After replacement of missing values with appropriate value, all features must be normalized to prevent factor with higher values influence on the classification result erroneously. There are different normalization methods such as Z-score normalization, Gaussian Normalization [1].

After preprocessing step, the proper machine learning can be applied to select critical features in the dataset [2]. Using grid search method in the algorithm, different combination of hyperparameters can be determined for each model. Then, classification algorithm is applied and best model is selected by taking into account of classification accuracy. There are many classification algorithms such as Artificial Neural Network (ANN), Gradient Boosting Tree (GBM), Support Vector Machine (SVM) [2–5]. The common goal of all classification algorithms is to minimize loss function and make the prediction more accurate. For example, in boosting algorithm, a strong learner is created by adding a new weak learner to each iteration. With each iteration, new models are built to overcome errors made in previous iterations and at the end, the loss function is minimized. In the classification algorithm, the grid search technique can also be used to create a model for each possible combination of all hyperparameter values such as the maximum depth of each tree, the number of trees, the learning rate, and the minimum number of observations at the terminal nodes of the trees in GBM. The accuracy of the grid search method is found by comparing the results according to different hyperparameter values. Each model in a different combination of parameters must be evaluated and the model that gives the most accurate result must be selected. Furthermore, k-fold cross-validation must be applied to evaluate the performance of the model. In k-fold cross validation, part of the data that is not used to train the model is then used to test this sample. Thus, every observation in the dataset has the opportunity to appear in the training and test set. After classification process, with the help of PCA cluster analysis, the selected features can be clustered and projected onto reduced 2D axes. (Bontempi et al. 2008; Hotelling 1936) [6, 7] PCA is a method for finding the projection of data onto a low-dimensional axis in such a way as to maximize variance. With the Kmeans clustering algorithm, the data points are divided into k sets, where each data point belongs to the set with the nearest average, and the data can be effectively clustered with decreasing axis size. This PCA cluster method provides virtual evidence for accuracy of classification result.

2.2 *Time Spanned Health Data Evaluation*

On the time-spanned health data evaluation, signal processing is one of the data collection methods, solving problems by making data meaningful for the correct interpretation, reducing noise, reconstructing the signal, data compression, and obtaining important information. They examine the activities of the organism, from gene-protein sequences to nerve and heart rhythms, tissue, and organ images. Signal processing includes a set of mathematical and statistical techniques used in the analysis, processing, and interpretation of biomedical signals. The methods of filter design of signal processing are the discrete-time filter design based on amplitude response, based on the length of the impulse response, and based on phase response to convert the signal from analog to digital [8–10]. These transformed signals are classified as continuous and discrete time signals according to the time variable, periodic and non-periodic according to their periodicity, and deterministic and random according to their statistical characteristics [8].

Biological signals are examined in two separate groups, electrical or non-electrical origin, which are detected by electrodes or transducers from the living body. These signals provide information on any pathological condition in the human body. Some of these signs and their sources are Electromyogram (EMG), Electrocardiogram (ECG), Electroencephalogram (EEG), Electrogastrogram (EGG), and Electrodermal activity (EDA) [11]. They are often corrupted by artifacts, noise, and missing data. Artifacts are generally divided into two groups which are physiological and non-physiological artifacts. Physiological artifacts come from a source other than the signal to be recorded from eye movement artifacts, muscle activity artifacts, motion artifacts, pulse artifacts, sweating artifacts, and respiratory artifacts. Non-physiological artifacts are produced by factors other than human anatomy, including environmental artifacts, recorder-induced artifacts, cable, and electrode-induced artifacts. In order to obtain important information to be used in the analysis of the signal, the effect of noises, and artifacts should be reduced or eliminated by different methods according to their source or characteristics, including Kalman filtering, median filtering Butterworth filter [12–15].

Biomedical diagnostic systems contain enormous data for analysis of signal processing. Time–frequency analysis methods allow the capture of hidden features that cannot be detected visually and numerically. The morphological features of the signals are extracted using mathematical functions on both the time domain and frequency domain, by carrying information from the time domain form to the frequency domain, or vice ver, using Fourier transform, wavelet transform, Hilbert transform, and periodicity transform [16–21].

At the feature extraction stage, it is ensured that the features that can represent that data are obtained from the raw data. In the feature selection phase, effective feature values are obtained from the existing feature set by using various feature selection algorithms. In this way, effective features are detected and the size of the feature vector is reduced. These features can be obtained both using the entire time series at the same time and splitting into appropriate window widths and each window width processes the data recorded at a certain time separately. The time and frequency domain features are extracted using statistical methods, energy, and entropy. As a morphological feature vector, features are obtained using common spatial patterns, local binary patterns as well as statistical time and frequency domain, and intrinsic energy features including variance, number of zero crossings, mean, median, mode, waveform length, root mean square, average absolute value, average frequency, median frequency, peak frequency, average power, total power, sample entropy, Shannon entropy, fuzzy entropy, permutation entropy, spectral entropy, Kolmogorov-Sinai entropy, approximate entropy, Renyi's Entropy, permutation entropy, Tsalli's entropy, wavelet entropy and Phase Entropy (PhEn), distribution entropy, Kraskov entropy (Millan et al. 2018; Kang et al. 2018; Xiaolin et al. 2018) [19, 22–25].

As well as the feature extraction methods, different feature selection algorithms are performed. The purpose of feature selection is to reduce the number of features by selecting the most qualified features for the related problem within the feature set under consideration. Thus, feature selection helps to reduce the number of dimensions. Some feature selection methods are principal component analysis (PCA), independent component analyses (ICA), mutual information, particle swarm optimization (PSO), and genetic algorithms [26–30].

In the modeling of nonlinear systems, other than the determination of the source of uncertainty in the data or related physical events, another factor we encounter is which techniques should be used to model depending on the problem of interest. The emergence of many situations such as class imbalance, class noise, outlier observation, and irrelevant features cause a decrease in model reliability and performance. In this context, the hybridization of artificial intelligence methods with appropriate signal transformations for the solution of different problems in the field of health allows flexible modeling and more effective solutions to be obtained.

Machine learning is a subset of artificial intelligence, to solve different types of problems, which are classification, clustering, and regression. Classification is a method used to categorize data into predetermined classes, by assigning data points to specific categories or classes. Clustering is a method that aims to form homogeneous groups by bringing together data points with similar characteristics, by discovering hidden structures and relationships in the data set. Regression is a method used to understand the relationship between variables and to estimate the value of a dependent variable, by determining the dependence of a dependent variable on independent variables and to predict future values. Some machine learning methods are support vector machine, decision trees, random forest, ensemble learning, long short-term memory, bidirectional long short-term memory, recurrent neural network, logistic regression, k-mean clustering, the naïve-Bayes classifier [16, 19, 31–36].

The effectiveness of the solutions obtained from the models determined by the use of model selection criteria should be determined by reliability analysis. For the methods used for classification, clustering, and regression problems, model selection criteria should be used to determine the best model, and reliability and effectiveness analyses should not be neglected. The artificial intelligence techniques used increase the complexity of the predicted models depending on both the number of inputs and the hyperparameters of the models. Effective approaches to control the complexity of models are feature selection, cross-validation, early stopping, training with noise, mixtures of networks, branching and pruning techniques (Tibshirani 1994) [16, 19, 30, 33, 35–38].

2.3 Health Image Data Evaluation

For analysis image data, different algorithms have convolutional neural network (CNN) structures, such as You Only Look Once (YOLO), RESNET, VGGNET, GOOGLENET(INCEPTION), Dense Convolutional Network (DenseNet). [39–42].

Imaged data must be preprocessed before the analysis. The preprocessed step contains standardization of images, adjustment of morphological conversions and pixel luminance conversions, normalization, taking average and standard deviation of input data and data augmentation.

Standardization scales images to the same size. Morphological conversions and pixel luminance conversions include thresholding, erosion and dilation, opening and closing steps. At thresholding step, all pixels with intensities above a certain threshold are taken and transformed. Pixels whose value is less than the threshold are converted to zero. This process results in binary image. In erosion process, bright areas are reduced and dark areas are enlarged. Dilation is the opposite, dark areas are reduced and bright areas are magnified. Opening step can remove small bright spots, connect small dark cracks. Closing process removes small dark spots in the image and connects small shiny cracks.

Normalization is one of the most important step in the preprocessing part. Pixel density are normalized so that their values fall within a limited range. By taking the mean and standard deviation of the input data, the average values for each pixel in all training samples are obtained. This process helps to get an idea of the basic structures in the image. Data augmentation is to increase data diversity without collecting new data and making a change. Especially if the amount of data we have is not enough to perform the classification task well enough, we should perform data augmentation. It should only be done on training data.

Convolutional learning, especially image data based on deep learning algorithms allows operations to be performed on it. By making transformations on the image data, the data is vectorized as shown in many figures. For this, some special convolution layers are used. Convolutional neural network architecture includes three layers in addition to the input and output layer. The first is the convolution layer which come after input layer. This layer is followed by the sampling layer and end with the full connection layer. Convolution is a conversion process which is filter-assisted moving of each moment of an image in a slider window. After convolution layer, a nonlinear function is used to check output of each layer. The purpose of the pooling layer is to reduce the size and resolution of the inputs from the convolution layer. Thus, the number of parameters in the network and the amount of computation can be reduced. After sampling of the convolutional network, the full link layer is activated. The output of the last convolution layer is flattened and converted to a vector here.

There are different algorithms which are used CNN structures. One of this algorithm is VGGNet. It consists of 16 convolutional layers and has a very smooth architecture. It is the most preferred architecture for feature extraction from images. It contains 3×3 convolution layer and many filters. VGGNet network consists of 138 million parameters.

ResNet architecture is called residual neural network. It has algorithm which transfer One ResNet module to another module. These transferred links together also known as ported gates or coupled repeating units. Although it has 152 layers, it has a lower complexity than VGGNet [41].

The GoogleNet architecture differs from other architectures by adding a new element called the starter module. Stack normalization, image distortion and

RMSprop optimization that is designated for neural networks are used in this module. This architecture uses very small size and large quantity convolution layer and greatly reduces the number of parameters.

In DenseNet architecture, which is called dense network, each layer is an additional layer from all previous layers. It transfers its own feature maps to all subsequent layers. Each layer receives collective information from all layers. Because each layer receives feature maps from all previous layers, the network can be thinner and more compact. Thus, it has higher computation efficiency and memory efficiency.

YOLO algorithm can do object tracking quickly and it is an effective algorithm in terms of accuracy. The reason why the YOLO algorithm is so fast is by passing the image through the neural network at one time, the class and coordinates of all the objects in the image can be guessed. The YOLO architecture divides the image into regions, then divides the objects in these regions and draws the boxes called bounding boxes. After that, the probability of the object being found in each region and the trust score are calculated.

3 Conclusion

The average human lifespan is increasing across the world. The importance of big data analytics application in healthcare is increasing day by day. Based on different format of health data, the analytics techniques may vary. In this study, the critical points in the analysis of different formatted health data are emphasized. In order to gain robust and accurate prediction or prevention of healthcare situations, all types of health data must be analyzed together. After understanding of advantages and pitfalls, in the future, it will be very useful to develop the big software platforms which contribute to evaluation of different data type together.

References

1. Abdi, H., Williams, L.J.: Normalizing data. Encycl. Res. Des. **1** (2010)
2. Kulan, H., Dag, T.: In silico identification of critical proteins associated with learning process and immune system for Down syndrome. Plos One. **14** (2019)
3. Natekin, A., Knoll, A.: Gradient boosting machines, a tutorial. Front. Neurorobot. **7**, 21 (2013)
4. Chicco, D.: Ten quick tips for machine learning in computational biology. BioData mining **10**(1), 35 (2017)
5. Alpaydin, E. (2010). *Introduction to machine learning*. MIT press.
6. Hotelling, H.: Analysis of a complex of statistical variables into principal components. J. Educ. Psychol. **24**, 498–520 (1933)
7. Leznik, M., Tofallis, C.: Estimating invariant principal components using diagonal regression (2005)
8. Haykin, S., Veen, B.V.: Signals and Systems. John Willey & Sons. Inc., New York (1999)
9. Piskorowski, J.: Time-efficient removal of power-line noise from EMG signals using IIR notch filters with non-zero initial conditions. Biocybern. Biomed. Eng. **33**(3), 171–178 (2013)

10. Sreelekha, K.R., Bindiya, T.S.: Design of cost effective variable bandwidth 2D low-pass, high-pass and band-pass filters with improved circularity. Digital Signal Process. **133**, 103842 (2023)
11. Shortlii, E.H., Cimino, J.J.: Biomedical Informatics Computer Applications in Health Care and Biomedicine, (Third Edition). Springer (2006)
12. Ahmad, M., Jung, L.T., Bhuiyan, A.A.: A biological inspired fuzzy adaptive window median filter (FAWMF) for enhancing DNA signal processing. Comput. Methods Progr. Biomed. **149**, 11–17 (2017)
13. Bougerol, P.: Kalman filtering with random coefficients and contractions. SIAM J. Control. Optim. **31**(4), 942–959 (1993)
14. Mutanen, T.P., Metsomaa, J., Makkonen, M., Varone, G., Marzetti, L., Ilmoniemi, R.J.: Source-based artifact-rejection techniques for TMS–EEG. J. Neurosci. Methods **382**, 109693 (2022)
15. Robertson, D.G.E., Dowling, J.J.: Design and responses of Butterworth and critically damped digital filters. J. Electromyogr. Kinesiol. **13**(6), 569–573 (2003)
16. Kocadagli, O., Ozer, E., Batista, A.G.: Preictal phase detection on EEG signals using hybridized machine learning classifiers with a novel feature selection procedure based GAs and ICOMP. Expert Syst. Appl. **212**, 118825 (2023)
17. Louis, A.K., Maass, D., Rieder, A.: Wavelets: Theory and Applications. John Wiley & Sons Ltd (1997)
18. Mallat, S.G.: A theory for multiresolution signal decomposition: the wavelet representation. IEEE Trans. Pattern Anal. Mach. Intell. **11**(7), 674–693 (1989)
19. Raghu, S., Sriraam, N., Temel, Y., Rao, S.V., Hegde, A.S., Kubben, P.L.: Performance evaluation of DWT based sigmoid entropy in time and frequency domains for automated detection of epileptic seizures using SVM classifier. Comput. Biol. Med. **110**, 127–143 (2019)
20. Sethares, W.A., Staley, T.W.: Periodicity transforms. IEEE Trans. Signal Process. **47**(11), 2953–2964 (1999)
21. Szczęsna, A., Augustyn, D.R., Josiński, H., Harężlak, K., Świtoński, A., Kasprowski, P.: Chaotic biomedical time signal analysis via wavelet scattering transform. J. Comput. Sci. **72**, 102080 (2023)
22. Zhang, T., Chen, W., Li, M.: Fuzzy distribution entropy and its application in automated seizure detection technique. Biomed. Signal Process. Control **39**, 360–377 (2018)
23. Luo, H., Qiu, T., Liu, C., Huang, P.: Research on fatigue driving detection using forehead EEG based on adaptive multi-scale entropy. Biomed. Signal Process. Control **51**, 50–58 (2019)
24. Luo, T.J.: Parallel genetic algorithm based common spatial patterns selection on time–frequency decomposed EEG signals for motor imagery brain-computer interface. Biomed. Signal Process. Control **80**, 104397 (2023)
25. Ozer, E., Kocadagli, O., Batista, A.G.: Time-frequency analysis of the EEG signals: visual identification of epileptic patterns. In: y-BIS 2019 Conference Book: Recent Advances in Data Science and Business Analytics (2019). ISBN- 978–605–5005–95–5
26. Buzzell, G.A., Niu, Y., Aviyente, S., Bernat, E.: A practical introduction to EEG time-frequency principal components analysis (TF-PCA). Dev. Cogn. Neurosci. **55**, 101114 (2022)
27. Cui, D., Pu, W., Liu, J., Bian, Z., Li, Q., Wang, L., Gu, G.: A new EEG synchronization strength analysis method: S-estimator based normalized weighted-permutation mutual information. Neural Netw. **82**, 30–38 (2016)
28. Judith, A.M., Priya, S.B., Mahendran, R.K.: Artifact removal from EEG signals using regenerative multi-dimensional singular value decomposition and independent component analysis. Biomed. Signal Process. Control **74**, 103452 (2022)
29. Li, H., Guo, W., Zhang, R., Xiu, C.: Variable length particle swarm optimization and multi-feature deep fusion for motor imagery EEG classification. Biochem. Biophys. Res. Commun. **571**, 131–136 (2021)
30. James, G., Witten, D., Hastie, T., Tibshirani, I.R.: An introduction to statistical learning with applications in R (2017)
31. Cortes, C., Vapnik, V.: Support-vector networks. Mach. Learn. **20**, 273–297 (1995)
32. Efron, B., Tibshirani, R.J.: An introduction to the bootstrap (Chapman & Hall/CRC monographs on statistics & applied probability). Chapman and Hall/CRC (1994)

33. Bishop, C.M., Nasrabadi, N.M.: Pattern recognition and machine learning, vol. 4, no. 4, p. 738. Springer, New York (2006)
34. Hochreiter, S., Schmidhuber, J.: Long short-term memory. Neural Comput. **9**(8), 1735–1780 (1997)
35. Tsiouris, KM, Pezoulas, V.C., Zervakis, M., Konitsiotis, S., Koutsouris, D.D., Fotiadis, D.I.: A long short-term memory deep learning network for the prediction of epileptic seizures using EEG signals. Comput. Biol. Med. **99**, 24–37 (2018)
36. Unanyan, N.N., Belov, A.A.: Design of upper limb prosthesis using real-time motion detection method based on EMG signal processing. Biomed. Signal Process. Control **70**, 103062 (2021)
37. Aggarwal, C.C.: Neural networks and deep learning. Springer **10**(978), 3 (2018)
38. Li, M., Chen, W., Zhang, T.: Classification of epilepsy EEG signals using DWT-based envelope analysis and neural network ensemble. Biomed. Signal Process. Control **31**, 357–365 (2017)
39. Sagar, A.: Convolutional neural network for breast cancer classification: deep learning for solving the most commonly diagnosed cancer in women. Towards Data Sci. Medium Publ. Shar. Concept. Ideas Codes
40. Hamed, G.: YOLO based breast masses detection and classification in full-field digital mammograms. Comput. Methods Progr. Biomed. 200 (2020). https://doi.org/10.1016/j.cmpb.2020.105823
41. Yılmaz, A., Kaya, U.: Derin Öğrenme. Kodlab, İstanbul (2021)
42. Özkan, Y.: Uygulamalı Derin Öğrenme. Papatya Yayıncılık, İstanbul (2021)
43. Hotelling, H.: Relations between two sets of variates. In Breakthroughs in Statistics: Methodology and Distribution, pp. 162–190. Springer New York, New York, NY (1992)
44. Mason, L., Baxter, J., Bartlett, P., Frean, M.: Boosting algorithms as gradient descent. Adv. Neural Inf. Process. Syst. **12** (1999)
45. Lotter, W., Diab, A.R., Haslam, B., Kim, J.G., Grisot, G., Wu, E. Gregory Sorensen, A.: Robust breast cancer detection in mammography and digital breast tomosynthesis using an annotation-efficient deep learning approach. Nat. Med. **27**(2), 244–249 (2021)
46. Millán, P.C., García-Ferrero, M.Á., Llanes-Estrada, F.J., Riojano, A.P., García, E.M.S.: Shannon entropy and particle decays. Nucl. Phys. B **930**, 583–596 (2018)
47. Kulan, H., Dag, T., : Using machine learning classifiers to identify the critical proteins in down syndrome. Proceedings of the 2018 2nd International Conference on Computational Biology and Bioinformatics. 51–54 (2018)
48. Mahmoodirad, A., Allahviranloo, T., Niroomand, S.: A new effective solution method for fully intuitionistic fuzzy transportation problem. Soft. Comput. **23**(12), 4521–4530 (2019)
49. Moloudzadeh, S., Allahviranloo, T., Darabi, P.: A new method for solving an arbitrary fully fuzzy linear system. Soft. Comput. **17**(9), 1725–1731 (2013)
50. Rahmani, A., Lotfi, F.H., Rostamy-Malkhalifeh, M., Allahviranloo, T.: A new method for defuzzification and ranking of fuzzy numbers based on the statistical beta distribution. Adv. Fuzzy Syst. **2016**, 1–8 (2016)

Evaluation of Hospitals and Health Care Centers with Ratio Data

Mehdi Soltanifar

Abstract One of the most important topics in healthcare management is the performance evaluation of hospitals and healthcare centers. This work is done with different models of decision analysis and after determining the evaluation criteria. One of the most up-to-date and widely used ways to evaluate performance is the use of non-parametric models such as Data Envelopment Analysis (DEA). In many evaluations, after determining the criteria and specifying the inputs and outputs for using DEA models, we are faced with ratio data. Traditional DEA models are not suitable models for handling this type of data, and it is necessary to use DEA models to handle this type of data. In this research, after examining some ratio criteria for evaluating public hospitals and health centers, DEA-R models are presented to handle these data both in cases of non-negative data and negative data.

Keywords Data envelopment analysis (DEA) · Ratio data · DEA-R models · Negative data · Public hospitals · Health care centres

1 Introduction and Motivation

Public health is actually the science of protecting and improving the health of people and their living places. Improving the level of public health is achieved by promoting a healthy lifestyle, research on the prevention of diseases and injuries and their timely diagnosis, prevention and treatment of infectious diseases. One of the tools to improve the quality of public health is public health centers and public hospitals that provide good health services. Health centers are community-based, patient-centered organizations that provide affordable, accessible, and high-quality primary health care services to individuals and families, including those experiencing homelessness, living in poverty, residents of public housing, the disabled, and Veterans offer. Public hospitals (public or government-supervised hospitals) provide free or low-cost

M. Soltanifar (✉)
Department of Mathematics, Semnan Branch, Islamic Azad University, Semnan, Iran
e-mail: soltanifarmahdi@gmail.com; mehdi.soltanifar@iau.ac.ir

T. Allahviranloo et al. (eds.), *Decision Making in Healthcare Systems*,
Studies in Systems, Decision and Control 513,
https://doi.org/10.1007/978-3-031-46735-6_4

health care to every citizen. These hospitals are usually run with government funds. However, there are also government-funded and government-supervised hospitals. Therefore, continuous monitoring of health centers and public hospitals is essential and one of the duties of the government. This monitoring requires the evaluation and ranking of public hospitals and health centers. In order to achieve this, it is necessary to determine evaluation criteria and indicators and then use decision analysis models. So far, researchers have presented and used many methods to evaluate public hospitals and health care centers. Many of these methods can be found in [1–3]. In this research, the focus is on the methods of decision analysis, which uses mathematical models and after determining the indicators and evaluation criteria, calculates the center's efficiency score or ranks them. Among these methods, non-parametric methods such as Data Envelopment Analysis can be mentioned.

Data Envelopment Analysis (DEA) is a technique based on linear programming to evaluate the performance of a set of homogeneous Decision-Making Units (DMUs) [4]. DEA is a suitable and efficient tool in the field of measuring and evaluating productivity, which is used as a non-parametric method to calculate the efficiency of DMUs. Today, the use of DEA technique is expanding rapidly and is used in the evaluation of various organizations and industries such as the banking industry, post office, hospitals, educational centers, power plants, refineries, etc. [5–18]. There have been many developments in theoretical and practical aspects in DEA models, which makes it indispensable to know its various aspects for more precise application [19]. The many advantages of the DEA technique, such as insensitivity to the units of measurement of inputs and outputs, calculating the relative efficiency of units, high generalizability and expansion, the possibility of hybridizing it with other decision-making methods such as Multi-Criteria Decision-Making (MCDM) methods and the existence of efficient methods for ranking the units prompted researchers to use this technique in healthcare management widely. Linna [20] measured hospital cost efficiency with panel data models. Banker et al. [21] conducted an illustrative study of hospital production using DEA and translog methods. Stefko et al. [22] applied the DEA technique to evaluate the efficiency of health care in the Slovak Republic. A network-DEA model to evaluate the impact of quality and access on hospital performance was presented by Afonso et al. [23]. Chiu et al. [24] used the DEA model to study the performance of hospitals through medical quality. Antunes et al. [25] evaluated performance and synergy in Chinese health care and showed that synergy has played a pivotal role in China's health care systems. Miszczynska and Miszczyński [26] presented a window-DEA evaluation to measure the efficiency of the healthcare sector in Poland. Hollingsworth [27] applied DEA policy to measure the efficiency and productivity of health care delivery. Kohl et al. [28] reviewed 262 papers on DEA applications in healthcare with a particular focus on hospitals. Arya and Yadav [29] applied DEA to assess the health sector by considering the logic of uncertainty. Recently, research trends from 2017 to 2022 have been presented by Jung et al. [30] regarding efficiency measurement using DEA in public health care.

Recent research points out that most mathematical models like dynamic systems and also linear systems get involved with real-world problems. Since their related information has different forms like certainty and uncertainty, the uncertain version of these models does have more importance in the applications. In health problems, two types of mathematical models; fuzzy dynamic systems and fuzzy linear programming problems even transportation problems, play an important role, on the other hand, the main and basic model of fuzzy linear programming problems is fuzzy linear systems.

In conclusion, fuzzy differential equations (as a special version of dynamic systems) [31, 32], and fuzzy linear systems (as a basic model of fuzzy linear programming problems) [33], have an important role in this research. Recently several research has been done on investigating the advanced version of the uncertain information [31, 34, 35], and moreover the above-mentioned basic models.

One of the techniques for decision making is Data Envelopment Analysis (DEA), and many researchers have conducted research on this topic. Several recent papers have been cited to mention their research area [4, 36, 37, 38]. Some authors have explored the topic in a different way: safety analysis and reliability [39, 40, 41].

In the studies carried out for the evaluation of public hospitals and health centers, first the effective evaluation criteria are extracted in the form of inputs and outputs, and then DEA models are used for evaluation, calculation of relative efficiency, ranking, etc. But in many cases, after determining the criteria and specifying the inputs and outputs, we are faced with ratio data, which traditional DEA models are not suitable models for evaluating this type of data. In this research, we intend to study the evaluation criteria of public hospitals and health centers, which are provided in the form of ratio data, and then use the appropriate DEA models, known as DEA-R models, to handle these data. Therefore, the continuation of the chapter is organized as follows. In Sect. 2, the introductions related to DEA models that are able to handle ratio data are presented. In Sect. 3, the motivation for presenting this research is presented by examining relative criteria in the evaluation of public hospitals and health centers. In Sect. 4, some management perspectives are presented with the healthcare management aspect, and finally, the conclusion of this chapter is presented in Sect. 5.

2 Literature Review

In the study of many organizations, especially public hospitals and health centers, inputs and outputs are presented in a ratio form. Therefore, it is necessary to provide DEA models to handle this form of data. In this section, ratio-based DEA (DEA-R) models are discussed in the presence of non-negative data as well as negative data.

2.1 Non-negative Data

Consider m-dimension positive input vector of $(x_{1j}, x_{2j}, \ldots, x_{mj}) > \mathbf{0}$ for DMU$_j$, $1 \leq j \leq n$ that is used for producing s-dimension positive output vector of

can only be used for non-negative data, and this is a limitation for their application in various problems. In the next section, DEA-R models for handling negative data are presented.

2.2 Negative Data

In the evaluation of many organizations and units, the possibility of negative data is a probable hypothesis. The DEA-R models mentioned in the previous section are not able to handle negative data. Therefore, in the continuation of the models of the previous part, models are rewritten in such a way that they are able to handle negative data. The models are presented for two cases of negative outputs or negative inputs. It should be noted that the simultaneous negative assumption of inputs and outputs is not a correct assumption due to the structure of the models.

First suppose the outputs of the problem are divided into two categories. The first category of outputs that are positive, and the second category of outputs can be negative ($\mathrm{Y_r}$). Variables $\mathrm{Y_r^P}$ and $\mathrm{Y_r^N}$ are defined as follows [47, 48]:

$$y_{rj}^P = \begin{cases} y_{rj} & if\ y_{rj} \geq 0 \\ 0 & Otherwise \end{cases} \qquad y_{rj}^N = \begin{cases} -y_{rj} & if\ y_{rj} < 0 \\ 0 & Otherwise \end{cases}, \forall j$$

In fact, $y_{rj} = y_{rj}^P - y_{rj}^N$ and $y_{rj}^P, y_{rj}^N \geq 0$. DEA-R input-oriented in the presence of negative outputs is presented in the model (9).

$$\begin{aligned}
&\max\ \theta \\
&s.t. \\
&\sum_j \lambda_j \frac{y_{rj}}{x_{ij}} \geq \theta \frac{y_{rp}}{x_{ip}}, \quad \forall i, \forall r \in O' \\
&\sum_j \lambda_j \frac{y_{rj}^P}{x_{ij}} \geq \theta \frac{y_{rp}^P}{x_{ip}}, \quad \forall i, \forall r \in O'' \\
&\sum_j \lambda_j \frac{y_{rj}^N}{x_{ij}} \leq \theta \frac{y_{rp}^N}{x_{ip}}, \quad \forall i, \forall r \in O'' \\
&\sum_j \lambda_j \left(\frac{x_{ip}}{x_{ij}}\right) = \theta, \quad \forall i \\
&\sum_j \lambda_j = 1 \\
&\lambda_j \geq 0, \forall j \\
&\theta \text{ is free.}
\end{aligned} \tag{9}$$

where the index set associated with the variables are specified with $O\prime$ and the index set associated with the variables Y^P are specified with O''. By presenting this model, Soltanifar et al. [16] showed that their model is always feasible.

In a similar way, Soltanifar et al. [16] assumed that inputs are divided into two categories. A positive group and another group that can be negative. Note that the second category can be positive or negative. The following variables can be defined for second category inputs.

$$x_{ij}^{P} = \begin{cases} x_{ij} & if\, x_{ij} \geq 0 \\ 0 & Otherwise \end{cases} \qquad x_{ij}^{N} = \begin{cases} -x_{ij} & if\, x_{ij} < 0 \\ 0 & Otherwise \end{cases}, \forall j$$

In fact, $x_{ij} = x_{ij}^{P} - x_{ij}^{N}$ and $x_{ij}^{P}, x_{ij}^{N} \geq 0$. DEA-R output-oriented in the presence of negative inputs is presented in model (10).

$$\begin{aligned}
&\min\ \theta \\
&s.t. \\
&\sum_j \lambda_j \frac{x_{ij}}{y_{rj}} \leq \theta \frac{x_{ip}}{y_{rp}}, \quad \forall r, \forall i \in I\prime \\
&\sum_j \lambda_j \frac{x_{ij}^{P}}{y_{rj}} \leq \theta \frac{x_{ip}^{P}}{y_{rp}}, \quad \forall r, \forall i \in I'' \\
&\sum_j \lambda_j \frac{x_{ij}^{N}}{y_{rj}} \geq \theta \frac{x_{ip}^{N}}{y_{rp}}, \quad \forall r, \forall i \in I'' \\
&\sum_j \lambda_j \left(\frac{y_{rp}}{y_{rj}}\right) = \theta, \quad \forall r \\
&\sum_j \lambda_j = 1 \\
&\lambda_j \geq 0, \quad \forall j \\
&\theta \text{ is free.}
\end{aligned} \tag{10}$$

where the index set associated with the variables I^P are specified with $I\prime$ and the index set associated with the variables I^P are specified with I''. By presenting this model, Soltanifar et al. [16] proved its feasibility.

Soltanifar et al. [16] also rewrote their DEA-R models with the modifications made by Kaffash et al. [49] on the models presented by Emrouznejad et al. [47, 48]. This rewriting is presented in models (11) and (12).

$$
\begin{aligned}
&\max\ \theta \\
&s.t. \\
&\sum_j \lambda_j \frac{y_{rj}}{x_{ij}} \geq (1+\theta)\frac{y_{rp}}{x_{ip}}, \quad \forall i, \forall r \in O' \\
&\sum_j \lambda_j \frac{y^P_{rj}}{x_{ij}} \geq (1+\theta)\frac{y^P_{rp}}{x_{ip}}, \quad \forall i, \forall r \in O'' \\
&\sum_j \lambda_j \frac{y^N_{rj}}{x_{ij}} \leq (1-\theta)\frac{y^N_{rp}}{x_{ip}}, \quad \forall i, \forall r \in O'' \\
&\sum_j \lambda_j \left(\frac{x_{ip}}{x_{ij}}\right) = (1+\theta), \quad \forall i \\
&\sum_j \lambda_j = 1 \\
&\lambda_j \geq 0, \forall j \\
&\theta \text{ is free.}
\end{aligned}
\tag{11}
$$

$$
\begin{aligned}
&\min\ \theta \\
&s.t. \\
&\sum_j \lambda_j \frac{x_{ij}}{y_{rj}} \leq (1+\theta)\frac{x_{ip}}{y_{rp}}, \quad \forall r, \forall i \in I' \\
&\sum_j \lambda_j \frac{x^P_{ij}}{y_{rj}} \leq (1+\theta)\frac{x^P_{ip}}{y_{rp}}, \quad \forall r, \forall i \in I'' \\
&\sum_j \lambda_j \frac{x^N_{ij}}{y_{rj}} \geq (1-\theta)\frac{x^N_{ip}}{y_{rp}}, \quad \forall r, \forall i \in I'' \\
&\sum_j \lambda_j \left(\frac{y_{rp}}{y_{rj}}\right) = (1+\theta), \quad \forall r \\
&\sum_j \lambda_j = 1 \\
&\lambda_j \geq 0, \quad \forall j \\
&\theta \text{ is free.}
\end{aligned}
\tag{12}
$$

The feasibility of these models was also proved by Soltanifar et al. [16]. In the next section, the motivation and necessity of using these models in the evaluation of public hospitals and health centers is presented.

3 Ratio Data in Healthcare Management and Motivation to Use DEA-R Models

In most of the performance evaluation and ranking methods, it is necessary to first determine the criteria affecting the quality and quantity of the services provided, and then determine the efficiency of each unit in each criterion. The criteria can be profit or cost type or presented in qualitative or quantitative form. Data related to these criteria can also be collected in different forms: in the form of a tree structure and pairwise comparison matrices, in the form of a decision matrix, in the form of an input/output table, etc. In fact, depending on what model is going to be used to evaluate the performance, the data collection form is different. To use non-parametric models such as DEA models, data are set in the form of input and output tables. Basic DEA models can be used for non-negative data, but these models are not suitable for ratio or negative ratio data [47, 48, 50]. In such cases, the DEA-R models presented in the previous section should be used. In this section, first, the criteria after presenting and constructing the inputs and outputs are presented in the form of non-negative ratio data and show the necessity of using DEA-R models for non-negative data. Then the case where ratio criteria are based on healthcare standards is discussed. In this case, ratio criterion is provided that can be negative and this shows the necessity of using DEA-R models for negative data.

Ghiyasi et al. [51] used the criteria of Table 1 in the evaluation of public hospitals.

They intended to use DEA models to evaluate public hospitals. Therefore, they presented the input/output table in the form of Table 2.

Therefore, they faced ratio inputs and outputs, which must be handled by DEA-R models.

[13] used the standard criteria of the World Health Organization to evaluate public hospitals and health centers, which were presented in a radio format (Table 3). "Bed occupancy rate risk" is a criterion that can have a negative value. Therefore, they inevitably used DEA-R models that have the ability to handle negative data for evaluation. In this way, the motivation and necessity of using the models presented in the previous section for the management of healthcare services is clear, and therefore, while using the many advantages of the DEA policy, the evaluation can be done considering the type of data.

Further managerial implications and applications regarding the use of DEA policy in healthcare management are presented in the next section.

4 Further Managerial Implications and Applications

In many real-world problems, especially those related to health care management, decision makers are faced with data on evaluation criteria that are only available in the form of ratios or converted to ratio form after conversion to inputs and outputs. This may have various reasons, including the confidentiality of criteria values in a

Table 1 Criteria for assessing hospitals [51]

Criterion number	Criterion title	Definition
C_1	Number of physicians	Total number of medical doctors (physicians) in the hospital
C_2	Number of surgeons	Total number of surgical specialists in the hospital (surgery is an invasive technique with the fundamental principle of physical intervention on organs/organ systems/tissues for diagnostic or therapeutic reasons)
C_3	Number of emergency physicians	A physician who directs emergency medical technicians in the emergency department and focuses on immediate decision-making and necessary actions to prevent death or any further disability in pre-hospital settings
C_4	Number of nurses	Persons who have completed a program of basic nursing education and are qualified and registered or authorized to provide responsible and competent service for the promotion of health, prevention of illness, care of the sick, and rehabilitation, and are actually working in the hospital. Nursing personnel includes professional nurses, auxiliary nurses, enrolled nurses and related occupations such as dental nurses and primary care nurses
C_5	Number of hospital beds	The number of hospital beds available in public and private hospitals. Hospital beds are regularly maintained and staffed for the accommodation and full-time care of a succession of inpatients and situated in the wards or a part of a hospital where continuous medical care for inpatients is provided. The total number of such beds constitutes the normally available bed complement of the hospital. Cribs and bassinets maintained for use by healthy newborn babies who do not require special care are not included
C_6	Number of active hospital beds	Hospital beds that are actively available
C_7	Number of special hospital beds	The number of beds regularly maintained and staffed for the accommodation and full-time care of a succession of inpatients and which are situated in the wards or a part of the hospital where continuous medical care for inpatients is provided. The total number of such beds constitutes the normally available bed complement of the hospital. Cribs and bassinets maintained for use by healthy newborn babies who do not require special care are not included
C_8	Number of emergency admission	Patients admitted to the hospital when admission is unpredictable and at short notice because of clinical needs
C_9	Number of hospital operating rooms	An operating room, also called a surgery center, is the unit of a hospital where surgical procedures are performed
C_{10}	Number of outpatients	The number of patients who are not hospitalized overnight but visit a hospital, clinic or associated facility for diagnosis or treatment

(continued)

Table 1 (continued)

Criterion number	Criterion title	Definition
C_{11}	Number of hospitalized patients	The number of patients who are hospitalized overnight
C_{12}	Number of surgical operations	Total number of surgical operations (surgery is an invasive technique with the fundamental principle of a physical intervention on organs/organ systems/tissues for diagnostic or therapeutic reasons)

Table 2 Inputs and outputs for evaluating hospitals [51]

Inputs/outputs	Calculation formula
Input 1	C_1/C_5
Input 2	C_4/C_5
Input 3	C_7/C_5
Output 1	C_{10}/C_1
Output 2	C_{11}/C_6
Output 3	C_{12}/C_9
Output 4	C_8/C_3
Output 5	C_{12}/C_2

public hospital or the standard definitions provided in the ratio form by competent organizations. In such cases, models capable of handling ratio data such as DEA-R models should be used to evaluate units. Also, sometimes some criteria are supplied with negative data and these models should have the ability to handle negative data as well. In the study of such public hospitals or health centers, managers sometimes face issues such as resource allocation, merging two or more centers, and similar issues for which the use of inverse DEA-R models can be very helpful [13, 16, 51–53]. In fact, the use of the models presented in this chapter is not limited to performance evaluation and ranking, and most DEA policy applications such as resource allocation, merger analysis, benchmarking, progress review, and the like are possible. Ratio data are important and very common in public hospital and health center management literature. Any kind of evaluation and planning of such centers is involved with such data. Due to the nature of ratio data, it is important to treat them accurately and logically.

Table 3 Criteria in the study of hospitals [13]

Criterion	Title	Criterion formula	Type of criterion	Description
I_1	Number of nurses to beds	$\frac{\text{Nursing staff number}}{\text{Total hospital beds}}$	Input	This criterion is used to supply nursing staff compared to the total hospital beds and is used in planning for proper human resource allocation. Total hospital beds include curative (or acute) care, rehabilitative, long-term, and other hospital beds
I_2	Number of generalist physicians to beds	$\frac{\text{Generalist physicians number}}{\text{Total hospital beds}}$	Input	General physicians are medical doctors who treat acute and chronic illnesses and provide preventive care and health education to patients of all ages. They are responsible for the provision of continuing care to individuals and families. The ratio of generalist physicians to the total hospital beds is a criterion for allocating hospital resources

(continued)

Table 3 (continued)

Criterion	Title	Criterion formula	Type of criterion	Description
I_3	Number of specialists physicians to beds	$\frac{\text{Specialist physicians number}}{\text{Total hospital beds}}$	Input	Specialist physicians are pediatricians, anesthesiologists, cardiologists, dermatologists, hematologists, internists, pathologists, orthopedists, ophthalmologists, neurologists, obstetricians/ gynecologists, psychiatrists, medical specialists, surgical specialists, and so on
I_4	Equipment to the population covered by hospital	$\frac{\text{Equipment score}}{\text{Total population covered by the hospital}}$	Input	This criterion shows access to hospital equipment, including Gamma Camera, Radiotherapy, Angiography, CT scan, MRI, etc. Geographical distribution and waiting time, particularly for these devices, are essential. In other words, this criterion is the score of each hospital due to the existence or absence of the above devices at that hospital

(continued)

Table 3 (continued)

Criterion	Title	Criterion formula	Type of criterion	Description
O_1	Bed occupancy rate risk	$85 - \left(\frac{\text{Utilized bed -days}}{\text{Available bed -days}} \times 100\right)$	Output	The bed occupancy rate is the average number of days when a hospital bed was occupied as % of available 365 days. Bed occupancy rate is one of the hospital productivity criteria. This rate is also used to interpret the sources of service providers and guides for planning and managing hospital beds. Studies have shown that a high occupancy rate (usually above 85%) can indicate bed deficiency and is generally associated with an increased risk of hospital infections
O_2	Bed turnover interval	$\frac{\text{Available bed days} - \text{Utilized bed days}}{\text{Inpatient discharges}}$	Output	This criterion shows the level of exploitation of the hospital beds. Short turnover intervals have been linked to increased methicillin-resistant Staphylococcus aureus (MRSA) infections

(continued)

Table 3 (continued)

Criterion	Title	Criterion formula	Type of criterion	Description
O_3	Inpatient admission rate	$\frac{\text{The number of hospital admissions}}{\text{Total population covered by the hospital}} \times 1000$	Output	This criterion shows the number of hospital admissions per person per year. This criterion represents inpatient care and utilization. Hospital records are the basis for statistics on performance related to inpatient activities, including the number of beds, admissions, discharges, deaths, and stay duration
O_4	Bed turnover rate	$\frac{\text{Number of discharges (including deaths)}}{\text{Total hospital beds}}$	Output	The hospital bed turnover rate measures the extent of hospital utilization. It is the number of times there is a change of occupant for a bed during a given period

5 Conclusion

The focus of this chapter is on the use of DEA policy in health care management and specifically the performance evaluation and ranking of public hospitals and health centers. Where evaluation criteria are available in the form of ratio data and sometimes, they take negative values. DEA-R models can provide researchers with DEA policy for handling relative data. Also, these models were presented in a form that has the ability to handle negative ratio data. Although the basic models provided for performance evaluation and ranking are provided, but by placing these models as a basis, it is possible to apply other management such as resource allocation, merging, benchmarking, progress review, and the like.

References

1. Diehr, P., Yanez, D., Ash, A., Hornbrook, M., Lin, D.Y.: Methods for analyzing health care utilization and costs. Annu. Rev. Public Health **20**(1), 125–144 (1999)
2. Fronczek-Munter, A.: Evaluation methods for hospital facilities. Int. J. Facil. Manag. **12**, 215–226 (2013)
3. Mbau, R., Musiega, A., Nyawira, L., Tsofa, B., Mulwa, A., Molyneux, S., Barasa, E.: Analysing the efficiency of health systems: a systematic review of the literature. Appl. Health Econ. Health Policy **21**(2), 205–224 (2023)
4. Akram, M., Shahzadi, S., Shah, S.M.U., Allahviranloo, T.: A fully Fermatean fuzzy multi-objective transportation model using an extended DEA technique. Granul. Comput. (2023). https://doi.org/10.1007/s41066-023-00399-6
5. Sharafi, H., Hosseinzadeh Lotfi, F., Jahanshahloo, G., Rostamy-malkhalifeh, M., Soltanifar, M., Razipour-GhalehJough, S.: Ranking of petrochemical companies using preferential voting at unequal levels of voting power through data envelopment analysis. Math. Sci. **13**, 287–297 (2019)
6. Sharafi, H., Soltanifar, M., Lotfi, F.H.: Selecting a green supplier utilizing the new fuzzy voting model and the fuzzy combinative distance-based assessment method. EURO J. Decis. Process. **10**, 100010 (2022)
7. Soltanifar, M.: A new interval for ranking alternatives in multi attribute decision making problems. J. Appl. Res. Indus. Eng. (2022)
8. Soltanifar, M.: A new group voting analytical hierarchy process method. J. Operat. Res. Appl. Appl. Math. Lahijan Azad Univ. **14**(3), 1–13 (2017)
9. Soltanifar, M.: The voting linear assignment method for determining priority and weights in solving MADM problems. J. Appl. Res. Indus. Eng. **8**(Special Issue), 1–17 (2021)
10. Soltanifar, M., Farhadi, F.: An application of data envelopment analysis for measuring the relative efficiency in banking industry. Manag. Sci. Lett. **4**(5), 1021–1026 (2014)
11. Soltanifar, M., Shahghobadi, S.: Selecting a benevolent secondary goal model in data envelopment analysis cross-efficiency evaluation by a voting model. Socioecon. Plann. Sci. **47**(1), 65–74 (2013)
12. Soltanifar, M., Sharafi, H.: Preferential voting in the presence of undesirable voters. Int. J. Appl. Decis. Sci. **15**(6), 753–766 (2022)
13. Soltanifar, M., Tavana, M., Ghiyasi M., Sharafi, H.: A new method for solving inverse data envelopment analysis problems with negative ratio data. OR Spectrum (vol. Submitted 2023)
14. Soltanifar, M., Jahanshahloo, G.R., Lotfi, F.H., Mansourzadeh, S.M.: On efficiency in convex hull of DMUs. Appl. Math. Model. **37**(4), 2267–2278 (2013)
15. Soltanifar, M., Shahghobadi, S.: Classifying inputs and outputs in data envelopment analysis based on TOPSIS method and a voting model. Int. J. Bus. Anal. (IJBAN) **1**(2), 48–63 (2014)
16. Soltanifar, M., Hosseinzadeh Lotfi, F., Sharafi, H., Lozano, S.: Resource allocation and target setting: a CSW–DEA based approach. Ann. Oper. Res. **318**(1), 557–589 (2022)
17. Lotfi, F.H., Jahanshahloo, G.R., Ebrahimnejad, A., Soltanifar, M., Mansourzadeh, S.M.: Target setting in the general combined-oriented CCR model using an interactive MOLP method. J. Comput. Appl. Math. **234**(1), 1–9 (2010)
18. Soltanifar, M., Lotfi, F.H.: The voting analytic hierarchy process method for discriminating among efficient decision-making units in data envelopment analysis. Comput. Ind. Eng. **60**(4), 585–592 (2011)
19. Emrouznejad, A., Yang, G.L.: A survey and analysis of the first 40 years of scholarly literature in DEA: 1978–2016. Socioecon. Plann. Sci. **61**, 4–8 (2018)
20. Linna, M.: Measuring hospital cost efficiency with panel data models. Health Econ. **7**(5), 415–427 (1998)
21. Banker, R.D., Conrad, R.F., Strauss, R.P.: A comparative application of data envelopment analysis and translog methods: an illustrative study of hospital production. Manage. Sci. **32**(1), 30–44 (1986)

22. Stefko, R., Gavurova, B., Kocisova, K.: Healthcare efficiency assessment using DEA analysis in the Slovak Republic. Heal. Econ. Rev. **8**(1), 1–12 (2018)
23. Afonso, G.P., Ferreira, D.C., Figueira, J.R.: A network-DEA model to evaluate the impact of quality and access on hospital performance. Annal. Operat. Res. 1–31 (2023)
24. Chiu, Y.H., Liu, H.H., Chang, M.C., Hsu, L.H.: Use DEA model to study hospitals' performance through medical quality. J. Stat. Manag. Syst. **11**(5), 823–846 (2008)
25. Antunes, J., Hadi-Vencheh, A., Jamshidi, A., Tan, Y., Wanke, P.: TEA-IS: a hybrid DEA-TOPSIS approach for assessing performance and synergy in Chinese health care. Decis. Support Syst. 113916 (2023)
26. Miszczynska, K., Miszczyński, P.M.: Measuring the efficiency of the healthcare sector in Poland–a window-DEA evaluation. Int. J. Product. Perform. Manag. **71**(7), 2743–2770 (2021)
27. Hollingsworth, B.: The measurement of efficiency and productivity of health care delivery. Health Econ. **17**(10), 1107–1128 (2008)
28. Kohl, S., Schoenfelder, J., Fügener, A., Brunner, J.O.: The use of Data Envelopment Analysis (DEA) in healthcare with a focus on hospitals. Health Care Manag. Sci. **22**, 245–286 (2019)
29. Arya, A., Yadav, S.P.: Development of intuitionistic fuzzy super-efficiency slack-based measure with an application to health sector. Comput. Ind. Eng. **115**, 368–380 (2018)
30. Jung, S., Son, J., Kim, C., Chung, K.: Efficiency measurement using data envelopment analysis (DEA) in public healthcare: research trends from 2017 to 2022. Processes **11**(3), 811 (2023)
31. Allahviranloo, T., Lotfi, F.H., Kiasari, M.K., Khezerloo, M.: On the fuzzy solution of LR fuzzy linear systems. Appl. Math. Model. **37**(3), 1170–1176 (2013). https://doi.org/10.1016/j.apm.2012.03.037
32. Chehlabi, M., Allahviranloo, T.: Concreted solutions to fuzzy linear fractional differential equations. Appl. Soft Comput. **44**, 108–116 (2016). https://doi.org/10.1016/j.asoc.2016.03.011
33. Mahmoodirad, A., Allahviranloo, T., Niroomand, S.: A new effective solution method for fully intuitionistic fuzzy transportation problem. Soft. Comput. **23**(12), 4521–4530 (2019). https://doi.org/10.1007/s00500-018-3115-z
34. Moloudzadeh, S., Allahviranloo, T., Darabi, P.: A new method for solving an arbitrary fully fuzzy linear system. Soft. Comput. **17**(9), 1725–1731 (2013). https://doi.org/10.1007/s00500-013-0986-x
35. Rahmani, A., Lotfi, F.H., Rostamy-Malkhalifeh, M., Allahviranloo, T.: A new method for defuzzification and ranking of fuzzy numbers based on the statistical beta distribution. Adv. Fuzzy Syst. **2016**, 1–8 (2016). https://doi.org/10.1155/2016/6945184
36. Amirteimoori, A., Allahviranloo, T., Kordrostami, S., Bagheri, S.F.: Improving decision-making units in performance analysis methods: a data envelopment analysis approach. Math. Sci. (2023). https://doi.org/10.1007/s40096-023-00512-5
37. Amirteimoori, A., Allahviranloo, T., Zadmirzaei, M.: Scale elasticity and technical efficiency analysis in the European forest sector: a stochastic value-based approach. Eur. J. Forest Res. (2023). https://doi.org/10.1007/s10342-023-01589-2
38. Amirteimoori, A., Allahviranloo, T., Zadmirzaei, M., Hasanzadeh, F.: On the environmental performance analysis: a combined fuzzy data envelopment analysis and artificial intelligence algorithms. Expert Syst. Appl. **224**, 119953 (2023). https://doi.org/10.1016/j.eswa.2023.119953
39. Abbasi, F., Allahviranloo, T.: The fuzzy arithmetic operations of transmission average on Pseudo-Hexagonal fuzzy numbers and its application in fuzzy system reliability analysis. Fuzzy Inf. Eng. **13**(1), 58–78 (2021). https://doi.org/10.1080/16168658.2021.1915449
40. Abbasi, F., Allahviranloo, T.: Realistic solution of fuzzy critical path problems, case study: the airport's cargo ground operation systems. Granul. Comput. **8**(3), 617–632 (2022). https://doi.org/10.1007/s41066-022-00347-w
41. Allahviranloo, T., Abbasi, F.: A new estimation of failure analysis in fuzzy Environment, case study: the electrical model failure for the football stadium. New Math. Nat. Comput. **18**(03), 791–817 (2022). https://doi.org/10.1142/s1793005722500387
42. Despić, O., Despić, M., Paradi, J.C.: DEA-R: ratio-based comparative efficiency model, its mathematical relation to DEA and its use in applications. J. Prod. Anal. **28**(1–2), 33–44 (2007)

43. Despić, O.: Some properties of geometric DEA models. Croat. Oper. Res. Rev. **4**(1), 2–18 (2013)
44. Mozaffari, M.R., Dadkhah, F., Jablonsky, J., Wanke, P.F.: Finding efficient surfaces in DEA-R models. Appl. Math. Comput. **386**, 125497 (2020)
45. Olesen, O.B., Petersen, N.C., Podinovski, V.V.: Efficiency measures and computational approaches for data envelopment analysis models with ratio inputs and outputs. Eur. J. Oper. Res. **261**(2), 640–655 (2017)
46. Mozaffari, M.R., Gerami, J., Wanke, P.F., Kamyab, P., Peyvas, M.: Ratio-based data envelopment analysis: an interactive approach to identify benchmark. Results Control Optim **6**, 100081 (2022)
47. Emrouznejad, A., Anouze, A.L., Thanassoulis, E.: A semi-oriented radial measure for measuring the efficiency of decision-making units with negative data, using DEA. Eur. J. Oper. Res. **200**(1), 297–304 (2010)
48. Emrouznejad, A., Amin, G.R., Thanassoulis, E., Anouze, A.L.: On the boundedness of the SORM DEA models with negative data. Eur. J. Oper. Res. **206**(1), 265–268 (2010)
49. Kaffash, S., Kazemi Matin, R., Tajik, M.: A directional semi-oriented radial DEA measure: an application on financial stability and the efficiency of banks. Ann. Oper. Res. **264**, 213–234 (2018)
50. Emrouznejad, A., Amin, G.R.: DEA models for ratio data: convexity consideration. Appl. Math. Model. **33**(1), 486–498 (2009)
51. Ghiyasi, M., Soltanifar, M., Sharafi, H.: A novel inverse DEA-R model with application in hospital efficiency. Socioecon. Plann. Sci. **84**, 101427 (2022)
52. Mahla, D., Agarwal, S., Amin, G.R., Mathur, T.: An inverse data envelopment analysis model to consider ratio data and preferences of decision-makers. IMA J. Manag. Math. (2022)
53. Sohrabi, A., Gerami, J., Mozaffari, M.R.: A novel inverse DEA-R model for inputs/output estimation. J. Math. Ext. **16** (2021)
54. Abbasi, F., Allahviranloo, T.: Conception and implementation of a new Data-Driven fuzzy method for reliability and safety analysis. New Math. Nat. Comput. **16**(02), 339–361 (2020). https://doi.org/10.1142/s1793005720500210
55. Allahviranloo, T., Abbasbandy, S., Rouhparvar, H.: The exact solutions of fuzzy wave-like equations with variable coefficients by a variational iteration method. Appl. Soft Comput. **11**(2), 2186–2192 (2011). https://doi.org/10.1016/j.asoc.2010.07.018
56. Allahviranloo, T., Ezadi, S.: Z-Advanced numbers processes. Inf. Sci. **480**, 130–143 (2019). https://doi.org/10.1016/j.ins.2018.12.012
57. Allahviranloo, T., Gouyandeh, Z., Armand, A.: A full fuzzy method for solving differential equation based on Taylor expansion. J. Intell. Fuzzy Syst. **29**(3), 1039–1055 (2015). https://doi.org/10.3233/ifs-151713
58. Allahviranloo, T.A., Kermani, M.: Numerical methods for fuzzy linear partial differential equations under new definition for derivative. Iran. J. Fuzzy Syst. **7**(3), 33–50 (2010). https://doi.org/10.22111/ijfs.2010.187.
59. Abbasbandy, S., Viranloo, T.A.: Numerical solution of fuzzy differential equation. Math. Comput. Appl. **7**(1), 41–52 (2002). https://doi.org/10.3390/mca7010041
60. Banker, R.D., Amirteimoori, A., Allahviranloo, T., Sinha, R.P.: Performance analysis and managerial ability in the general insurance market: a study of India and Iran. Inf. Technol. Manage. (2023). https://doi.org/10.1007/s10799-023-00405-y
61. Charnes, A., Cooper, W.W., Rhodes, E.: Measuring the efficiency of decision-making units. Eur. J. Oper. Res. **2**(6), 429–444 (1978)
62. Lotfi, F.H., Jahanshahloo, G.R., Soltanifar, M., Ebrahimnejad, A., Mansourzadeh, S.M.: Relationship between MOLP and DEA based on output-orientated CCR dual model. Expert Syst. Appl. **37**(6), 4331–4336 (2010)
63. Seyyedabbasi, A.: WOASCALF: a new hybrid whale optimization algorithm based on sine cosine algorithm and levy flight to solve global optimization problems. Adv. Eng. Softw. **173**, 103272 (2022). https://doi.org/10.1016/j.advengsoft.2022.103272

64. Seyyedabbasi, A.: A reinforcement learning-based metaheuristic algorithm for solving global optimization problems. Adv. Eng. Softw. **178**, 103411 (2023). https://doi.org/10.1016/j.advengsoft.2023.10341
65. Seyyedabbasi, A.: Binary sand cat swarm optimization algorithm for wrapper feature selection on biological data. Biomimetics **8**(3), 310 (2023)
66. Seyyedabbasi, A., Kiani, F., Allahviranloo, T., Fernandez-Gamiz, U., Noeiaghdam, S.: Optimal data transmission and pathfinding for WSN and decentralized IoT systems using I-GWO and Ex-GWO algorithms. Alex. Eng. J. **63**, 339–357 (2023)
67. Soltanifar, M.: A n ew voting model for groups with members of unequal power and proficiency. Int. J. Indus. Math. **12**(2), 121–134 (2020)
68. Soltanifar, M., Krylovas, A., Kosareva, N.: Voting-KEmeny Median Indicator Ranks Accordance method for determining criteria priority and weights in solving multi-attribute decision-making problems. Soft Comput. 1–16 (2023)
69. Soltanifar, M., Tavana, M., Santos-Arteaga, F.J., Sharafi, H.: A hybrid multi-attribute decision-making and data envelopment analysis method for solving problems with heterogeneous attributes. Environ. Sci. Policy (vol. Submitted 2022)
70. Soltanifar, M., Ghiyasi, M., Sharafi, H.: Inverse DEA-R models for merger analysis with negative data. IMA J. Manag. Math. (2022)

Multiple Attribute Decision Making in Ranking the Criteria in Health (with Certain and Uncertain Data)

Mansour Soufi

Abstract Multi Attribute Decision Making techniques are used to evaluate the performance of the healthcare system with several attributes and sub-attributes. By using MADM, we can identify the best solutions to improve the performance of the healthcare system. This method allows us to compare and rank various factors such as the quality of medical services, access to treatment, healthcare costs, and so on. Given the breadth and complexity of the healthcare system, evaluating its performance based on a single attribute is usually not sufficient. For example, we can refer to the issue of access to treatment. In this case, we can use attributes such as the distance between the hospital and the place of residence, the number of hospital beds, and the number of specialist physicians to evaluate it. In short, MADM can be useful in improving the performance of the healthcare system and achieving health goals. Using this method, one can easily identify the necessary attributes and propose appropriate solutions to improve them. In this section, we intend to use some MADM methods to rank the performance evaluation attributes of the smart healthcare management system. The smart healthcare system refers to a set of technologies and information systems that are designed and implemented to improve the performance of the healthcare system and promote public health. This system is built based on wireless communications, social networks, sensors, robots, artificial intelligence, cloud, and smart health data. Using the smart healthcare system, health resources can be used more effectively, efficiently, and beneficially.

Keywords Multi attribute decision making · Evaluate the performance · Healthcare · Smart healthcare system · Certain and uncertain data

M. Soufi (✉)
Department of Industrial Management, Rasht Branch, Islamic Azad University, Rasht, Iran
e-mail: msoufi45@gmail.com

T. Allahviranloo et al. (eds.), *Decision Making in Healthcare Systems*,
Studies in Systems, Decision and Control 513,
https://doi.org/10.1007/978-3-031-46735-6_5

1 Introduction and Motivation

The word "decision-making" means to cut off, and its general concept is to cut off intentions and aims and to reach a conclusion and a solution. Decision-making is defined as choosing one solution among several options. So far, various theories and methods have been proposed for decision-making in research issues. Effective decision-making is an integral part of organizational management. Managers, team leaders, and even employees are involved in structured, semi-structured, and non-structured decision-making every day. According to the organizational levels introduced by Henry Mintzberg, decisions at the operational manager level are structured and planned, decisions at the middle manager level are semi-structured, and decisions at the senior manager level are unstructured and unplanned. Undoubtedly, proper choices and approaches help to achieve organizational goals more effectively, resulting in optimizing operational decisions for the growth of products (goods, services, and ideas).

Herbert Simon, an American economist and popular scientist, was one of the first theorists to highlight the importance of decision-making in the business environment. He became famous for his numerous contributions in the fields of psychology, statistics, and mathematics, and received the Nobel Prize in Economics in 1978. However, he is best known for his work in the area of decision-making in organizations, which is also called behaviorism. Herbert Simon's decision-making theory was first introduced in his famous book "Administrative Behavior" in 1947. Simon emphasized strategic decisions because if they are not made in a timely manner, they will have a negative influence on the organization's goals. This concept can be divided into two parts: one is a decision that individuals reach based on experience (intuitive decision-making), and the other is a decision that is made through a logical process. Also, the results of decisions should be measurable. One of the techniques for decision making is Data Envelopment Analysis (DEA), and many researchers have conducted research on this topic. Several recent papers have been cited to mention their research area [6, 13, 14, 15]. Some authors have explored the topic in a different way: safety analysis and reliability [4, 5, 7].

Contrary to classical theorists, Simon's view is that there is no best decision, because decision-makers are never able to have complete information, therefore there will always be a better action or decision. Simon's decision-making theory takes into account psychological aspects that have been overlooked by classical economists. Factors such as stress and incentives limit an individual's capacity to solve complex problems. Generally, logical decision-making is very limited and humans exhibit different behaviors in the presence of risks and uncertainty. At the core of this theory is the concept of "Utility" which suggests that individuals should pursue goals or make decisions that minimize risks and drawbacks instead of solely focusing on maximizing the objective function.

There are three stages in the decision-making process:

A: Awareness or information gathering stage

In this stage, the decision-making area must be identified and the decision issue must be specified. The problems and issues of the organization are identified to analyze and find solutions for managing the organizational environment.

B: Design stage

In this stage, various solutions are created, developed, and analyzed. Management is looking for appropriate strategies. Internal environmental analysis is done to identify strengths and weaknesses, and external environmental analysis is done to identify opportunities and threats. Ultimately, operational strategies are determined in this stage. There are two types of thinking in this stage: 1—Option thinking, and 2—Value thinking. Option thinking means choosing one option from among several options, and value thinking means focusing on generating new options for decision making. In the definition of design, the concepts of creation and development are related to value thinking, and the analysis of solutions is related to option thinking.

C: Selection Stage

After preparing a list of options, the selection stage begins, in which the different consequences of all options are critically examined and evaluated to choose the most appropriate option. This stage requires creativity, judgment, and quantitative analysis skills.

The decision-making environment is a set of factors and conditions that affect the decision-making process. These factors can be internal or external to the organization and can include political, economic, social, technological, legal, and environmental factors. Understanding the decision-making environment is essential for making effective and informed decisions. It requires a thorough analysis of the factors that may influence the decision, as well as an understanding of their interrelationships and potential influence s. By considering these factors and their potential effects, decision-makers can make more informed and effective decisions.

Familiarity and mastery of the "science and art of decision-making" is one of the very important prerequisites for effective studies and research. Undoubtedly, the ultimate goal of such research is to achieve a deeper and better understanding for aligning actions with each other and even aligning actions with "inaction". Actions that are ultimately formulated and implemented in the form of specific and coherent programs and plans must generally be identified, evaluated and selected based on a systematic, scientific and valid method.

As Simon mentioned in the decision-making stages, in the awareness or informational stage, the decision-making environment must be identified. Generally, three types of environmental conditions for decision-making have been identified:

1. Certainty: When the decision maker has complete information about the problem and the available alternatives, and can accurately predict the outcome of each alternative. Modeling for these decision-making conditions is mostly based on

mathematical and specific models such as cost–benefit analysis, classical optimization models, inventory control, substitution models, job allocation, linear programming, and some cases of dynamic programming.
2. Risk: When the decision maker has incomplete information about the problem and the available alternatives, and cannot accurately predict the outcome of each alternative, but can estimate the probability of success for each alternative. For example, designing attack scenarios during wartime is a risky decision-making process, although a commander tries to gather most of the information about the enemy in advance. The models used for decision making in such conditions may be various mathematical and probabilistic models. All mathematical models can be introduced in the framework of operations research, which, in addition to the models presented for decision making under certainty conditions, uses probabilistic models such as expected value, linear programming, break-even analysis, return on investment, Bayesian analysis, probability distribution curves, queuing models, Markov chain analysis, decision tree analysis, game theory, and queuing theory.
3. Uncertainty: When the decision maker has very little or no information about the problem and the available alternatives, and cannot accurately predict the outcome of each alternative or estimate the probability of success for each alternative. Modeling for this type of decision-making is mostly done through decision matrices. In this case, decision-makers also resort to intuitive or creative methods. Creativity is itself an agent for better understanding the problem and identifying options.
4. Conflicting: Decision making in conflicting situations involves making a choice between two or more options, each of which has its own advantages and disadvantages. In such situations, the decision maker may need to balance conflicting goals and objectives in order to arrive at the best possible solution.

To make decisions in conflicting situations, various techniques and methods can be used. These may include multi-criteria decision analysis (MCDA), game theory, decision trees, and sensitivity analysis, among others. MCDA involves considering multiple criteria or factors in the decision-making process and assigning weights to each criterion to reflect their relative importance. Game theory involves analyzing the choices of multiple parties with conflicting interests and predicting the outcome of the decision based on the strategies chosen by each party. Decision trees involve mapping out the possible outcomes of different decisions and their associated probabilities. Sensitivity analysis involves testing the robustness of a decision by varying different parameters and assessing their influence on the decision outcome.

Effective decision making in conflicting situations requires a clear understanding of the goals and objectives involved, as well as a comprehensive analysis of the available options and their associated risks and benefits. It may also involve collaboration and negotiation with other stakeholders to arrive at a mutually acceptable solution.

2 Literature Review

During the era of industrial revolution around the world, and especially after World War II, optimization models gained the attention of many mathematicians and industry professionals. The main emphasis of classical optimization models is to have a criterion or objective function that can be linear, non-linear, or a combination of both. The algorithms used for such decisions are different, but most of them do not consider many environmental factors and consider them as uncontrollable factors. For this reason, the power of these algorithms is limited to the use of various criteria and they differ from each other. These algorithms have drawbacks such as the inability to use multiple and continuous criteria, uncertainty and risk, considering the project's relationship with the value share and optimal use of resources, non-monetary attributes, and the decision maker's knowledge and expertise. These weaknesses have led to the emergence of various multi-criteria decision-making (MCDM) algorithms in the last 50 years [26]. MCDM algorithms can provide more flexibility and adaptability in the decision-making process. Multi-criteria decision-making methods are divided into two categories: multiple objective decision-making (MODM) and multiple attribute decision-making (MADM). The purpose of multi-criteria decision-making is to sort, rank, select, and describe criteria and options. Data sorting refers to arranging data in a particular format. Sorting algorithms determine a specific order for arranging data. Common orderings are often numerical or alphabetical. The importance of sorting lies in the fact that searching for data can be optimized at a higher level if it is sorted. Sorting can also help to represent data in more readable formats based on one or more predefined features such as skin color, race, gender, objects, or variables and attributes. In ranking, options are ranked, and the highest and lowest preferences are identified. In selection, one or more options are selected together. They determine what should be and prescribe it, rather than describe it. In description, they describe how the changes or features of a variable should be or are, and there is no prescription. In all of these, we are faced with four tasks and two general states: (A) Variable values are the criterion for action. (B) The desirability of the variable value is the criterion for action. The desirability is a mental and relative concept that varies for different individuals [37].

In many reviewed articles, it was found that multi-criteria decision-making techniques are used regardless of their specific application, and after implementation, no specific framework is followed for model validation. Each decision-making method has its own specific application, such as AHP, ANP, PROMETHEE, TOPSIS, MAUT/UTA, MACBETH, and DEA for selection and ranking, AHP Sort, UTADIS, ELECTRE Tri, and FowSort for sorting, and GAIA and FU-Gaia for description. Some techniques have specific applications, for example, ELECTREI is only used for selection and ELECTREII&III are only used for ranking.

In multi-criteria decision-making models, different criteria are considered to evaluate various options. These models can be classified based on different classification methods, such as:

Combination methods: In these methods, different criteria are combined using combination methods to calculate an overall score for each option. For example, AHP, ANP, and TOPSIS are methods in this category.

Outranking methods: In these methods, options are ranked based on the different scores assigned to them according to various criteria. For example, ELECTRE and PROMETHEE are methods in this category.

Disaggregation methods: In these methods, different criteria are evaluated separately, and then scores are assigned to the options using grouping methods. For example, MAUT/UTA and MACBETH are methods in this category.

Combination and Outranking methods: In these methods, different criteria are combined using combination methods, and then options are ranked using outranking methods. For example, GAIA is a method in this category [38].

Table 1 shows the types of classification of MCDM methods based on the type of decision-making problem. Table 2 shows the Required inputs for MCDM ranking or choice methods. Table 5 indicates the required inputs for ranking or choice methods in multi-criteria decision making. This table examines multiple alternatives based on various criteria using different decision-making techniques. Different outputs are generated using various methods. The "Effort Input" column represents the level of effort required for each step, where a higher level indicates more effort and a lower level indicates less effort [17].

The Inputs column lists the main inputs required for MCDM, including the criteria, alternatives, performance scores, and weights. The MCDM Methods column lists the specific methods chosen for each step, including TOPSIS for ranking alternatives, SAW for aggregating performance scores, AHP for calculating weighted scores, and ELECTRE for determining dominance.

The Outputs column lists the specific outputs generated by each step, including a ranking of alternatives, a numerical score for each alternative, a weighted score for each alternative, and a determination of which alternatives dominate the others.

Note that the specific inputs, methods, and outputs chosen will depend on the specific characteristics of the decision problem and the preferences of the decision maker. This is just an example to illustrate the different steps involved in MCDM.

In another case, MCDM can be classified into two categories: compensatory and non-compensatory. Based on this, in compensatory models, the decision maker is willing to trade-off between criteria and attribute, and a change in one attribute is compensated by an opposing change in other attributes. However, in non-compensatory models, the decision maker is not willing to trade-off between criteria. A weakness in one attribute cannot be compensated by an advantage in another attribute. Each attribute is the basis for evaluating competing options.

Compensatory methods are also classified into three categories: scoring methods, compromising methods, and non-ranking methods.

Scoring methods: the preferred option has the highest score. In these methods, the top-scoring option is selected using various algorithms.

Table 1 MCDM method classification according to type of decision problem

Type of problem	MCDM methods
Choice problem	1. Multi-attribute utility theory (MAUT) 2. Simple multi-attribute rating technique (SMART) 3. Preference ranking organization method for enrichment evaluations (PROMETHEE) 4. Elimination and choice expressing reality (ELECTRE) 5. Analytic hierarchy process (AHP) 6. Technique for order preference by similarity to ideal solution (TOPSIS) 7. Goal programming (GP) 8. Multi-objective linear programming (MOLP) 9. Genetic algorithms (GA)
Ranking problem	1. Analytic hierarchy process (AHP) 2. Technique for order preference by similarity to ideal solution (TOPSIS) 3. Preference ranking organization method for enrichment evaluations (PROMETHEE) 4. Elimination and choice expressing reality (ELECTRE) 5. Multi-attribute utility theory (MAUT) 6. Simple multi-attribute rating technique (SMART) 7. Grey relational analysis (GRA)
Sorting problem	1. Multi-attribute utility theory (MAUT) 2. Simple multi-attribute rating technique (SMART) 3. Analytic hierarchy process (AHP) 4. Technique for order preference by similarity to ideal solution (TOPSIS) 5. Preference ranking organization method for enrichment evaluations (PROMETHEE) 6. Elimination and choice expressing reality (ELECTRE) 7. Grey relational analysis (GRA)
Description problem	1. Data envelopment analysis (DEA) 2. Free disposal hull (FDH)

Compromising methods: the preferred option has the highest proximity and similarity to the ideal option.

Non-ranking methods: the preferred option has the best situation according to a defined consistent criterion (Table 3).

Non-compensatory models are decision-making models that do not allow for trade-offs between different criteria. In other words, these models do not permit a high score on one criterion to compensate for a low score on another. Non-compensatory models are often used when the decision being made is important, complex, and has a high level of risk, as they allow for a more structured and rigorous decision-making process. Examples of non-compensatory models include the lexicographic model, the conjunctive model, and the disjunctive model. In the lexicographic model, decision-makers first rank the criteria in order of importance and then choose the option that performs best on the most important criterion. In the conjunctive model,

Table 2 Required inputs for MCDM ranking or choice methods

Inputs	Input level	MCDM methods	Outputs
Criteria	Low	Analytic hierarchy process (AHP)	Weighted criteria scores
Alternative	Low	Simple additive weighting (SAW)	Score for each alternative
Performance	High	Technique for order of preference by similarity to ideal solution (TOPSIS)	Distance from ideal solution and negative ideal solution, relative closeness
Weights	Low	Electre I	Dominance matrix
Performance	High	Promethee II	Preference degree and net flow
Weights	Low	Analytic network process (ANP)	Overall priority and importance of each criterion
Performance	High	Grey relational analysis (GRA)	Grey relational grade
Weights	Low	Technique for order preference by similarity to ideal solution–grey relation analysis (TOPSIS-GRA)	Grey relational distance and relative closeness
Performance	High	Preference ranking organization method for enrichment evaluations (PROMETHEE)	Preference degree and net flow
Performance	High	Grey decision-making trial and evaluation laboratory (DEMATEL)	Direct and indirect influences of criteria
Weights	Low	Elimination et choix traduisant la realité (ELECTRE III)	Credibility and stability indices

decision-makers set minimum acceptable standards for each criterion and choose the option that meets all of these standards. In the disjunctive model, decision-makers set minimum acceptable standards for each criterion and choose the option that meets any of these standards [22].

Figure 1 depicts a classification of Operation Research (OR) techniques in the field of decision making.

Multiple Attribute Decision Making (MADM) is a widely used approach in various fields, including healthcare, to support decision-making processes involving multiple criteria [27]. MADM methods assist decision-makers in ranking and prioritizing alternatives based on their performance on various attributes. A Comprehensive Review of MADM Techniques in Healthcare Decision Making provides an overview of various MADM techniques and their applications in healthcare decision-making. It discusses the use of certain and uncertain data and highlights the challenges and limitations faced by decision-makers in the health domain.

A Fuzzy MADM Approach for Ranking Health Criteria [18] presents a fuzzy MADM approach for ranking health criteria by considering the uncertainty associated with the evaluation of alternatives. The proposed method utilizes fuzzy logic to handle vague and imprecise information.

Table 3 A number of compensatory and non-compensatory techniques

Method	Type	Features
Analytical hierarchy process (AHP)	Compensatory	Multiple criteria, hierarchical structure
Technique for order preference by similarity to ideal solution (TOPSIS)	Compensatory	Ranking alternatives, distance to ideal solution
Preference ranking organization method for enrichment evaluation (PROMETHEE)	Compensatory	Ranking alternatives, pairwise comparison
Simple additive weighting (SAW)	Compensatory	Weighted sum approach
Elimination and choice expressing reality (ELECTRE)	Non-compensatory	Categorical criteria, outranking approach
Grey relational analysis (GRA)	Compensatory	Multiple criteria, degree of similarity
VlseKriterijumska Optimizacija I Kompromisno Resenje (VIKOR)	Compensatory	Ranking alternatives, distance to ideal and anti-ideal solutions
Technique for order preference by similarity to ideal solution for complex proportional assessment (TOPSIS-COPRAS)	Compensatory	Ranking alternatives, distance to ideal solution, proportional preferences
Multi-attribute global inference of quality (MAGIQ)	Compensatory	Multiple criteria, fuzzy logic approach

Note that this is not an exhaustive list and there are many other MCDM methods that may be used in different decision-making contexts.

Interval-Valued Intuitionistic Fuzzy MADM Method for Health Technology Assessment introduces an interval-valued intuitionistic fuzzy MADM method for health technology assessment. The method combines interval-valued intuitionistic fuzzy sets with a MADM approach to handle uncertain and imprecise data.

An Integrated Approach for Ranking Health Criteria Using Dempster-Shafer Theory and Technique for Order of Preference by Similarity to Ideal Solution proposes an integrated approach for ranking health criteria based on Dempster-Shafer theory and Technique for Order of Preference by Similarity to Ideal Solution (TOPSIS). The Dempster-Shafer theory is utilized to handle uncertain and imprecise data, while TOPSIS is employed for ranking alternatives.

A Hybrid MADM Method for Ranking Health Criteria with Hesitant Fuzzy Information presents a hybrid MADM method for ranking health criteria using hesitant fuzzy information. The proposed method combines the hesitant fuzzy linguistic term set with the VIKOR method to handle uncertainty and hesitancy in decision-making.

Fuzzy Analytic Hierarchy Process for Ranking Health Criteria with Uncertain Data proposes a fuzzy Analytic Hierarchy Process (AHP) for ranking health criteria when faced with uncertain data. The fuzzy AHP extends the traditional AHP by incorporating fuzzy numbers to represent uncertain judgments.

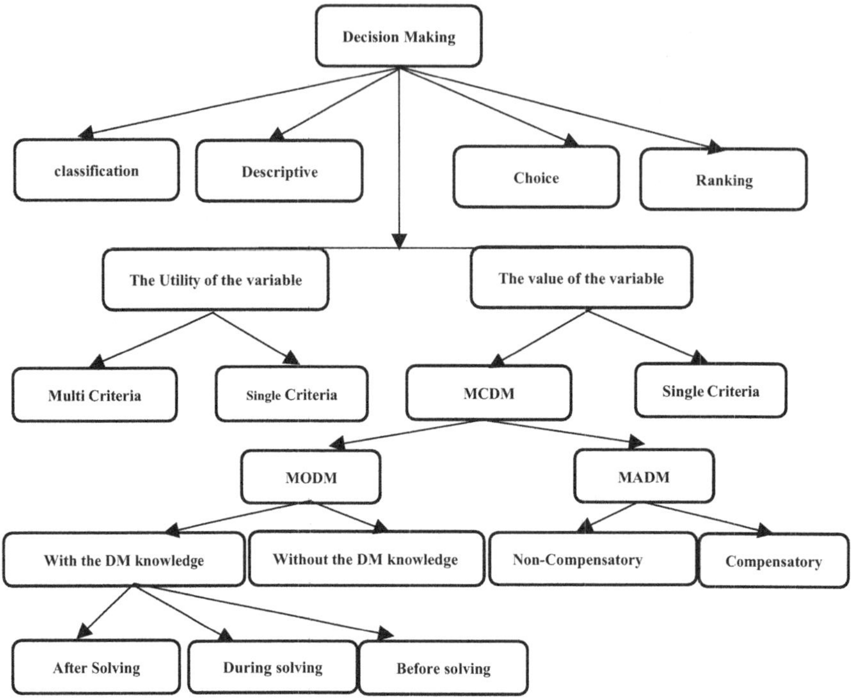

Fig. 1 Classification of operation research techniques in the field of decision making

Recent research points out that most mathematical models like dynamic systems and also linear systems get involved with real-world problems. Since their related information has different forms like certainty and uncertainty, the uncertain version of these models does have more importance in the applications.

In health problems, two types of mathematical models; fuzzy dynamic systems and fuzzy linear programming problems even transportation problems, play an important role, on the other hand, the main and basic model of fuzzy linear programming problems is fuzzy linear systems.

In conclusion, fuzzy differential equations (as a special version of dynamic systems) [1, 11, 20], and fuzzy linear systems (as a basic model of fuzzy linear programming problems) [33], have an important role in this research. Recently several research has been done on investigating the advanced version of the uncertain information [11, 34, 36], and moreover the above-mentioned basic models.

In conclusion, the literature review spanning from 2013 to 2023 demonstrates the progress made in applying MADM techniques to rank health criteria with both certain and uncertain data. These techniques have shown promise in supporting decision-making processes in healthcare, enabling stakeholders to make informed choices and allocate resources. However, further research is needed to address the challenges associated with robust modeling, handling diverse data, and incorporating stakeholder preferences effectively [27].

3 Smart Healthcare System Management

The existential philosophy of the healthcare system is to produce health through providing services to patients, and if it does not have the acceptance and trust of patients, it will lose its identity. Complexity, increasing costs, and the vital nature of healthcare are among the factors that encourage health organizations to transform their performance evaluation. On the other hand, there is a growing population in cities and metropolises worldwide, and migration or frequent travel requires special attention to adopt better healthcare policies and management. Additionally, the massive influx of other diseases is uncontrollable, and the patients' condition does not improve every day with traditional methods.

Due to the constant increase in patients with chronic diseases and long-term medical treatments, the medical sector has faced considerable pressure in recent years. Some clinical applications have evolved to overcome the burden of chronic hospital patients. In science and technology, the concept of smart healthcare has recently gained a lot of attention and has shown great promise. Technology-based healthcare generally refers to a type of service design that provides healthcare to individuals anywhere, anytime, and with electronic devices such as laptops, tablets, or smartphones. The concept of smart healthcare includes electronic health.

In the conceptual model of smart health, all elements of the healthcare system and health insurance such as hospitals, clinics, other medical and para-clinical centers, medical offices, pharmacies, laboratories, imaging centers, etc. are equipped with intelligent systems that are interconnected in a unified and comprehensive system architecture, and fulfill the current and future needs of stakeholders at various levels. Smart healthcare is actually one of the benefits of technological advancements and communication, which has emerged to improve the quality of healthcare and hygiene services with the help of humans. Smart healthcare is defined by technology, which includes better diagnostic tools, better treatment for patients, and devices that improve the quality of life for everyone.

The key concept of smart healthcare includes health and hygiene services, electronic record management, smart home services, and smart medical devices and connections. In smart healthcare, not only in the field of treatment, but throughout the entire health value chain, whether in the field of health and prevention or in the field of monitoring, health attributes are measured and, if necessary, the system will intelligently provide the necessary alerts. Smart healthcare in the health sector will focus more on disease prevention, and individuals' health attributes will be continuously measured, recorded, and maintained and updated on dedicated servers. In other words, an intelligent health file has been created and a specialist continuously examines the individual's health attributes. By informing the person and providing necessary consultations, the specialist always guides the individual.

For long-term medical care and clinical access to accurate physiological performance measurements, a numerical scale is a tool that measures the quality of performed activities. It is considered an essential part of any activity as it leads to the improvement of services by using measurable information. Timely and relevant information and performance evaluation lead to awareness among healthcare decision-makers, enable monitoring the implementation of policies, and move towards goals. It also increases stakeholders' trust in service providers. Measurement and performance evaluation lead to motivating individuals towards desirable behavior. Avoiding this process is like abandoning valuable and scarce resources to an unknown fate. This process helps managers evaluate the results and, with the necessary feedback, choose and implement corrective and remedial actions based on the level of success in goals and plans. Given the importance of performance evaluation, it is important to prioritize factors in performance evaluation. This is also important due to the competition present in the healthcare organization industry. The factors that have priority in performance evaluation include setting precise and achievable goals, measuring the quality and quantity of performance, providing appropriate feedback to individuals and organizations, and developing and implementing corrective plans to improve performance.

The high cost and economic pressure of medical care, aging population, increasing prevalence of chronic diseases, and shortage of skilled personnel justify the need for smart healthcare. The use of intelligent technologies can overcome many of the limitations of the healthcare sector and adopting information and communication technology in healthcare as a way to bridge the supply–demand gap and based on its strategic goals, which are based on increasing efficiency, improving service quality, equitable access, and optimal management and monitoring, can have positive effects on improving health attributes in society as one of the fundamental pillars of growth and development. The World Health Organization (WHO) also stated in its 2018 statement that the use of digital health solutions can revolutionize how people access better healthcare standards and services for the promotion and protection of their health and well-being.

By implementing the intelligent automation process in the healthcare network and the treatment sector, the evaluation criteria will undoubtedly change based on the nature of the virtual system. What is important in achieving the desirable performance of the health sector is usability, accessibility, responsiveness, and standardization. Unfortunately, due to the infrastructural weaknesses in the field of healthcare system intelligence, precise attention and evaluation of these parameters are important and necessary, especially with the prevalence of emerging and pervasive diseases in the present era, such as the bitter experience of the COVID-19 pandemic. In many cases, in-person treatment conditions carry a very high risk, and even for many patients, it is not possible. In this case, if the ground for non-in-person treatments is provided adequately, it will save a lot of healthcare costs. Therefore, the need to pay attention to the infrastructural performance management of intelligent healthcare is of double importance.

4 Ranking Healthcare Attributes with Madm Technique

Multi Attribute Decision Making techniques are used to evaluate the performance of the healthcare system with several attributes and sub-attributes. By using MADM, we can identify the best solutions to improve the performance of the healthcare system. This method allows us to compare and rank various factors such as the quality of medical services, access to treatment, healthcare costs, and so on. Given the breadth and complexity of the healthcare system, evaluating its performance based on a single attribute is usually not sufficient. For example, we can refer to the issue of access to treatment. In this case, we can use attributes such as the distance between the hospital and the place of residence, the number of hospital beds, and the number of specialist physicians to evaluate it. In short, MADM can be useful in improving the performance of the healthcare system and achieving health goals. Using this method, one can easily identify the necessary attributes and propose appropriate solutions to improve them. In this section, we intend to use some MADM methods to rank the performance evaluation attributes of the smart healthcare management system. The smart healthcare system refers to a set of technologies and information systems that are designed and implemented to improve the performance of the healthcare system and promote public health. This system is built based on wireless communications, social networks, sensors, robots, artificial intelligence, cloud, and smart health data. Using the smart healthcare system, health resources can be used more effectively, efficiently, and beneficially.

Due to the multi attribute nature of the issue of managing health in educational and medical centers, one of the main challenges in any research is identifying a set of evaluation attributes and sub-attributes.

5 Identifying the Attributes and Sub-attributes for Evaluating the Performance of Smart Healthcare Management

To accomplish this task, after studying and reviewing the background of the subject, a set of criteria and sub-criteria used in previous studies were extracted and made available to experts through an online questionnaire. Considering the large number of criteria, in this stage, a set of criteria and sub-criteria were extracted for the implementation of the Delphi method and the next screening stage by eliminating some of them that were unimportant or lacked the necessary data and also by merging them and adding some specific criteria under study. These mentioned criteria are presented in Table 4.

Table 4 Attribute and sub-attribute for evaluating the health management performance of educational and medical centers

Main attribute	Sub-attribute	Definition of attribute
Responsiveness	Handling problems	Refers to the ability of a healthcare system to respond promptly and appropriately to the needs and expectations of its patients and other stakeholders
	Easy platform	
Suitability	Closeness to personal preferences	Refers to the appropriateness and compatibility of the healthcare services provided with the needs and preferences of the patients
	Easy access to facilities	
	Closeness to needs	
Standardization	Global standards	Refers to the extent to which healthcare practices, processes, and outcomes are consistent, uniform, and adhere to established guidelines or standards
	Fit with successful samples	
	Ease of use	
Efficiency	Time and resource management	Refers to the ability of a healthcare system to maximize the outputs it generates from the available resources
	Use of technology	
	Workforce productivity	
	Cost-effectiveness	
Effectiveness	Clinical outcomes	Refers to the extent to which a healthcare system or intervention achieves its intended goals and objectives
	Patient satisfaction	
	Quality of life	
	Adverse events	
Safety	Incidence of adverse events	Refers to the ability of a healthcare system to ensure the prevention of errors, harm, or injury to patients during the provision of healthcare services
	Patient safety culture	
	Error reporting	
	Infection control	
Sustainability	Environmental influence	Refers to the ability of the healthcare system to meet the current and future healthcare needs of the population while also ensuring that the resources are used in a way that promotes long-term environmental, social, and economic sustainability
	Resource conservation	
	Cost containment	
	Social responsibility	
	Cultural sustainability	
Equity	Access of the underprivileged	Refers to the fairness and justice in the distribution of healthcare resources, services, and outcomes among different population groups, regardless of their social, economic, or demographic characteristics
	Fairness in resource allocation	
	Equal treatment for all patients	
	Elimination of discrimination	
	Rural and urban health disparities	

5.1 Execution of Delphi Process

In the Delphi method used in this research, 10 experts were selected to rate 30 criteria and sub-criteria extracted from the literature based on their importance. In the first questionnaire, the experts were asked to add any other criteria they thought were important besides the mentioned ones. Accordingly, two sub-criteria, "excellent performance" and "quality of work," were added for evaluating the effectiveness criterion in the second round. The results of the first round are presented in Fig. 2 and Table 5.

After analyzing the results of the first round, by adding two proposed sub-attributes by experts, the second questionnaire along with the results of the first round was made available to the experts. Also, attributes that had extreme differences of opinion among respondents were identified. The results of the second round of the Delphi method can be seen in Fig. 3 and Table 6.

Based on the results obtained in the second round, in order to ensure the results and obtain consensus among the experts, the third round was also conducted. In this round, if the difference in the average of each criterion becomes zero, it means that the experts have reached a consensus on that criterion. The results of the third round are presented in Fig. 3 and Table 7 (Fig. 4).

As shown in Table 7, the experts have reached a consensus on most criteria, meaning that the difference in the average between the second and third rounds is zero. Figure 5 shows the results of the third round and a comparison of the second and third rounds.

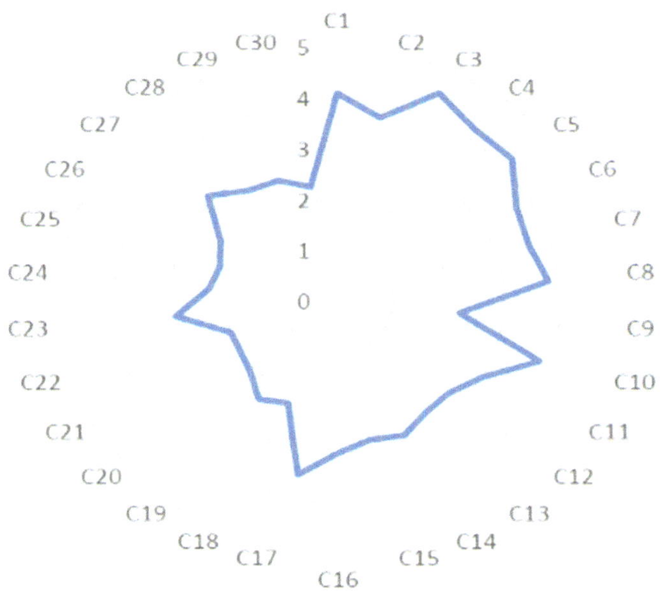

Fig. 2 First round results of expert survey in Delphi method

Table 5 The results obtained in the first round of the Delphi method

Main attribute	Sub-attribute	Mean	Standard deviation
Responsiveness	Handling problems	2	0.816
	Easy platform	2	1.033
Suitability	Closeness to personal preferences	2	0.816
	Easy access to facilities	2	1.033
	Closeness to needs	2.9	0.994
Standardization	Global standards	2	0.816
	Fit with successful samples	2	1.033
	Ease of use	2.9	0.994
Efficiency	Time and resource management	4.1	0.876
	Use of technology	3.7	1.16
	Workforce productivity	4.5	0.707
	Cost-effectiveness	4.2	0.789
Effectiveness	Clinical outcomes	4.3	0.675
	Patient satisfaction	3.7	0.675
	Quality of life	3.6	0.699
	Adverse events	3.8	0.632
Safety	Incidence of adverse events	2.2	1.033
	Patient safety culture	3.8	0.919
	Error reporting	3	1.155
	Infection control	2.7	1.059
Sustainability	Environmental influence	2.7	1.059
	Resource conservation	2.9	1.197
	Cost containment	2.8	0.632
	Social responsibility	3	0.949
	Cultural sustainability	3.5	0.527
Equity	Accessibility for disadvantaged groups	2.3	1.059
	Fairness in resource allocation	2.2	0.632
	Equal treatment for all patients	2.7	1.252
	Elimination of discrimination	3.1	1.370
	Rural and urban health disparities	2.7	0.675

It is clear from Table 8 that the Kendall's coefficient of concordance has improved in each round compared to the previous round. After achieving desirable values of the Kendall's coefficient and reaching agreement on the importance of the criteria, the Delphi process can be terminated. Table 9 shows the final agreed-upon criteria and sub-criteria extracted by the Delphi method.

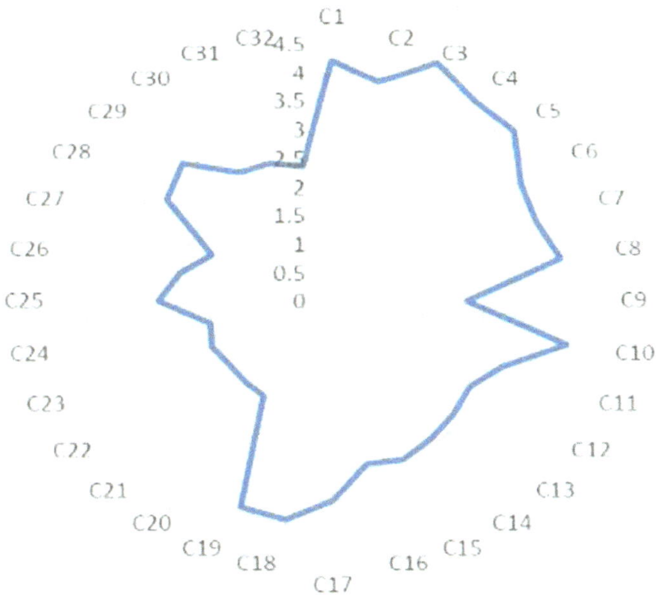

Fig. 3 Second round results of expert survey in Delphi method

6 Ranking Healthcare Attributes with Certain Data

6.1 Ranking Using Dematel Technique

To rank the attributes and sub-attributes, we will use the DEMATEL (Decision-Making Trial and Evaluation Laboratory) technique, which is a method that can help determine the causal relationships and the interdependencies between different attributes and sub-attributes DEMATEL is one of the multi-criteria decision-making methods used to identify the pattern of interrelationships among the variables under study. This method is used to identify the pattern of relationships among a set of criteria and attributes.

The term DEMATEL stands for Decision Making Trial and Evaluation. This method was introduced by Fonetla and Gabus. The goal of the DEMATEL technique is to identify the pattern of interrelationships among a set of criteria. This technique examines the intensity of relationships by scoring them, explores their importance together with feedback, and accepts non-transferable relationships.

The applications of the DEMATEL method include:

1. Considering mutual relationships: The advantage of this method over network analysis techniques is its clarity and transparency in reflecting the mutual relationships among a wide range of components. Experts are able to express their opinions on the effects (direction and intensity of effects) among factors with

Table 6 The results of expert survey in Delphi method

Main attribute	Sub-attribute	Mean	Standard deviation
Responsiveness	Handling problems	2.6	0.0
	Easy platform	2.4	0.0
Suitability	Closeness to personal preferences	2	0.2
	Easy access to facilities	2	0.4
	Closeness to needs	2	0.1
Standardization	Global standards	2.1	0.1
	Fit with successful samples	2	0.0
	Ease of use	2.8	0.1
Efficiency	Time and resource management	4.2	0.1
	Use of technology	3.9	0.2
	Workforce productivity	4.5	0.0
	Cost-effectiveness	4.2	0.0
Effectiveness	Clinical outcomes	4.2	0.1
	Patient satisfaction	3.7	0.0
	Quality of life	3.6	0.0
	Adverse events	3.8	0.0
	Excellent performance	3.9	0.0
	Quality of work	3.9	0.0
Safety	Incidence of adverse events	2.2	0.0
	Patient safety culture	3.9	0.1
	Error reporting	3	0.0
	Infection control	2.7	0.0
Sustainability	Environmental influence	2.8	0.1
	Resource conservation	2.9	0.0
	Cost containment	3	0.2
	Social responsibility	2.9	0.1
	Cultural sustainability	3.5	0.0
Equity	Accessibility for disadvantaged groups	2.5	0.2
	Fairness in resource allocation	2.1	0.1
	Equal treatment for all patients	2.6	0.1
	Elimination of discrimination	3.4	0.3
	Rural and urban health disparities	2.7	0.0

more mastery. The internal relationship matrix can be used as part of the primary supermatrix in the process of network analysis method.

2. Structuring complex factors into cause-and-effect groups: This is one of the most important functions and reasons for the widespread use of the DEMATEL method in problem-solving processes. By dividing a wide range of complex factors into

Table 7 The results obtained in the third round of the Delphi method

Main attribute	Sub-attribute	Mean	Standard deviation
Responsiveness	Handling problems	4.2	0.0
	Easy platform	3.9	0.0
Suitability	Closeness to personal preferences	4.5	0.0
	Easy access to facilities	4	0.2
	Closeness to needs	4.2	0.0
Standardization	Global standards	3.9	0.2
	Fit with successful samples	3.9	0.3
	Ease of use	4	0.2
Efficiency	Time and resource management	2	0.2
	Use of technology	4	0.1
	Workforce productivity	3	0.0
	Cost-effectiveness	2.7	0.0
Effectiveness	Clinical outcomes	3	0.2
	Patient satisfaction	3	0.1
	Quality of life	3	0.0
	Adverse events	2.8	0.1
	Excellent performance	3.5	0.0
	Quality of work	2	0.0
Safety	Incidence of adverse events	2	0.0
	Patient safety culture	2	0.0
	Error reporting	2.1	0.0
	Infection control	2	0.0
Sustainability	Environmental influence	3.9	0.0
	Resource conservation	3	0.2
	Cost containment	3	0.5
	Social responsibility	2.1	0.0
	Cultural sustainability	2.6	0.0
Equity	Accessibility for disadvantaged groups	3.4	0.0
	Fairness in resource allocation	3	0.3
	Equal treatment for all patients	2.6	0.0
	Elimination of discrimination	3.9	0.0
	Rural and urban health disparities	2.4	0.0

cause-and-effect groups, the decision-maker is placed in a more suitable condition to understand the relationships. This leads to a better understanding of the position and role of the factors involved in mutual influence.

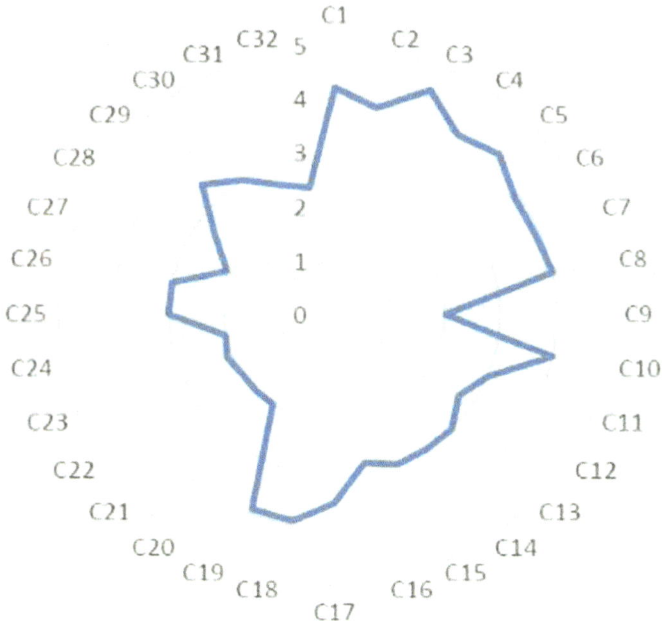

Fig. 4 Third round results of expert survey in Delphi method

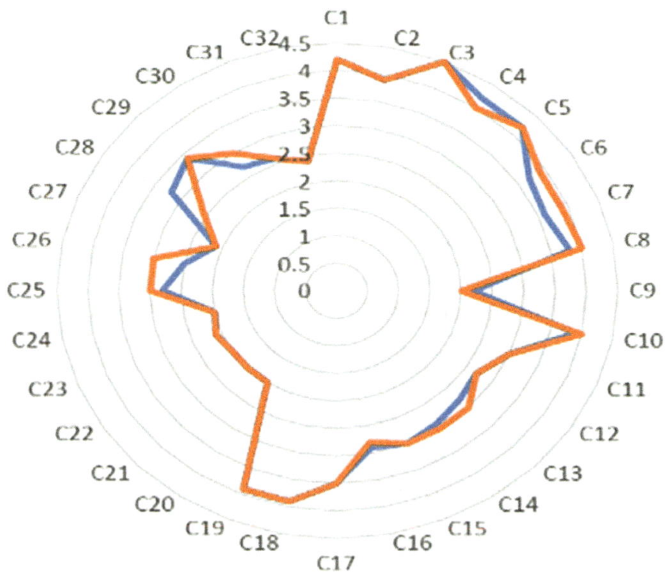

Fig. 5 Experts' disagreement in the second and third rounds of the Delphi method

Table 8 Kendall's coefficient of concordance values for three rounds of Delphi method

Expert code	Round 1	Round 2	Round 3
1	0.269	0.586	0.706
2	0.283	0.634	0.710
3	0.179	0.628	0.741
4	0.009	0.549	0.707
5	0.130	0.572	0.761
6	0.045	0.549	0.706
7	0.330	0.668	0.710
8	0.009	0.655	0.749
9	0.068	0.685	0.761
10	0.418	0.601	0.736

Table 9 Final criteria extracted by the Delphi method

Main attribute	Sub-attribute	Mean	Standard deviation
Responsiveness	Handling problems	4.2	0.0
	Easy platform	3.9	0.0
Suitability	Closeness to personal preferences	4.5	0.0
	Closeness to needs	4.2	0.0
Standardization	Global standards	3.9	0.0
	Ease of use	4	0.0
Efficiency	Workforce productivity	3	0.0
	Cost-effectiveness	2.7	0.0
Effectiveness	Quality of life	3	0.0
	Excellent performance	3.5	0.0
	Quality of work	2	0.0
Safety	Incidence of adverse events	2	0.0
	Patient safety culture	2	0.0
	Error reporting	2.1	0.0
	Infection control	2	0.0
Sustainability	Environmental influence	3.9	0.0
	Social responsibility	2.1	0.0
	Cultural sustainability	2.6	0.0
Equity	Accessibility for disadvantaged groups	3.4	0.0
	Equal treatment for all patients	2.6	0.0
	Elimination of discrimination	3.9	0.0
	Rural and urban health disparities	2.4	0.0

Performance evaluation attributes and sub-attributes of smart health management are ranked using a numerical spectrum {0, 1, 2, 3, 4} in order to determine the influence of each option on other options in the following order:

Step 1: The aggregate matrix of expert opinions is calculated.

Influence matrix, which is completed using experts' opinions, represents the relationships between attributes. This matrix is always square and its dimensions are equal to the number of attributes. The element in row (a) and column (b) of this matrix indicates the degree of influence of attribute A_l on attribute A_h. The number zero indicates no influence of the row attribute on the column attribute, and the higher this number, the greater the influence. The spectrum used can be formed arbitrarily, but in any case, zero must be a member of the spectrum. An example of acceptable spectra includes [0, 1, 2, 3, 4], [0, 1, 2, 3, 4 5], [0, 1, 2, …, 10], [0, 1, 2, …, 100], or any similar spectra. In this case, we use the spectrum from 0 to 4.

The influence matrix is represented by F, and its element in row (l) and column (h) is represented by $F_{l,h}$. If multiple experts' opinions are used, each element of the influence matrix is obtained by using the geometric mean of the corresponding elements.

The first step in the DEMATEL analysis is to construct the influence matrix, which shows the direct and indirect relationships between the attributes and sub-attributes. To do this, we calculate the "influence degree" (ID) for each pair of attributes/sub-attributes, which represents the extent to which one attribute/sub-attribute influences another.

To calculate the ID, we use the following formula:

$$\mathrm{ID} = (\mathrm{A} \times \mathrm{B})/(\mathrm{A} + \mathrm{B})$$

where A is the number of attributes/sub-attributes that directly influence the row attribute/sub-attribute, and B is the number of attributes/sub-attributes that indirectly influence the row attribute/sub-attribute through the column attribute/sub-attribute.

For example, let's calculate the ID for the pair of sub-attributes Handling problems and Easy platform under the attribute Responsiveness:

$$\mathrm{ID}\ (\text{Handling problems} \rightarrow \text{Easy platform}) = (1 \times 1)/(1 + 1) = 0.5$$

$$\mathrm{ID}\ (\text{Easy platform} \rightarrow \text{Handling problems}) = (1 \times 1)/(1 + 1) = 0.5$$

The influence matrix is then constructed by organizing the ID values into a matrix, with the row attributes/sub-attributes listed on the left and the column attributes/sub-attributes listed on the top. The diagonal elements of the matrix are set to zero, as an attribute/sub-attribute cannot directly influence itself.

To form the influence matrix, the opinions of 10 experts have been used. For example, the opinion of the first expert regarding the influence of attributess on each other is shown in Table 10. M = 0, VL = 1, L = 2, H = 3, VH = 4.

Similarly, nine other expert opinions were obtained and then combined using the geometric mean. The aggregation matrix of expert opinions is shown in Table 11.

Table 10 The opinions of the first expert regarding the influence of attributes on each other

Expert 1	Responsiveness	Suitability	Standardization	Efficiency	Effectiveness	Safety	Sustainability	Equity
Responsiveness	0	VL	L	M	M	H	H	VL
Suitability	L	0	VL	L	L	M	L	L
Standardization	H	VH	0	M	M	H	VH	H
Efficiency	H	M	H	0	VL	L	M	M
Effectiveness	M	H	M	L	0	M	L	H
Safety	H	L	H	L	VL	0	L	VH
Sustainability	L	M	H	H	VH	L	0	H
Equity	VH	VH	H	M	M	H	H	0

Table 11 The aggregate influence matrix of expert opinions

Influence matrix	Responsiveness	Suitability	Standardization	Efficiency	Effectiveness	Safety	Sustainability	Equity
Responsiveness	0	0	0	1	1	1	3	1
Suitability	1	0	0	3	0	1	3	1
Standardization	2	1	0	1	0	0	2	0
Efficiency	2	0	2	0	1	0	0	0
Effectiveness	0	4	0	2	0	0	0	2
Safety	1	3	1	1	1	0	1	2
Sustainability	3	1	2	0	1	1	0	0
Equity	4	2	1	0	0	2	2	0

Step 2: The row sum of the matrix and the value of S are calculated.

The value of α is obtained from the inverse of the maximum row sum (Table 12).

Step 3: The elements of matrix F are divided by α to obtain matrix M (Table 13).

Step 4: The matrix of overall effects (C) is calculated.

To calculate this matrix, the following steps are performed in order:
a: Matrix M is divided by a unity matrix (I) (Table 14).
b: The inverse of matrix I-M is calculated (Table 15).
c: Matrix C is calculated by multiplying matrix M by the inverse of matrix I-M (Table 16).

Step 5: The overall influence or R is calculated for each attribute. To do this, the sum of the rows is calculated (Table 17).

Step 6: The overall responsiveness or D of each index is calculated by summing each column (Table 18).

Step 7: The overall dependence ($R_i + D_i$) and independence ($R_i - D_i$) are calculated (Table 19).

Step 8: The threshold of influences is calculated.

It calculated from the arithmetic mean of the elements of matrix C. The threshold for the influences of matrix C is equal to 0.210. Therefore, in the effects diagram, only the effects with intensity greater than 0.210 are displayed.

Now, based on the overall dependency and overall non-dependency, we can rank and interpret the type of relationships according to the influence threshold (Table 20).

Based on the diagram, we can see that Responsiveness, Suitability, Equity and Safety are the most influential attributes, as they have the most arrows pointing towards them. These attributes should be given the most attention when making decisions or taking actions related to the system being evaluated.

According to Table 18, the Responsiveness index has the highest value of D, making it the most influential factor. The Equity index also has the highest value of R, making it the most susceptible factor. Additionally, the Responsiveness index has the highest value of $D + R$, indicating the strongest correlation with other system factors.

To determine the relationships between the criteria, a threshold value of 0.210 is used. If a value is greater than this threshold, it is assigned a value of 1, indicating a relationship, and if it is less than the threshold, it is assigned a value of 0, indicating no relationship. In this way, a matrix of zeros and ones is formed, where ones indicate the influence of a row index on a column criterion. That is, if the intersection of a row index with a column index is one, it means that the row index has an influence on the column index, and when drawing a graph, a arrow is drawn from the row index to the column index. Table 21 shows the types of relationships between the attributes.

To rank the sub-attributes, calculations can be done in the same way based on the ranking of the main attributes, and the result can be seen in Table 22.

Table 12 The row sum of the matrix and α

F	Responsiveness	Suitability	Standardization	Efficiency	Effectiveness	Safety	Sustainability	Equity	Sum
Responsiveness	0	0	0	1	1	1	3	1	7
Suitability	1	0	0	3	0	1	3	1	9
Standardization	2	1	0	1	0	0	2	0	6
Efficiency	2	0	2	0	1	0	0	0	5
Effectiveness	0	4	0	2	0	0	0	2	8
Safety	1	3	1	1	1	0	1	2	10
Sustainability	3	1	2	0	1	1	0	0	8
Equity	4	2	1	0	0	2	2	0	11
								$\alpha =$	0.091

Table 13 Calculating matrix M by scalar multiplication of α*F

M	Responsiveness	Suitability	Standardization	Efficiency	Effectiveness	Safety	Sustainability	Equity
Responsiveness	0.000	0.000	0.000	0.091	0.091	0.091	0.273	0.091
Suitability	0.091	0.000	0.000	0.273	0.000	0.091	0.273	0.091
Standardization	0.182	0.091	0.000	0.091	0.000	0.000	0.182	0.000
Efficiency	0.182	0.000	0.182	0.000	0.091	0.000	0.000	0.000
Effectiveness	0.000	0.364	0.000	0.182	0.000	0.000	0.000	0.182
Safety	0.091	0.273	0.091	0.091	0.091	0.000	0.091	0.182
Sustainability	0.273	0.091	0.182	0.000	0.091	0.091	0.000	0.000
Equity	0.364	0.182	0.091	0.000	0.000	0.182	0.182	0.000

Table 14 Matrix I-M

I-M	Responsiveness	Suitability	Standardization	Efficiency	Effectiveness	Safety	Sustainability	Equity
Responsiveness	1.000	0.000	0.000	−0.091	−0.091	−0.091	−0.273	−0.091
Suitability	−0.091	1.000	0.000	−0.273	0.000	−0.091	−0.273	−0.091
Standardization	−0.182	−0.091	1.000	−0.091	0.000	0.000	−0.182	0.000
Efficiency	−0.182	0.000	−0.182	1.000	0.959	0.002	0.024	0.004
Effectiveness	0.000	−0.364	0.000	−0.182	1.000	0.000	0.000	−0.182
Safety	−0.091	−0.273	−0.091	−0.091	−0.091	1.000	−0.091	−0.182
Sustainability	−0.273	−0.091	−0.182	0.000	−0.091	−0.091	1.000	0.000
Equity	−0.364	−0.182	−0.091	0.000	0.000	−0.182	−0.182	1.000

Table 15 Inverse matrix of I-M

$(I\text{-}M)^{-1}$	Responsiveness	Suitability	Standardization	Efficiency	Effectiveness	Safety	Sustainability	Equity
Responsiveness	1.276	0.139	0.150	0.185	−0.002	0.199	0.456	0.164
Suitability	0.370	1.055	0.169	0.316	−0.211	0.193	0.452	0.125
Standardization	0.361	0.133	1.104	0.162	−0.083	0.084	0.347	0.044
Efficiency	0.019	−0.333	0.094	0.775	−0.760	−0.075	−0.127	−0.184
Effectiveness	0.273	0.390	0.130	0.295	0.775	0.123	0.249	0.222
Safety	0.458	0.406	0.259	0.269	−0.071	1.168	0.433	0.277
Sustainability	0.514	0.230	0.292	0.160	0.029	0.205	1.291	0.109
Equity	0.741	0.370	0.286	0.217	−0.054	0.365	0.593	1.156

Table 16 C matrix (M* $(I - M)^{-1}$)

C	Responsiveness	Suitability	Standardization	Efficiency	Effectiveness	Safety	Sustainability	Equity
Responsiveness	0.276	0.139	0.150	0.185	−0.002	0.199	0.456	0.164
Suitability	0.370	0.055	0.169	0.316	−0.211	0.193	0.452	0.125
Standardization	0.361	0.133	0.104	0.162	−0.083	0.084	0.347	0.044
Efficiency	0.322	0.085	0.240	0.090	0.055	0.063	0.169	0.058
Effectiveness	0.273	0.390	0.130	0.295	−0.225	0.123	0.249	0.222
Safety	0.458	0.406	0.259	0.269	−0.071	0.168	0.433	0.277
Sustainability	0.514	0.230	0.292	0.160	0.029	0.205	0.291	0.109
Equity	0.741	0.370	0.286	0.217	−0.054	0.365	0.593	0.156

Table 17 Weighted value of R

	R
Responsiveness	1.566
Suitability	1.469
Standardization	1.152
Efficiency	1.081
Effectiveness	1.458
Safety	2.197
Sustainability	1.830
Equity	2.673

Table 18 Weighted value of D

	D
Responsiveness	3.313
Suitability	1.807
Standardization	1.629
Efficiency	1.695
Effectiveness	−0.562
Safety	1.399
Sustainability	2.989
Equity	1.156

Table 19 Weighted value of overall dependence and independence

	$R_i + D_i$	$R_i - D_i$
Responsiveness	4.879	−1.747
Suitability	3.276	−0.339
Standardization	2.781	−0.477
Efficiency	2.776	−0.613
Effectiveness	0.897	2.020
Safety	3.596	0.798
Sustainability	4.819	−1.160
Equity	3.829	1.518

6.2 *Determining the Weights of the Attributes Using the "Swara" Technique*

This technique is among the mental methods for determining the weights of attributes. In this method, first, the attributess are prioritized using experts' opinions, and then the weights are determined. It is necessary for each expert to identify their important attributes, and then the following steps should be taken:

Table 20 Ranking based on overall dependency and overall non-dependency

	R + D	Rank	R − D	Rank
Responsiveness	4.879	1	−1.747	8
Suitability	3.276	5	−0.339	4
Standardization	2.781	6	−0.477	5
Efficiency	2.776	7	−0.613	6
Effectiveness	0.897	8	2.020	1
Safety	3.596	4	0.798	3
Sustainability	4.819	2	−1.160	7
Equity	3.829	3	1.518	2

Step 1: The percentage of votes for each attribute is calculated by dividing the number of votes for that attribute by the number of experts. The percentage of votes represents the relative frequency of each attributes. The attributes are ranked in descending order based on the percentage of votes. Table 23 shows the opinions of 10 experts about the attributes.

Step 2: In a new table, the attributes are written in order of priority (Table 24).

Step 3: The relative difference of the scores of each attribute compared to the next attribute, i.e. S_j, is calculated for each attribute (except the first attribute) (Table 25).

Step 4: The growth value K_j is equal to 1 for the first attribute and equal to $1 + S_j$ for the other attributes (Table 26).

Step 5: We set the value of the first recovered attribute, q_1, equal to 1, and by dividing the previous attribute q_j by its coefficient k_j, we can calculate the values of the other attributes q_j (Table 27).

Step 6: The QJ's are divided by their sum to calculate the weight of each attribute (Tables 28 and 29).

6.3 Ranking of Performance Evaluation Attributes for Smarthealthcare Management Using "Waspas" Technique

Given that the ranking of sub-attributes is similar to the ranking of indices, in other MADM methods explained, only the main indices are ranked.

The WASPAS[1] technique was introduced in 2012 and is a combination of the SAW and WPM techniques. At first, the opinions of 10 experts on the importance of

[1] Weighted Aggregate Sum Product Assessment.

Table 21 Relationships between the attributes

	Responsiveness	Suitability	Standardization	Efficiency	Effectiveness	Safety	Sustainability	Equity
Responsiveness	1	0	0	0	0	0	1	0
Suitability	1	0	0	1	0	0	1	0
Standardization	1	0	0	0	0	0	0	0
Efficiency	1	0	1	0	0	0	0	0
Effectiveness	1	1	0	1	0	0	1	1
Safety	1	1	1	1	0	0	1	1
Sustainability	1	1	1	0	0	0	1	0
Equity	1	1	1	1	0	1	1	0

Table 22 Ranking of sub-attributes

Main attribute	Sub-attribute	Rank
Responsiveness	Easy platform	1
	Handling problems	2
Sustainability	Cultural sustainability	3
	Environmental influence	4
	Social responsibility	4
Equity	Rural and urban health disparities	5
	Accessibility for disadvantaged groups	6
	Elimination of discrimination	7
	Equal treatment for all patients	8
Safety	Error reporting	9
	Incidence of adverse events	10
	Patient safety culture	11
	Infection control	12
Suitability	Closeness to personal preferences	13
	Closeness to needs	14
Standardization	Ease of use	15
	Global standards	16
Efficiency	Workforce productivity	17
	Cost-effectiveness	18
Effectiveness	Excellent performance1	19
	Quality of life	20
	Quality of work	21

attributess are taken pairwise compared and on a nine-point spectrum. For example, the opinions of the expert 1 are presented in the matrix Table 30.

It is possible to convert qualitative attributes to quantitative attributes using various methods. One of the best methods is to use distance scales or bipolar scales. A common method for measuring a qualitative attributes using a distance scale is to use a distance bipolar scale based on a point yield scale. In this scale, zero assigns the lowest value and 10 assigns the highest value. In positive attributes, the higher the attributes is the more desirable it is. In negative attributes, this value is reversed. Performance evaluation attributes for smart health management all have positive aspects.

Matrix Table 31 show the quantified attributes.

Similarly, the opinions of 9 other experts were also obtained and combined with the geometric mean of the opinions of 10 experts, as shown in matrix Table 32. It is reminded that the weights of the attributes (W_j) were calculated using the SWARA method.

Table 23 Prioritization of attributes by 10 experts

	Expert1	Expert2	Expert3	Expert4	Expert5	Expert6	Expert7	Expert8	Expert9	Expert10	Average	Rank
Responsiveness	3	5	2	3	1	3	3	1	1	2	2.4	2
Suitability	2	2	3	2	3	1	2	2	3	3	2.3	1
Standardization	1	7	6	1	2	2	4	3	4	4	3.4	3
Efficiency	5	6	4	4	5	6	6	5	15	6	6.2	6
Effectiveness	8	3	8	5	7	7	8	8	6	7	6.7	8
Safety	6	4	1	8	8	8	7	6	8	5	6.1	5
Sustainability	4	8	7	7	6	5	5	7	7	8	6.4	7
Equity	7	1	5	6	4	4	1	4	2	1	3.5	4

Table 24 Priority of attributes

Rank	1	2	3	4	5	6	7	8
Attributes	Suitability	Respon-siveness	Standard-ization	Equity	Safety	Efficiency	Sustain-ability	Effective-ness
Average priority	2.3	2.4	3.4	3.5	6.1	6.2	6.4	6.7

Table 25 Calculated S_j

Attributes	Suitability	Respon-siveness	Standard-ization	Equity	Safety	Efficiency	Sustain-ability	Effective-ness
S_j	–	0.1	1	0.1	2.6	0.1	0.2	0.3

Table 26 Calculated K_j

Attributes	Suitability	Respon-siveness	Standard-ization	Equity	Safety	Efficiency	Sustain-ability	Effective-ness
K_j	1	1.1	2	1.1	3.6	1.1	1.2	1.3

Table 27 Calculated q_j

Attributes	Suit-ability	Respon-siveness	Stan-dardiza-tion	Equity	Safety	Effi-ciency	Sustain-ability	Effec-tiveness	SUM
q_j	1	0.909	0.455	0.413	0.115	0.104	0.087	0.067	3.150

Table 28 Calculated W_j

Attributes	Suit-ability	Respon-siveness	Stan-dardiza-tion	Equity	Safety	Effi-ciency	Sustain-ability	Effec-tiveness	SUM
W_j	0.317	0.289	0.144	0.131	0.036	0.033	0.028	0.021	1

Table 29 The weight of the attributes in order of priority

Attributes	Respon-siveness	Suitability	Standard-ization	Efficiency	Effective-ness	Safety	Sustain-ability	Equity
Wj	0.289	0.317	0.144	0.033	0.021	0.036	0.028	0.131

The implementation steps of this technique are as follows:

Step 1. The decision matrix is normalized using a dimensionless linear method (Matrix Table 33).

Step 2. The dimensionless values obtained in step 1 are multiplied by the weights of the attributes.

Step 3. The row sum of the weighted dimensionless matrix are calculated $\left(U_i^1\right)$ (Table 34).

Table 30 Pairwise comparison of attributes by expert 1

Expert 1	Responsiveness	Suitability	Standardization	Efficiency	Effectiveness	Safety	Sustainability	Equity
Responsiveness	–	VH	H	M	MH	MH	H	M
Suitability	ML	–	VL	L	M	L	VL	M
Standardization	H	VH	–	M	M	VL	M	L
Efficiency	L	M	MH	–	VL	ML	M	M
Effectiveness	M	ML	L	ML	–	M	VL	M
Safety	M	ML	H	L	VL	–	L	M
Sustainability	H	VH	M	M	M	H	–	H
Equity	M	MH	M	L	M	MH	H	–

Table 31 Quantified attributes matrix.docx

Expert 1	Responsiveness	Suitability	Standardization	Efficiency	Effectiveness	Safety	Sustainability	Equity
Responsiveness	–	9	7	5	6	6	7	5
Suitability	2	–	1	3	5	3	1	5
Standardization	7	9	–	5	5	1	5	3
Efficiency	3	5	6	–	1	2	5	5
Effectiveness	5	2	3	2	–	5	1	5
Safety	5	2	7	3	2	–	3	5
Sustainability	7	9	5	5	5	7	–	7
Equity	5	6	5	3	5	6	7	–

Table 32 Aggregated decision matrix

	Responsiveness	Suitability	Standardization	Efficiency	Effectiveness	Safety	Sustainability	Equity
Responsiveness	–	3.820	4.615	5.225	5.584	5.589	6.567	7.204
Suitability	3.094	–	2.577	3.717	5.207	7.969	5.028	6.708
Standardization	7.579	6.468	–	5.115	5.687	7.172	5.753	5.939
Efficiency	3.962	4.562	3.904	–	3.519	5.146	5.555	6.470
Effectiveness	5.335	4.345	5.536	3.266	–	6.052	3.956	5.603
Safety	4.543	3.787	5.268	4.228	3.702	–	4.427	4.997
Sustainability	5.125	5.359	5.046	4.555	6.268	5.803	–	6.584
Equity	6.583	5.649	5.844	5.612	6.804	7.326	7.175	–
Wj	0.021	0.019	0.043	0.186	0.290	0.169	0.223	0.047

Table 33 Normalized matrix

NM	Responsiveness	Suitability	Standardization	Efficiency	Effectiveness	Safety	Sustainability	Equity
Responsiveness		3.820	4.615	5.225	5.584	5.589	6.567	7.204
Suitability	3.094		2.577	3.717	5.207	7.969	5.028	6.708
Standardization	7.579	6.468		5.115	5.687	7.172	5.753	5.939
Efficiency	3.962	4.562	3.904		3.519	5.146	5.555	6.470
Effectiveness	5.335	4.345	5.536	3.266		6.052	3.956	5.603
Safety	4.543	3.787	5.268	4.228	3.702		4.427	4.997
Sustainability	5.125	5.359	5.046	4.555	6.268	5.803		6.584
Equity	6.583	5.649	5.844	5.612	6.804	7.326	7.175	
Wj	0.021	0.019	0.043	0.186	0.290	0.169	0.223	0.047

Table 34 Weighted normalized matrix and row sum

WNM	Responsiveness	Suitability	Standardization	Efficiency	Effectiveness	Safety	Sustainability	Equity	(U_i^1)
Responsiveness	0.000	0.011	0.034	0.173	0.238	0.119	0.205	0.047	0.827
Suitability	0.009	0.000	0.019	0.123	0.222	0.169	0.157	0.044	0.743
Standardization	0.021	0.019	0.000	0.170	0.243	0.152	0.179	0.039	0.824
Efficiency	0.011	0.014	0.029	0.000	0.150	0.109	0.173	0.042	0.528
Effectiveness	0.015	0.013	0.040	0.108	0.000	0.129	0.123	0.037	0.465
Safety	0.013	0.011	0.039	0.140	0.158	0.000	0.138	0.033	0.532
Sustainability	0.014	0.016	0.037	0.151	0.268	0.123	0.000	0.043	0.652
Equity	0.019	0.017	0.043	0.186	0.290	0.156	0.223	0.000	0.934

Step 4: The values of the normalized matrix calculated in Step 1 reach to the power of the attributes weight.

Step 5: The row-wise product of the power-normalized matrix from Step 4 is calculated $\left(U_i^2\right)$ (Table 35).

Step 6: The row-wise sum and the row-wise product average of the normalized weighted matrix are calculated. Then the attributes are ranked in descending order (Table 36).

Step 5: Obtaining alternative selection criteria function for the matrix. The permanent of this matrix, is defined as the alternative selection criteria function. The permanent of a matrix was introduced by Cauchy in 1812. At that time, while developing the theory of determinants, he also defined a certain subclass of symmetric functions which later Muir named permanents. The permanent is a standard matrix function and is used in combinatorial mathematics. The permanent function is obtained in a similar manner as the determinant but unlike in a determinant where a negative sign appears in the calculation, in a variable permanent function positive signs replace these negative signs. Application of the permanent concept will lead to a better appreciation of selection attributes. Moreover, using this no negative sign will appear in the expression (unlike determinant of a matrix in which a negative sign can appear) and hence no information will be lost. The per(CS) contains terms arranged in (M + 1) groups, and these groups represent the measures of criteria and the relative importance loops. The first group represents the measures of M criteria. The second group is absent as there is no self-loop in the digraph. The third group contains 2-criterion relative importance loops and measures of (M-2) criteria. Each term of the fourth group represents a set of a 3-criterion relative importance loop, or its pair, and measures of (M − 3) criteria. The fifth group contains two sub-groups. The terms of the first sub-group is a set of two 2-criterion relative importance loops and the measures of (M − 4) criteria. Each term of second sub-group is a set of a 4-attribute relative importance loop, or its pair, and the measures of (M − 4) criteria. The sixth group contains two subgroups. The terms of the first sub-group are a set of a 3-criterion relative importance loop, or its pair, and 2-criterion importance loop and the measures of (M − 5) criteria. Each term of the second sub-group is a set of a 5-criterion relative importance loop, or its pair, and the measures of (M − 5) criteria. Similar other terms of the equation are defined. Thus, the CS fully characterizes the considered alternative selection evaluation problem, as it contains all possible structural components of the criteria and their relative importance. It may be mentioned that this equation is nothing but the determinant of an M _ M matrix but considering all the terms as positive.

Step 6: Evaluation and ranking of the alternatives, in this step all alternatives are ranked according to their permanent values calculated in the previous step.

Table 35 Weighted power-normalized matrix and its row-wise product

	Responsiveness	Suitability	Standardization	Efficiency	Effectiveness	Safety	Sustainability	Equity	(U_i^2)
Responsiveness	0.000	0.990	0.990	0.987	0.944	0.942	0.980	1.000	0.843
Suitability	0.981	0.000	0.966	0.926	0.925	1.000	0.924	0.997	0.747
Standardization	1.000	1.000	0.000	0.983	0.949	0.982	0.952	0.991	0.864
Efficiency	0.986	0.993	0.983	0.000	0.826	0.929	0.944	0.995	0.694
Effectiveness	0.993	0.992	0.998	0.904	0.000	0.954	0.875	0.988	0.734
Safety	0.989	0.990	0.996	0.949	0.838	0.000	0.898	0.983	0.684
Sustainability	0.992	0.996	0.994	0.962	0.976	0.948	0.000	0.996	0.870
Equity	0.997	0.997	1.000	1.000	1.000	0.986	1.000	0.000	0.980

$M \quad M-1 \quad M \quad M$

per (Cs) = $\prod A_i + \sum\sum \ldots \sum (a_{ij}\, a_{ji})\, A_k A_l A_m A_n A_o \ldots A_t A_M$

$i=1 \quad i=1 \quad j=i+1 \quad M=t+1$

$M-2 \quad M-1 \quad M \quad M$

$+ \sum\sum\sum \ldots \sum (\, a_{ij} a_{jk}\, a_{ki} + a_{ik}\, a_{kj}\, a_{ji})\, A_l\, A_m\, A_n\, Ao \ldots A_t\, A_M$

$i=1 \quad j=i+1\ k=i+1 \quad M=t+!$

$M-3 \quad M \quad M-1 \quad M \quad M$

$+ \sum\sum\sum\sum \ldots \sum (\, aij\ a\ ji + akl\ alk)\ Am\ An\ Ao\ \ldots At\ AM$

$i=1 \quad j=i+1\ k=i+1\ l=i+2 \quad M=t+1$

$M-3 \quad M \quad M-1 \quad M \quad M$

$+ \sum\sum\sum\sum \ldots \sum (\, aij\ a\ jk\ akl\ ali + ail\ alk\ akj\ a\ ji)\ Am\ An\ Ao \ldots At\ AM +$

$i=1 \quad j=i+1\ k=i+1\ l=i+2 \quad M=t+1$

$M-2\ M-1 \quad M \quad M-1\ M-2 \quad M$

$\sum\sum\sum\sum\sum \ldots\ldots \sum (\, aija\ jk\ aki + aik\ akj\ a\ ji)(\, alm\ am)\ An\ Ao\ \ldots At\ Am +$

$i=1 \quad j=1\ j=i+1\ l=1\ m=l+1 \quad m=t+1$ (1)

$M-4\ M-1 \quad M \quad M \quad M \quad M$

$\sum\sum\sum\sum\sum \ldots\ldots \sum (aij\ a\ jk\ akl\ alm\ ami + a\text{Ʒ}amj\ alk\ akj\ a\ ji)\ An\ Ao \ldots\ldots At\ Am +$

$i=1 \quad j=i+1\ k=j+1\ l=1\ m=l+1 \quad M=t+1$

$M-3\ M-1 \quad M \quad M \quad M-1 \quad M \quad M$

$\sum\sum\ \sum\sum\sum\ \sum \ldots\ldots \sum (\, aija\ jk\ aki + aik\ akja\ ji)(\, alm\ amn\ anl + \mathrm{aln}\ anmaml)\ Ao \ldots.\ At\ Am$

$i=1 \quad j=i+1\ k=j+1\ l=1\ m=l+1\ n=m+1 \quad M=t+1$

$M-5\ M-1 \quad M \quad M-2\ M-1 \quad M \quad M$

$+ \sum\sum\ \sum\sum\sum\ \sum \ldots\ldots \sum (\ aij\ a\ jk\ akl\ alm\ ami + a\text{Ʒ}amj\ alk\ akj\ a\ ji) + (\ alm\ a_{mn}\ anl + \mathrm{aln}\ a_{nm} a_{ml})\ A_o \ldots At\ AM$

$i=1 \quad j=i+1\ k=j+1\ l=1\ m=l+1\ n=m+1 \quad M=t+1$

$M-5\ M-1 \quad M \quad M \quad M \quad M \quad M$

$+ \sum\sum\sum\sum\sum\sum \ldots\ldots \sum (\ aij + a\ jk\ akl\ alm\ amn\ anj + a\text{¿}anmaml\ alk\ akj\ a\ ji)\ Ao \ldots At\ AM$

$i=1 \quad j=i+1\ k=j+1\ l=1\ m=l+1\ n=m+1 \quad M=t+1$

Table 36 Average of row-wise sum and row-wise product

U_i	Rank
0.835	3
0.745	5
0.844	2
0.611	6
0.599	8
0.608	7
0.761	4
0.957	1

The ranking of performance evaluation attributes for intelligent healthcare management with GTMA is being reviewed. The sub- attributes ranking is presented to the readers.

- The expert opinion aggregation matrices and their normalization matrices, which were calculated using the WASPAS method, are utilized (Tables 37 and 38).
- A separate importance degree matrix is formed for each of the attributes. For this purpose, the weights corresponding to each attributes are divided by each other. The normalized values of each attribute, for which the importance degree matrix has been calculated, are placed on the main diagonal. As an example, Table 39 is provided for the Responsiveness attribute and Table 40 for the Suitability attribute. The same method is used to calculate the matrices for the other six indicators (Table 40).
- The constant value of the matrix is calculated for each attributes. The constant matrix is the determinant of the matrix, where only negative entries are transformed into positive to preserve the information. The highest obtained value represents the best option. Other attributes are also ranked based on the obtained constant value of their matrices (Table 41).

7 Ranking Strategies

Table 42 demonstrates the ranking of main indicators using three methods: DEMATEL, WASPAS, and GTMA. As seen, the rankings differ from one another. This situation is common in real-world problems. For this reason, decision-makers do not limit themselves to a single method when making important decisions. Instead, they employ different methods for ranking and, in cases where the results are not consistent, use “integration methods” such as 1–average ranking, 2–BORDA, and 3–COPELAND.

Table 37 Aggregated decision matrix

	Responsiveness	Suitability	Standardization	Efficiency	Effectiveness	Safety	Sustainability	Equity
Responsiveness	–	3.820	4.615	5.225	5.584	5.589	6.567	7.204
Suitability	3.094	–	2.577	3.717	5.207	7.969	5.028	6.708
Standardization	7.579	6.468	–	5.115	5.687	7.172	5.753	5.939
Efficiency	3.962	4.562	3.904	–	3.519	5.146	5.555	6.470
Effectiveness	5.335	4.345	5.536	3.266	–	6.052	3.956	5.603
Safety	4.543	3.787	5.268	4.228	3.702	–	4.427	4.997
Sustainability	5.125	5.359	5.046	4.555	6.268	5.803	–	6.584
Equity	6.583	5.649	5.844	5.612	6.804	7.326	7.175	–
Wj	0.021	0.019	0.043	0.186	0.290	0.169	0.223	0.047

Table 38 Normalized matrix

	Responsiveness	Suitability	Standardization	Efficiency	Effectiveness	Safety	Sustainability	Equity
Responsiveness	–	3.820	4.615	5.225	5.584	5.589	6.567	7.204
Suitability	3.094	–	2.577	3.717	5.207	7.969	5.028	6.708
Standardization	7.579	6.468	–	5.115	5.687	7.172	5.753	5.939
Efficiency	3.962	4.562	3.904	–	3.519	5.146	5.555	6.470
Effectiveness	5.335	4.345	5.536	3.266	–	6.052	3.956	5.603
Safety	4.543	3.787	5.268	4.228	3.702	–	4.427	4.997
Sustainability	5.125	5.359	5.046	4.555	6.268	5.803	–	6.584
Equity	6.583	5.649	5.844	5.612	6.804	7.326	7.175	–

Table 39 Importance degree matrix for responsiveness

Responsiveness	Responsiveness	Suitability	Standardization	Efficiency	Effectiveness	Safety	Sustainability	Equity
Responsiveness	1.000	1.100	0.500	0.115	0.074	0.126	0.096	0.455
Suitability	0.909	0.591	0.455	0.104	0.067	0.115	0.087	0.413
Standardization	2.00	2.200	0.790	0.230	0.147	0.253	0.191	0.909
Efficiency	8.712	9.583	4.356	0.931	0.641	1.100	0.833	3.960
Effectiveness	13.591	14.950	6.795	1.560	0.821	1.716	1.300	6.178
Safety	7.920	8.712	3.960	0.909	0.583	0.701	0.758	3.600
Sustainability	10.454	11.500	5.227	1.200	0.769	1.320	0.915	4.752
Equity	2.200	2.420	1.100	0.253	0.162	0.278	0.210	1.000

Table 40 Importance degree matrix for suitability

Suitability	Responsiveness	Suitability	Standardization	Efficiency	Effectiveness	Safety	Sustainability	Equity
Responsiveness	0.408	1.10	0.50	0.11	0.07	0.13	0.10	0.45
Suitability	0.909	1.000	0.45	0.10	0.07	0.11	0.09	0.41
Standardization	2.00	2.200	0.441	0.230	0.147	0.253	0.191	0.909
Efficiency	8.712	9.583	4.356	0.662	0.641	1.100	0.833	3.960
Effectiveness	13.591	14.950	6.795	1.560	0.765	1.716	1.300	6.178
Safety	7.920	8.712	3.960	0.909	0.583	1.000	0.758	3.600
Sustainability	10.454	11.500	5.227	1.200	0.769	1.320	0.701	4.752
Equity	2.200	2.420	1.100	0.253	0.162	0.278	0.210	0.931

Table 41 Constant value and rank of attributes

Attributes	PV	Rank
Responsiveness	10.776	2
Suitability	10.051	6
Standardization	8.571	8
Efficiency	10.702	3
Effectiveness	8.742	7
Safety	10.189	5
Sustainability	10.991	1
Equity	10.201	4

Table 42 Ranking obtained from three methods of DEMATEL, WASPAS, and GTMA

Attributes	GTMA	WASPAS	DEMATEL
Responsiveness	2	3	1
Suitability	6	5	5
Standardization	8	2	6
Efficiency	3	6	7
Effectiveness	7	8	8
Safety	5	7	4
Sustainability	1	4	2
Equity	4	1	3

7.1 Average Ranking Method

This method re-ranks the indicators based on the average rankings obtained from different MADM methods (Table 43).

Table 43 Ranking using average method

Attributes	GTMA	WASPAS	DEMATEL	Average	Rank
Responsiveness	2	3	1	2	1
Suitability	6	5	5	5.33	4
Standardization	8	2	6	5.33	4
Efficiency	3	6	7	5.33	4
Effectiveness	7	8	8	7.67	5
Safety	5	7	4	5.33	4
Sustainability	1	4	2	2.33	2
Equity	4	1	3	2.66	3

Based on the averages, it can be concluded that: Responsiveness > Sustainability > Equity > Safety = Suitability = Standardization = Efficiency > Effectiveness.

The result of ranking using the mean method is similar to the ranking using the DEMATEL method, with the difference being that Suitability, Standardization, and Efficiency have all achieved a rank of 4 instead of ranks 5 to 7, placing them in the same rank.

7.2 BORDA Method

This method is based on the majority rule. In this method, the number of times that one method is preferred over another or, in other words, the row has dominance over the column, is denoted by M. If there is no majority vote in pairwise comparisons or if the votes are tied, it is encoded as X. X indicates column dominance over the row. The priority attribute in this method is how many times the attribute losers (M) have a majority in the row (Table 44).

Based on the BORDA, it can be concluded that: Responsiveness > Sustainability > Equity > Suitability > Safety = Standardization = Efficiency > Effectiveness.

7.3 COPELAND Method

This method begins where the BORDA method ends. The Copeland method considers not only the number of "wins" but also the number of "losses" for each attribute. The score that COPELAND assigns to each option is calculated by subtracting the number of "losses" ($\sum$R) from the number of "wins" ($\sum$C) (Table 45).

Based on the COPELAND, it can be concluded that: Responsiveness > Sustainability > Equity Suitability > Safety > Standardization = Efficiency > Effectiveness.

8 Integration Stage

In this stage, an agreement can be reached through the formation of a partially ordered set (POSET). According to this integration, a consensus can be achieved based on linear priorities through POSET. The set of priorities has been obtained as follows:

AVERAGE: Responsiveness > Sustainability > Equity > Safety = Suitability = Standardization = Efficiency > Effectiveness.

BORDA: Responsiveness > Sustainability > Equity > Safety = Suitability > Standardization = Efficiency > Effectiveness.

COPELAND: Responsiveness > Sustainability > Equity > Suitability > Safety > Standardization = Efficiency > Effectiveness.

Table 44 Ranking using BORDA method

Attributes	Responsiveness	Suitability	Standardization	Efficiency	Effectiveness	Safety	Sustainability	Equity	$\sum C$	Rank
Responsiveness	–	M	M	M	M	M	M	M	7	1
Suitability	X	–	M	M	M	M	X	X	4	4
Standardization	X	X	–	M	M	X	X	X	2	5
Efficiency	X	X	X	–	M	M	X	X	2	5
Effectiveness	X	X	X	X	–	X	X	X	0	6
Safety	X	M	M	M	M	–	X	X	4	4
Sustainability	X	M	M	M	M	M	–	M	6	2
Equity	X	M	M	M	M	M	X		5	3

Table 45 Ranking using COPELAND method

Attributes	$\sum C$	$\sum R$	$\sum C - \sum R$	Rank
Responsiveness	7	0	7	1
Suitability	4	3	1	4
Standardization	2	5	−3	6
Efficiency	2	5	−3	6
Effectiveness	0	7	−7	7
Safety	4	5	−1	5
Sustainability	6	1	5	2
Equity	5	2	3	3

Based on the similarity between the AVERAGE and BORDA strategies, the partial ranking (P_1) can be described. Accordingly, Effectiveness always has less preference compared to any other attributes. Safety, Suitability, Standardization and Efficiency have no preference compared to each other in P1, but always have less preference compared to Responsiveness, Sustainability and Equity. Therefore, it can be said that the highest preference is for Responsiveness among all attributes.

9 Ranking Healthcare Attributes with Uncertain Data

Uncertain data refers to data points or sets that are incomplete, ambiguous, or uncertain. These types of data can arise in various fields such as finance, healthcare, and engineering, and can be caused by factors such as measurement error, missing values, or subjective interpretations.

Uncertain data can be classified into three main categories: probabilistic, possibilistic, and fuzzy data. Probabilistic uncertain data is data for which the degree of uncertainty is quantified by probability distributions. Possibilistic uncertain data is data for which the degree of uncertainty is quantified by possibility distributions. Fuzzy uncertain data is data for which the degree of uncertainty is quantified by fuzzy sets.

Various techniques can be used to deal with uncertain data, including probability theory, possibility theory, fuzzy logic, and rough sets. These techniques can be used to model uncertainty and make predictions or decisions based on uncertain data.

One example of uncertain data is weather forecasting. Weather forecasts are based on numerous uncertain factors such as temperature, humidity, and wind speed. Weather forecasters use probabilistic models to predict the likelihood of different weather patterns, but there is always some degree of uncertainty in the forecasts.

There are various types of uncertain data, including:

1. Probabilistic uncertain data: Probabilistic uncertain data is data for which the degree of uncertainty is quantified by probability distributions. This type of

data is commonly encountered in fields such as finance, where stock prices are predicted using probabilistic models based on historical data. Another example is in medical diagnosis, where probabilistic models are used to estimate the likelihood of a certain disease given various symptoms.

2. Possibilistic uncertain data: Possibilistic uncertain data is data for which the degree of uncertainty is quantified by possibility distributions. This type of data is commonly encountered in fields such as artificial intelligence, where fuzzy logic and possibility theory are used to handle uncertain data. For example, in facial recognition systems, possibilistic uncertain data can be used to handle variations in lighting, angle, and facial expression.
3. Fuzzy uncertain data: Fuzzy uncertain data is data for which the degree of uncertainty is quantified by fuzzy sets. Fuzzy sets are used to handle data that is not clearly defined, such as when assigning a numerical value to a subjective concept like "large" or "small". For example, fuzzy uncertain data can be used in decision-making processes, where various factors may have different degrees of importance.
4. Interval uncertain data: Interval uncertain data is data for which the degree of uncertainty is quantified by a range of values. This type of data is commonly encountered in fields such as engineering, where measurements may have a certain degree of error. For example, if a measurement is taken to be 10 m with an error of plus or minus 0.5 m, then the interval uncertain data would be [9.5, 10.5] meters.
5. Missing data: Missing data refers to data points that are incomplete or missing. This type of uncertain data can arise for various reasons, such as data entry errors or sensor malfunctions. Missing data can be handled using techniques such as imputation, which involves estimating missing values based on other available data points.

In summary, uncertain data is a broad category that includes various types of incomplete, ambiguous, or uncertain data. Different techniques can be used to handle these types of data, depending on the specific context and the degree of uncertainty involved.

One of the methods for modeling uncertain data is the use of neural networks. In this method, uncertain information is input into the neural network and the network has the ability to learn and predict automatically based on its training data.

Considering that uncertain data usually includes low-quality and inaccurate information, it is necessary to use methods with high accuracy and the ability to improve data quality for analyzing and making decisions based on this type of data.

Fuzzy logic and rough set-based methods can be useful in complex decision-making processes where uncertain data is important and critical. For example, we can rank the performance evaluation attributes of smart healthcare management using fuzzy DEMATEL. The ranking of sub-attributes is also similar to the main attributes and can be calculated separately, and then based on the ranking of the main attributes, the sub-attributes are also ranked, like Crisp DEMATEL, which is calculated above. Triangular Chung fuzzy numbers are used for fuzzification.

9.1 Fuzzy Sets and Fuzzy Numbers

Fuzzy set theory, which was introduced by Zadeh (1965) to deal with problems in which a source of vagueness is involved, has been utilized for incorporating imprecise data into the decision framework. A fuzzy set $\tilde{A}$ can be defined mathematically by a membership function $\mu_{\tilde{A}}(X)$, which assigns each element x in the universe of discourse X a real number in the interval [0, 1]. A triangular fuzzy number $\tilde{A}$ can be defined by a triplet (a, b, c) as illustrated in Fig. 6.

The membership function $\mu_{\tilde{A}}(X)$ is defined as

$$\frac{x-a}{b-a} \quad a_{\leq x \leq b}$$

$$\mu_A(x) = \underline{-\bar{c}_x} \quad b \leq \quad x \leq \quad c \;\Big|$$

$$b - c$$

$$0 \quad otherwise$$

Basic arithmetic operations on triangular fuzzy numbers $A_1 = (a_1, b_1, c_1)$, where $a_1 \leq b_1 \leq c_1$, and $A_2 = (a_2, b_2, c_2)$, where $a_2 \leq b_2 \leq c_2$, can be shown as follows:

Addition:

$$A_1 \oplus A_2 = (a_1 + a_2, b_1 + b_2, c_1 + c_2)$$

Subtraction:

$$A_1 \oplus A_2 = (a_1 - a_2, b_1 - b_2, c_1 - c_2)$$

Multiplication: if k is a scalar

$$K \otimes A \quad 1 = \begin{cases} (ka_1, kb_1, kc_1), k > 0 \\ (kc_1, kb_1, ka_1), k < 0 \end{cases}$$

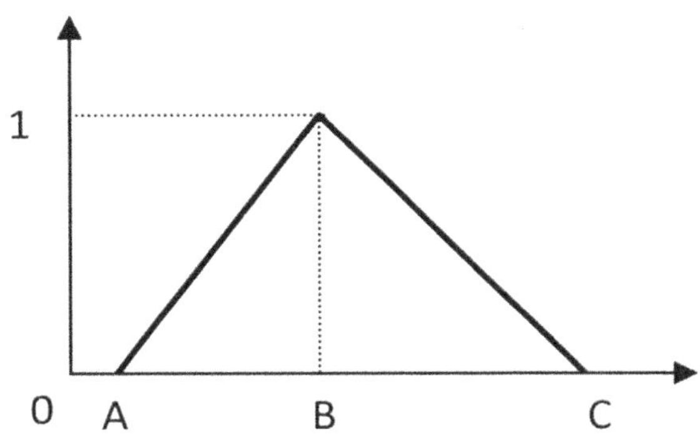

Fig. 6 A triangular fuzzy number $\tilde{A}$

Division:

$$A_1 \emptyset A_2^{\approx\left(\frac{a_1}{c_2}, \frac{b_1}{b_2}, \frac{c_1}{a_2}\right)}$$

Although multiplication and division operations on triangular fuzzy numbers do not necessarily yield a triangular fuzzy number, triangular fuzzy number approximations can be used for many practical applications. Triangular fuzzy numbers are appropriate for quantifying the vague information about most decision problems including personnel selection (e.g. rating for creativity, personality, leadership, etc.). The primary reason for using triangular fuzzy numbers can be stated as their intuitive and computational-efficient representation. A linguistic variable is defined as a variable whose values are not numbers, but words or sentences in natural or artificial language. The concept of a linguistic variable appears as a useful means for providing approximate characterization of phenomena that are too complex or ill-defined to be described in conventional quantitative terms.

9.2 Using Fuzzy DEMATEL

Fuzzy DEMATEL (Decision Making Trial and Evaluation Laboratory) is a method used for solving complex decision-making problems by identifying and analyzing the causal relationships between factors involved in the problem. The steps involved in fuzzy DEMATEL are:

Step 1. Problem Definition: The first step is to clearly define the decision problem and identify the factors involved. This stage was explained at the beginning of the chapter, and with three rounds of Delphi method, 8 main attributes and 22 sub- attributes were selected by experts for evaluating the performance of smart healthcare management. The attributes and sub- attributes were ranked using the DEMATEL method with crisp data. However, here, assuming the uncertainty and fuzziness of the data, only the main attributes are ranked. Due to the similarity of the DEMATEL technique stages for ranking the sub- attributes, the calculations are assigned to the readers.

Step 2. Constructing a Fuzzy DEMATEL Matrix: The next step is to construct a Fuzzy DEMATEL matrix. The matrix is a square matrix where the rows and columns represent the factors involved in the decision problem. Each cell in the matrix represents the causal relationship between the two factors. The relationship is represented by a fuzzy number between 0 and 1. In this stage, pairwise comparison opinions of 10 experts are received separately, and after being transformed into triangular fuzzy numbers using Chang's fuzzy numbers, they are aggregated using the geometric mean to initiate the computational phase of the Fuzzy DEMATEL technique based on it.

Step 3. Fuzzy Set Operations: Fuzzy set operations are performed on the fuzzy numbers in the matrix to derive the influence degrees of each factor on the other

Table 46 Pairwise comparison of attributes by expert 1

Expert 1	Responsiveness	Suitability	Standardization	Efficiency	Effectiveness	Safety	Sustainability	Equity
Responsiveness	–	VH	H	M	MH	MH	H	M
Suitability	ML	–	VL	L	M	L	VL	M
Standardization	H	VH	–	M	M	VL	M	L
Efficiency	L	M	MH	–	VL	ML	M	M
Effectiveness	M	ML	L	ML	–	M	VL	M
Safety	M	ML	H	L	VL	–	L	M
Sustainability	H	VH	M	M	M	H	–	H
Equity	M	MH	M	L	M	MH	H	–

Table 47 Fuzzy pairwise comparison of attributes by expert 1

Expert 1	Responsiveness			Suitability			Standardization			Efficiency			Effectiveness			Safety			Sustainability			Equity		
Responsiveness	1	1	1	0	0	0.2	0.1	0.2	0.3	0.4	0.5	0.6	0.4	0.5	0.6	0.7	0.8	0.9	0.7	0.8	0.9	0	0	0.2
Suitability	0.2	0.35	0.5	1	1	1	0	0	0.2	0.1	0.2	0.3	0.1	0.2	0.3	0.4	0.5	0.6	0.2	0.35	0.5	0.1	0.2	0.3
Standardization	0.7	0.8	0.9	0.8	0.9	1	1	1	1	0.4	0.5	0.6	0.4	0.5	0.6	0.7	0.8	0.9	0.8	0.9	1	0.7	0.8	0.9
Efficiency	0.7	0.8	0.9	0.4	0.5	0.6	0.5	0.65	0.8	1	1	1	0	0	0.2	0.1	0.2	0.3	0.4	0.5	0.6	0.4	0.5	0.6
Effectiveness	0.4	0.5	0.6	0.5	0.65	0.8	0.4	0.5	0.6	0.1	0.2	0.3	1	1	1	0.4	0.5	0.6	0.2	0.35	0.5	0.7	0.8	0.9
Safety	0.7	0.8	0.9	0.2	0.35	0.5	0.7	0.8	0.9	0.1	0.2	0.3	0	0	0.2	1	1	1	0.2	0.35	0.5	0.8	0.9	1
Sustainability	0.1	0.2	0.3	0.4	0.5	0.6	0.5	0.65	0.8	0.7	0.8	0.9	0.8	0.9	1	0.2	0.35	0.5	1	1	1	0.7	0.8	0.9
Equity	0.7	0.8	0.9	0.1	0.2	0.3	0.2	0.4	0.5	0.2	0.35	0.5	0.4	0.5	0.6	0.8	0.9	1	0	0	0.2	1	1	1

Table 48 Aggregate fuzzy pairwise comparison of attributes by 10 experts

Aggregate	Responsiveness			Suitability			Standardization			Efficiency			Effectiveness			Safety			Sustainability			Equity		
Responsiveness	1	1	1	0.56	0.67	0.78	0.72	0.82	0.93	0.45	0.57	0.67	0.43	0.55	0.669	0.56	0.67	0.78	0.53	0.6	0.73	0.56	0.67	0.78
Suitability	0.29	0.41	0.54	1	1	1	0.46	0.59	0.71	0.28	0.42	0.56	0.569	0.671	0.786	0.57	0.67	0.78	0.17	0.26	0.37	0.63	0.72	0.83
Standardization	0.09	0.17	0.3	0.47	0.61	0.75	1	1	1	0.25	0.36	0.469	0.2	0.255	0.4	0.22	0.37	0.51	0.483	0.59	0.697	0.57	0.67	0.78
Efficiency	0.53	0.63	0.73	0.16	0.27	0.38	0.68	0.79	0.89	1	1	1	0.16	0.44	0.54	0.56	0.67	0.78	0.22	0.37	0.51	0.09	0.17	0.30
Effectiveness	0.09	0.17	0.3	0.47	0.61	0.75	0.46	0.58	0.69	0.25	0.36	0.469	1	1	1	0.25	0.36	0.469	0.2	0.255	0.4	0.22	0.37	0.51
Safety	0.71	0.81	0.91	0.3	0.39	0.55	0.39	0.51	0.63	0.22	0.37	0.51	0.303	0.369	0.524	1	1	1	0.56	0.6	0.78	0.56	0.67	0.78
Sustainability	0.22	0.37	0.51	0.15	0.22	0.35	0.71	0.81	0.91	0.4	0.5	0.6	0.483	0.59	0.697	0.71	0.81	0.91	1	1	1	0.56	0.67	0.78
Equity	0.71	0.81	0.91	0.3	0.39	0.55	0.39	0.51	0.63	0.56	0.67	0.786	0.303	0.369	0.524	0.22	0.37	0.51	0.56	0.6	0.78	1	1	1
ALPHA	3.64	4.37	5.2	3.41	4.16	5.11	4.81	5.61	6.39	3.35	4.88	5.554	4.288	4.244	5.14	3.31	4.29	5.249	3.723	4.275	5.267	4.19	4.94	5.78

Table 49 L-infinity norm

Attributes	ALPHA		
Responsiveness	4.81	5.55	6.345
Suitability	3.58	4.34	5.133
Standardization	3.28	4.025	4.909
Efficiency	3.97	4.741	5.577
Effectiveness	2.94	3.705	4.588
Safety	4.04	4.719	5.69
Sustainability	4.23	4.97	5.763
Equity	4.04	4.719	5.69
Maximum of row and column	4.81	5.61	6.39

Table 50 Normalized attributes matrix

NX~	Responsiveness			Suitability			Standardization			Efficiency			Effectiveness			Safety			Sustainability			Equity		
Responsiveness	0.16	0.18	0.21	0.09	0.12	0.16	0.11	0.15	0.19	0.07	0.10	0.14	0.07	0.10	0.14	0.09	0.12	0.16	0.08	0.11	0.15	0.09	0.12	0.16
Suitability	0.08	0.11	0.15	0.16	0.18	0.21	0.11	0.14	0.19	0.03	0.05	0.08	0.05	0.08	0.11	0.09	0.12	0.16	0.03	0.07	0.11	0.01	0.03	0.06
Standardization	0.01	0.03	0.06	0.07	0.11	0.16	0.16	0.18	0.21	0.04	0.06	0.10	0.03	0.05	0.08	0.03	0.07	0.11	0.08	0.11	0.14	0.09	0.12	0.16
Efficiency	0.05	0.07	0.11	0.04	0.07	0.12	0.07	0.11	0.15	0.16	0.18	0.21	0.09	0.12	0.16	0.09	0.12	0.16	0.03	0.05	0.08	0.10	0.13	0.17
Effectiveness	0.01	0.03	0.06	0.07	0.11	0.16	0.07	0.10	0.14	0.04	0.06	0.10	0.16	0.18	0.21	0.04	0.06	0.10	0.03	0.05	0.08	0.03	0.07	0.11
Safety	0.11	0.14	0.19	0.05	0.07	0.11	0.06	0.09	0.13	0.16	0.18	0.21	0.05	0.07	0.11	0.03	0.07	0.11	0.09	0.11	0.16	0.09	0.12	0.16
Sustainability	0.03	0.07	0.11	0.02	0.04	0.07	0.11	0.14	0.19	**0.06**	0.09	0.12	0.08	0.11	0.14	0.11	0.14	0.19	0.16	0.18	0.21	0.09	0.12	0.16
Equity	0.11	0.14	0.19	0.05	0.07	0.11	0.06	0.09	0.13	0.09	0.12	0.16	0.05	0.07	0.11	0.03	0.07	0.11	0.09	0.11	0.16	0.16	0.18	0.21

Table 51 Identity Matrix

I	Responsiveness			Suitability			Standardization			Efficiency			Effectiveness			Safety			Sustainability			Equity		
Responsiveness	1	1	1	0	0	0	0	0	0	0	0	0	0	0	0	0	0	0	0	0	0	0	0	0
Suitability	0	0	0	1	1	1	0	0	0	0	0	0	0	0	0	0	0	0	0	0	0	0	0	0
Standardization	0	0	0	0	0	0	1	1	1	0	0	0	0	0	0	0	0	0	0	0	0	0	0	0
Efficiency	0	0	0	0	0	0	0	0	0	1	1	1	0	0	0	0	0	0	0	0	0	0	0	0
Effectiveness	0	0	0	0	0	0	0	0	0	0	0	0	1	1	1	0	0	0	0	0	0	0	0	0
Safety	0	0	0	0	0	0	0	0	0	0	0	0	0	0	0	1	1	1	0	0	0	0	0	0
Sustainability	0	0	0	0	0	0	0	0	0	0	0	0	0	0	0	0	0	0	1	1	1	0	0	0
Equity	0	0	0	0	0	0	0	0	0	0	0	0	0	0	0	0	0	0	0	0	0	1	1	1

Table 52 Contrast between identity matrix and normalized matrix

I-NX ~	Responsiveness			Suitability			Standardization			Efficiency			Effectiveness			Safety			Sustainability			Equity		
Responsiveness	0.79	0.82	0.84	−0.16	−0.12	−0.09	−0.19	−0.15	−0.11	−0.14	−0.10	−0.07	−0.14	−0.10	−0.07	−0.16	−0.12	−0.09	−0.15	−0.11	−0.08	−0.16	−0.12	−0.09
Suitability	−0.15	−0.11	−0.08	0.79	0.82	0.84	−0.19	−0.14	−0.11	−0.08	−0.05	−0.03	−0.11	−0.08	−0.05	−0.16	−0.12	−0.09	−0.11	−0.07	−0.03	−0.06	−0.03	−0.01
Standardization	−0.06	−0.03	−0.01	−0.16	−0.11	−0.07	0.79	0.82	0.84	−0.10	−0.06	−0.04	−0.08	−0.05	−0.03	0.11	−0.07	−0.03	−0.14	−0.11	−0.08	−0.16	−0.12	−0.09
Efficiency	−0.11	−0.07	−0.05	−0.12	−0.07	−0.04	−0.15	−0.11	−0.07	0.79	0.82	0.84	−0.16	−0.12	−0.09	−0.16	−0.12	−0.09	−0.08	−0.05	−0.03	−0.17	−0.13	−0.10
Effectiveness	−0.06	−0.03	−0.01	−0.16	−0.11	−0.07	−0.14	−0.10	−0.07	−0.10	−0.06	−0.04	0.79	0.82	0.84	−0.10	−0.06	−0.04	−0.08	−0.05	−0.03	−0.11	−0.07	−0.03
Safety	−0.19	−0.14	−0.11	−0.11	−0.07	−0.05	−0.13	−0.09	−0.06	−0.21	−0.18	−0.16	−0.11	−0.07	−0.05	0.89	0.93	0.97	−0.16	−0.11	−0.09	−0.16	−0.12	−0.09
Sustainability	−0.11	−0.07	−0.03	−0.07	−0.04	−0.02	−0.19	−0.14	−0.11	−0.12	−0.09	−0.06	−0.14	−0.11	−0.08	−0.19	−0.14	−0.11	0.79	0.82	0.84	−0.16	−0.12	−0.09
Equity	−0.19	−0.14	−0.11	−0.11	−0.07	−0.05	−0.13	−0.09	−0.06	−0.16	−0.12	−0.09	−0.11	−0.07	−0.05	−0.11	−0.07	−0.03	−0.16	−0.11	−0.09	0.79	0.82	0.84

Table 53 Lower bound of the normalized matrix

NX ~ L	Responsiveness	Suitability	Standardization	Efficiency	Effectiveness	Safety	Sustainability	Equity
Responsiveness	0.156	0.088	0.113	0.070	0.067	0.088	0.083	0.088
Suitability	0.083	0.156	0.106	0.025	0.053	0.088	0.034	0.014
Standardization	0.014	0.074	0.156	0.039	0.031	0.034	0.076	0.089
Efficiency	0.045	0.044	0.072	0.156	0.089	0.089	0.027	0.099
Effectiveness	0.014	0.074	0.072	0.039	0.156	0.039	0.031	0.034
Safety	0.111	0.047	0.061	0.156	0.047	0.034	0.088	0.088
Sustainability	0.034	0.023	0.111	0.063	0.076	0.111	0.156	0.088
Equity	0.111	0.047	0.061	0.088	0.047	0.034	0.088	0.156

Table 54 Lower bound of Contrast between IM and NM

I-NX ~ L	Responsiveness	Suitability	Standardization	Efficiency	Effectiveness	Safety	Sustainability	Equity
Responsiveness	0.792	−0.162	−0.193	−0.139	−0.139	−0.162	−0.152	−0.163
Suitability	−0.152	0.792	−0.185	−0.079	−0.112	−0.162	−0.106	−0.063
Standardization	−0.062	−0.156	0.792	−0.098	−0.083	−0.106	−0.145	−0.163
Efficiency	−0.112	−0.116	−0.148	0.792	−0.163	−0.162	−0.077	−0.173
Effectiveness	−0.062	−0.156	−0.143	−0.098	0.792	−0.098	−0.083	−0.106
Safety	−0.189	−0.114	−0.131	−0.208	−0.109	0.894	−0.162	−0.163
Sustainability	−0.106	−0.073	−0.189	−0.125	−0.145	−0.189	0.792	−0.163
Equity	−0.189	−0.114	−0.131	−0.163	−0.109	−0.106	−0.162	0.792

Table 55 Reverse matrix of I-NX ~ L

(I-NX ~ L)^−1	Responsiveness	Suitability	Standardization	Efficiency	Effectiveness	Safety	Sustainability	Equity
Responsiveness	−0.122	−1.206	−1.467	−1.248	−1.175	−1.187	−1.217	−1.348
Suitability	−0.910	0.128	−1.132	−1.035	−0.938	−0.912	−0.986	−1.153
Standardization	−0.955	−0.884	−0.050	−0.960	−0.921	−0.919	−0.890	−0.983
Efficiency	−1.045	−1.071	−1.301	0.016	−0.969	−1.013	−1.121	−1.135
Effectiveness	−0.867	−0.777	−1.000	−0.866	0.313	−0.836	−0.869	−0.945
Safety	−1.017	−1.134	−1.378	−1.042	−1.077	−0.113	−1.082	−1.201
Sustainability	−1.104	−1.177	−1.314	−1.121	−1.039	−1.032	−0.020	−1.192
Equity	−1.015	−1.136	−1.381	−1.091	−1.082	−1.117	−1.080	−0.157

Table 56 Fuzzy importance score of lower bound

TL	Responsiveness	Suitability	Standardization	Efficiency	Effectiveness	Safety	Sustainability	Equity
Responsiveness	−0.608	−0.701	−0.844	−0.731	−0.693	−0.690	−0.706	−0.784
Suitability	−0.468	−0.398	−0.575	−0.559	−0.495	−0.470	−0.535	−0.624
Standardization	−0.495	−0.442	−0.464	−0.488	−0.470	−0.475	−0.435	−0.477
Efficiency	−0.575	−0.594	−0.706	−0.476	−0.515	−0.541	−0.619	−0.599
Effectiveness	−0.423	−0.355	−0.457	−0.411	−0.253	−0.396	−0.414	−0.457
Safety	−0.540	−0.628	−0.754	−0.514	−0.591	−0.621	−0.586	−0.646
Sustainability	−0.637	−0.672	−0.719	−0.625	−0.579	−0.563	−0.518	−0.659
Equity	−0.538	−0.633	−0.759	−0.590	−0.599	−0.628	−0.583	−0.579

Table 57 Middle bound of the normalized matrix

NX ~ M	Responsiveness	Suitability	Standardization	Efficiency	Effectiveness	Safety	Sustainability	Equity
Responsiveness	0.178	0.119	0.146	0.102	0.098	0.119	0.107	0.119
Suitability	0.112	0.178	0.141	0.048	0.078	0.119	0.066	0.030
Standardization	0.030	0.109	0.178	0.064	0.045	0.066	0.105	0.119
Efficiency	0.073	0.075	0.105	0.178	0.120	0.119	0.046	0.128
Effectiveness	0.030	0.109	0.103	0.064	0.178	0.064	0.045	0.066
Safety	0.144	0.070	0.091	0.178	0.066	0.066	0.107	0.119
Sustainability	0.066	0.039	0.144	0.089	0.105	0.144	0.178	0.119
Equity	0.144	0.070	0.091	0.119	0.066	0.066	0.107	0.178

Table 58 Middle bound of Contrast between IM and NM

I-NX ~ M	Responsiveness	Suitability	Standardization	Efficiency	Effectiveness	Safety	Sustainability	Equity
Responsiveness	0.822	−0.119	−0.146	−0.102	−0.098	−0.119	−0.107	−0.119
Suitability	−0.112	0.822	−0.141	−0.048	−0.078	−0.119	−0.066	−0.030
Standardization	−0.030	−0.109	0.822	−0.064	−0.045	−0.066	−0.105	−0.119
Efficiency	−0.073	−0.075	−0.105	0.822	−0.120	−0.119	−0.046	−0.128
Effectiveness	−0.030	−0.109	−0.103	−0.064	0.822	−0.064	−0.045	−0.066
Safety	−0.144	−0.070	−0.091	−0.178	−0.066	0.934	−0.107	−0.119
Sustainability	−0.066	−0.039	−0.144	−0.089	−0.105	−0.144	0.822	−0.119
Equity	−0.144	−0.070	−0.091	−0.119	−0.066	−0.066	−0.107	0.822

Table 59 Reverse matrix of I-NX ~ L

(I-NX ~ M)^−1	Responsiveness	Suitability	Standardization	Efficiency	Effectiveness	Safety	Sustainability	Equity
Responsiveness	1.710	0.647	0.839	0.675	0.601	0.637	0.631	0.732
Suitability	0.516	1.593	0.676	0.479	0.460	0.516	0.465	0.486
Standardization	0.394	0.478	1.670	0.463	0.392	0.429	0.479	0.553
Efficiency	0.511	0.512	0.676	1.670	0.546	0.548	0.474	0.645
Effectiveness	0.345	0.444	0.533	0.413	1.502	0.381	0.362	0.437
Safety	0.600	0.516	0.683	0.681	0.502	1.515	0.555	0.653
Sustainability	0.524	0.490	0.754	0.602	0.551	0.600	1.651	0.669
Equity	0.606	0.516	0.683	0.619	0.500	0.513	0.560	1.716

Table 60 Fuzzy importance score of middle bound

TM	Responsiveness	Suitability	Standardization	Efficiency	Effectiveness	Safety	Sustainability	Equity
Responsiveness	0.710	0.647	0.839	0.675	0.601	0.637	0.631	0.732
Suitability	0.516	0.593	0.676	0.479	0.460	0.516	0.465	0.486
Standardization	0.394	0.478	0.670	0.463	0.392	0.429	0.479	0.553
Efficiency	0.511	0.512	0.676	0.670	0.546	0.548	0.474	0.645
Effectiveness	0.345	0.444	0.533	0.413	0.502	0.381	0.362	0.437
Safety	0.600	0.516	0.683	0.681	0.502	0.515	0.555	0.653
Sustainability	0.524	0.490	0.754	0.602	0.551	0.600	0.651	0.669
Equity	0.606	0.516	0.683	0.619	0.500	0.513	0.560	0.716

Table 61 Upper bound of the normalized matrix

NX ~ U	Responsiveness	Suitability	Standardization	Efficiency	Effectiveness	Safety	Sustainability	Equity
Responsiveness	0.208	0.162	0.193	0.139	0.139	0.162	0.152	0.163
Suitability	0.152	0.208	0.185	0.079	0.112	0.162	0.106	0.063
Standardization	0.062	0.156	0.208	0.098	0.083	0.106	0.145	0.163
Efficiency	0.112	0.116	0.148	0.208	0.163	0.162	0.077	0.173
Effectiveness	0.062	0.156	0.143	0.098	0.208	0.098	0.083	0.106
Safety	0.189	0.114	0.131	0.208	0.109	0.106	0.162	0.163
Sustainability	0.106	0.073	0.189	0.125	0.145	0.189	0.208	0.163
Equity	0.189	0.114	0.131	0.163	0.109	0.106	0.162	0.208

Table 62 Upper bound of contrast between IM and NM

I-NX ~ U	Responsiveness	Suitability	Standardization	Efficiency	Effectiveness	Safety	Sustainability	Equity
Responsiveness	0.844	−0.088	−0.113	−0.070	−0.067	−0.088	−0.083	−0.088
Suitability	−0.083	0.844	−0.106	−0.025	−0.053	−0.088	−0.034	−0.014
Standardization	−0.014	−0.074	0.844	−0.039	−0.031	−0.034	−0.076	−0.089
Efficiency	−0.045	−0.044	−0.072	0.844	−0.089	−0.089	−0.027	−0.099
Effectiveness	−0.014	−0.074	−0.072	−0.039	0.844	−0.039	−0.031	−0.034
Safety	−0.111	−0.047	−0.061	−0.156	−0.047	0.966	−0.088	−0.088
Sustainability	−0.034	−0.023	−0.111	−0.063	−0.076	−0.111	0.844	−0.088
Equity	−0.111	−0.047	−0.061	−0.088	−0.047	−0.034	−0.088	0.844

Table 63 Reverse matrix of I-NX ~ L

(I-NX ~ U)^-1	Responsiveness	Suitability	Standardization	Efficiency	Effectiveness	Safety	Sustainability	Equity
Responsiveness	1.297	0.222	0.300	0.220	0.198	0.212	0.226	0.249
Suitability	0.182	1.265	0.246	0.126	0.145	0.177	0.132	0.119
Standardization	0.094	0.160	1.284	0.131	0.112	0.112	0.171	0.198
Efficiency	0.151	0.146	0.213	1.290	0.201	0.185	0.131	0.233
Effectiveness	0.078	0.153	0.175	0.115	1.241	0.104	0.102	0.115
Safety	0.226	0.154	0.215	0.292	0.162	1.143	0.206	0.230
Sustainability	0.143	0.126	0.270	0.197	0.191	0.217	1.289	0.233
Equity	0.232	0.154	0.215	0.218	0.159	0.140	0.211	1.303

Table 64 Fuzzy importance score of upper bound

TU	Responsiveness	Suitability	Standardization	Efficiency	Effectiveness	Safety	Sustainability	Equity
Responsiveness	0.446	0.393	0.516	0.400	0.368	0.376	0.397	0.443
Suitability	0.339	0.403	0.448	0.281	0.293	0.333	0.298	0.274
Standardization	0.232	0.331	0.456	0.291	0.252	0.266	0.334	0.378
Efficiency	0.313	0.312	0.418	0.446	0.369	0.343	0.279	0.418
Effectiveness	0.212	0.322	0.365	0.270	0.377	0.241	0.243	0.289
Safety	0.403	0.316	0.418	0.453	0.320	0.304	0.384	0.423
Sustainability	0.309	0.267	0.477	0.367	0.354	0.379	0.438	0.423
Equity	0.407	0.317	0.418	0.405	0.318	0.302	0.388	0.470

Table 65 Fuzzy importance score

T ~	Responsiveness			Suitability			Standardization			Efficiency			Effectiveness			Safety			Sustainability			Equity		
Responsiveness	−0.6	0.7	0.4	−0.7	0.6	0.4	−0.8	0.8	0.5	−0.7	0.7	0.4	−0.7	0.6	0.4	−0.7	0.6	0.4	−0.7	0.6	0.4	−0.8	0.7	0.4
Suitability	−0.5	0.5	0.3	−0.4	0.6	0.4	−0.6	0.7	0.4	−0.6	0.5	0.3	−0.5	0.5	0.3	−0.5	0.5	0.3	−0.5	0.5	0.3	−0.6	0.5	0.3
Standardization	−0.5	0.4	0.2	−0.4	0.5	0.3	−0.5	0.7	0.5	−0.5	0.5	0.3	−0.5	0.4	0.3	−0.5	0.4	0.3	−0.4	0.5	0.3	−0.5	0.6	0.4
Efficiency	−0.6	0.5	0.3	−0.6	0.5	0.3	−0.7	0.7	0.4	−0.5	0.7	0.4	−0.5	0.5	0.4	−0.5	0.5	0.3	−0.6	0.5	0.3	−0.6	0.6	0.4
Effectiveness	−0.4	0.3	0.2	−0.4	0.4	0.3	−0.5	0.5	0.4	−0.4	0.4	0.3	−0.3	0.5	0.4	−0.4	0.4	0.2	−0.4	0.4	0.2	−0.5	0.4	0.3
Safety	−0.5	0.6	0.4	−0.6	0.5	0.3	−0.8	0.7	0.4	−0.5	0.7	0.5	−0.6	0.5	0.3	−0.6	0.5	0.3	−0.6	0.6	0.4	−0.6	0.7	0.4
Sustainability	−0.6	0.5	0.3	−0.7	0.5	0.3	−0.7	0.8	0.5	−0.6	0.6	0.4	−0.6	0.6	0.4	−0.6	0.6	0.4	−0.5	0.7	0.4	−0.7	0.7	0.4
Equity	−0.5	0.6	0.4	−0.6	0.5	0.3	−0.8	0.7	0.4	−0.6	0.6	0.4	−0.6	0.5	0.3	−0.6	0.5	0.3	−0.6	0.6	0.4	−0.6	0.7	0.5
SUMC	−4.3	4.2	2.7	−4.4	4.2	2.7	−5.3	5.5	3.5	−4.4	4.6	2.9	−4.2	4.1	2.7	−4.4	4.1	2.5	−4.4	4.2	2.8	−4.8	4.9	3.1

Table 66 Fuzzy importance score and ranking based on R

Attributes	Sum of R			Defuzzification	Rank
Responsiveness	−5.758	5.473	3.339	3.802	1
Suitability	−4.124	4.192	2.670	2.962	5
Standardization	−3.746	3.859	2.541	2.744	7
Efficiency	−4.625	4.582	2.897	3.220	6
Effectiveness	−3.166	3.417	2.319	2.457	8
Safety	−4.880	4.706	3.021	3.297	4
Sustainability	−4.973	4.842	3.014	3.386	2
Equity	−4.909	4.714	3.025	3.300	3

Table 67 Fuzzy importance score and ranking based on C, R + C And R–C

Attributes	Sum of C			Defuzzification	Rank
Responsiveness	−4.272	4.208	2.629	2.951	4
Suitability	−4.217	4.007	2.556	2.798	8
Standardization	−5.256	5.516	3.487	3.916	1
Efficiency	−4.671	4.735	2.602	3.292	3
Effectiveness	−4.042	4.012	2.918	2.869	6
Safety	−4.363	4.125	2.509	2.862	7
Sustainability	−4.373	4.172	2.744	2.926	5
Equity	−4.768	4.813	3.075	3.398	2
	R + C			Defuzzification	Rank
Responsiveness	−10.067	9.664	5.932	6.731	1
Suitability	−8.861	8.569	5.418	5.996	7
Standardization	−9.043	9.376	6.007	6.652	3
Efficiency	−8.511	8.909	5.230	6.272	5
Effectiveness	−7.253	7.435	5.220	5.322	8
Safety	−9.187	8.768	5.471	6.112	6
Sustainability	−9.333	8.970	5.712	6.275	4
Equity	−9.667	9.486	6.052	6.663	2
	R − C			Defuzzification	Rank
Responsiveness	−8.424	1.248	7.574	0.830	1
Suitability	−7.200	0.554	7.079	0.401	3
Standardization	−7.274	−1.657	7.776	−1.180	8
Efficiency	−6.441	−0.560	7.299	−0.313	6
Effectiveness	−6.129	−0.589	6.344	−0.415	7
Safety	−7.333	0.519	7.325	0.388	4
Sustainability	−7.705	0.625	7.340	0.423	2
Equity	−7.974	−0.140	7.745	−0.134	5

factors. The operations include fuzzy addition, subtraction, multiplication, and division (Table 46).

Similarly, opinions of nine other experts were also obtained, and they were aggregated in the matrix Table 47 (Table 48).

Step 4. Normalization: The influence degrees obtained from the fuzzy set operations are normalized using the L-infinity or Supremum method. The next steps are the same as DEMATEL with crisp data, which were explained at the beginning of this chapter. In fuzzy logic calculations, each of the lower, middle, and upper bounds are calculated separately and the ranking is performed after their aggregation. Therefore, only the matrix calculations are mentioned in the following (Tables 49, 50 and 51).

In fuzzy number subtraction, the upper limit of the second number is subtracted from the lower limit of the first number. In fuzzy number division, the lower limit of the first number is divided by the upper limit of the second number (Tables 52, 53, 54, 55, 56, 57, 58, 59, 60, 61, 62, 63, 64, 65, 66 and 67).

References

1. Abbasbandy, S., Allahviranloo, T.A.: Numerical solutions of fuzzy differential equations by Taylor method. Comput. Methods Appl. Math. **2**(2), 113–124 (2002)
2. AlKhalifa, S.H., Althunibat, A.: Smart healthcare: reviewing cybersecurity challenges and approaches. Healthc. Inform. Res. **26**(1), 7–15 (2020)
3. Abbasi, F., Allahviranloo, T.: Conception and implementation of a new data-driven fuzzy method for reliability and safety analysis. New Math. Nat. Comput. **16**(02), 339–361 (2020). https://doi.org/10.1142/s1793005720500210
4. Abbasi, F., Allahviranloo, T.: The fuzzy arithmetic operations of transmission average on Pseudo-Hexagonal fuzzy numbers and its application in fuzzy system reliability analysis. Fuzzy Inf. Eng. **13**(1), 58–78 (2021). https://doi.org/10.1080/16168658.2021.1915449
5. Abbasi, F., Allahviranloo, T.: Realistic solution of fuzzy critical path problems, case study: the airport's cargo ground operation systems. Granul. Comput. **8**(3), 617–632 (2022). https://doi.org/10.1007/s41066-022-00347-w
6. Akram, M., Shahzadi, S., Shah, S.M.U., Allahviranloo, T.: A fully Fermatean fuzzy multi-objective transportation model using an extended DEA technique. Granul. Comput. (2023). https://doi.org/10.1007/s41066-023-00399-6
7. Allahviranloo, T., Abbasi, F.: A new estimation of failure analysis in fuzzy environment, case study: the electrical model failure for the football stadium. New Math. Nat. Comput. **18**(03), 791–817 (2022). https://doi.org/10.1142/s1793005722500387
8. Allahviranloo, T., Abbasbandy, S., Rouhparvar, H.: The exact solutions of fuzzy wave-like equations with variable coefficients by a variational iteration method. Appl. Soft Comput. **11**(2), 2186–2192 (2011)
9. Allahviranloo, T., Ezadi, S.: Z-advanced numbers processes. Inf. Sci. **480**, 130–143 (2019)
10. Allahviranloo, T., Gouyandeh, Z., Armand, A.: A full fuzzy method for solving differential equation based on Taylor expansion. J. Intell. Fuzzy Syst. **29**(3), 1039–1055 (2015)
11. Allahviranloo, T., Lotfi, F.H., Kiasari, M.K., Khezerloo, M.: On the fuzzy solution of LR fuzzy linear systems. Appl. Math. Model. **37**(3), 1170–1176 (2013)
12. Allahviranloo, T., Afshar Kermani, M.: Numerical methods for fuzzy linear partial differential equations under new definition for derivative. Iran. J. Fuzzy Syst. **7**(3), 33–50 (2010)

13. Amirteimoori, A., Allahviranloo, T., Kordrostami, S., Bagheri, S.F.: Improving decision-making units in performance analysis methods: a data envelopment analysis approach. Math. Sci. (2023). https://doi.org/10.1007/s40096-023-00512-5
14. Amirteimoori, A., Allahviranloo, T., Zadmirzaei, M.: Scale elasticity and technical efficiency analysis in the European forest sector: a stochastic value-based approach. Eur. J. Forest Res. (2023). https://doi.org/10.1007/s10342-023-01589-2
15. Amirteimoori, A., Allahviranloo, T., Zadmirzaei, M., Hasanzadeh, F.: On the environmental performance analysis: a combined fuzzy data envelopment analysis and artificial intelligence algorithms. Expert Syst. Appl. **224**, 119953 (2023). https://doi.org/10.1016/j.eswa.2023.119953
16. Banker, R.D., Amirteimoori, A., Allahviranloo, T., Sinha, R.P.: Performance analysis and managerial ability in the general insurance market: a study of India and Iran. Inf. Technol. Manage. (2023). https://doi.org/10.1007/s10799-023-00405-y
17. Bell, D.E.: Decision Making: Descriptive, Normative, and Prescriptive Interactions. Cambridge University Press (2017)
18. Chen, X., Ren, Z., Guo, S.: A fuzzy MADM approach for ranking health criteria. Expert Syst. Appl. **42**(4), 2355–2363 (2015)
19. Chen, Y., Fan, Z., Zhu, J.: Multi-criteria decision-making with incomplete preference information: a review. Omega **104**, 102387 (2021)
20. Chehlabi, M., Allahviranloo, T.: Concreted solutions to fuzzy linear fractional differential equations. Appl. Soft Comput. **44**, 108–116 (2016)
21. Dubossarsky, E., Wilder, B., Martin, T.: Uncertainty-aware self-supervised learning for medical image segmentation. Med. Image Anal. **72**, 102126 (2021)
22. Ishizaka, A., Nemery, P.: Multi-Criteria Decision Analysis: Methods and Software. John Wiley & Sons (2013)
23. Jafarnejad, A., Soufi, M., Bayati, A.: Prioritizing critical barriers of computerized maintenance management system (CMMS) by fuzzy multi attribute decision making (F-MADM)(Using LFPP). Kuwait Chapter Arab. J. Bus. Manag. Rev. **4**(3), 11 (2014)
24. Jones, J., Hunter, D., Considine, J.: Application of the Delphi technique in healthcare maintenance. Eng. Manag. J. **26**(4), 31–39 (2014)
25. Kahraman, C., Oztaysi, B., Kaya, İ: A comprehensive review of multi-criteria decision-making methods with applications in engineering. J. Clean. Prod. **276**, 124202 (2020)
26. Koulinas, G.K., Demesouka, O.E., Bougelis, G.G., Koulouriotis, D.E.: Risk prioritization in a natural gas compressor station construction project using the analytical hierarchy process. Sustainability **14**(20), 13172 (2022)
27. Li, D., Deng, Y., Zhou, D.: An integrated MADM approach based on interval type-2 fuzzy sets for medical equipment selection. Knowl.-Based Syst. **108**, 116–127 (2016)
28. Liao, Y., Gao, L., Chen, X.: Improving the quality of uncertain data for effective decision making: a probabilistic approach. Inf. Sci. **56**(3), 186–202 (2021)
29. Lin, R., Xu, Y.: A hybrid decision-making approach for multi-criteria decision-making problems based on 2-tuple linguistic information. Inf. Fusion **56**, 1–11 (2020)
30. Liu, Y., Zhang, Y.: Multi-criteria decision-making methods for assessing the sustainability of urban development. J. Clean. Prod. **341**, 130727 (2022)
31. Linstone, H.A., Turoff, M. (Eds.).: The Delphi method: techniques and applications. Addison-Wesley (2011)
32. Lu, Y., Chen, J., Hao, Q., et al.: Handling uncertain data in recommender systems: a review. Inf. Process. Manag. **58**(1), 102437 (2021)
33. Mahmoodirad, A., Allahviranloo, T., Niroomand, S.: A new effective solution method for fully intuitionistic fuzzy transportation problem. Soft. Comput. **23**(12), 4521–4530 (2019)
34. Moloudzadeh, S., Allahviranloo, T., Darabi, P.: A new method for solving an arbitrary fully fuzzy linear system. Soft. Comput. **17**(9), 1725–1731 (2013)
35. Ngan, T.N., Al-Ani, A.: A novel integrated fuzzy MCDM model for supplier selection with sustainability criteria. J. Clean. Prod. **279**, 123821 (2021)

36. Rahmani, A., Hosseinzadeh Lotfi, F., Rostamy-Malkhalifeh, M., Allahviranloo, T.: A new method for defuzzification and ranking of fuzzy numbers based on the statistical beta distribution. Adv. Fuzzy Syst. 2016 (2016)
37. Safari, H., Soufi, M.: Select a hypermarket location based on fuzzy multi criteria decision making (F-MCDM) techniques (hybrid of F-Delphi, F-Ahp, F-Llsm and F-Promethee). Kuwait Chap. Arab. J. Bus. Manag. Rev. **4**(1), 76–95 (2014)
38. Safari, H., Soufi, M.: Prioritize barriers of E-Factories in Iran's industries with hybrid multi criteria decision. Indian J. Fundam. Appl. Life Sci. **5**(1), 1329–1344 (2015)
39. Seyed-Hosseini, S.M., Amiri, M.: A multi-criteria decision-making approach for supplier selection using a new hybrid method based on interval type-2 fuzzy sets. J. Clean. Prod. **254**, 120146 (2020)
40. Wu, Y., Lu, Y., Liu, Y.: A fuzzy clustering approach for uncertain data in wireless sensor networks. IEEE Access **9**, 48717–48729 (2021)
41. Yeung, M.S., Lapinsky, S.E., Granton, J.T.: Critical care medicine and technology: the future is now. Crit. Care **23**(1), 342 (2019)

Healthcare Facility Location

Hamed Zhiani Rezai and Alireza Davoodi

Abstract Considering the importance of people's use of healthcare centers, locating these centers is one of the most critical issues to discuss. Several factors, such as accessibility and proximity to potential centers, the cost of construction and maintenance, and the quality of services provided, need to be taken into account while determining the best possible location for healthcare centers. In this chapter, we propose a novel method that utilizes the concepts of efficiency and Data Envelopment Analysis models to identify the optimal location for healthcare centers. The proposed model is non-linear and can be solved using a two-step Lexicographic method. Moreover, we demonstrate how to allocate population centers to each healthcare site, in addition to selecting which sites are chosen.

Keywords Healthcare facility location · Date envelopment analysis · Non-linear programming · Assignment

1 Introduction

Healthcare facility location is an important aspect of healthcare planning and management. By carefully selecting the optimal location for healthcare facilities, organizations can improve access to care, enhance patient outcomes, and optimize the use of available resources.

Recent research points out that most mathematical models like dynamic systems and also linear systems get involved with real-world problems. Since their related information has different forms like certainty and uncertainty, the uncertain version of these models does have more importance in the applications.

H. Z. Rezai (✉)
Department of Mathematics, Mashhad Branch, Islamic Azad University, Mashhad, Iran
e-mail: hz_rezai@hotmail.com

A. Davoodi
Department of Mathematics, Neyshabur Branch, Islamic Azad University, Neyshabur, Iran

T. Allahviranloo et al. (eds.), *Decision Making in Healthcare Systems*,
Studies in Systems, Decision and Control 513,
https://doi.org/10.1007/978-3-031-46735-6_6

In health problems, two types of mathematical models; fuzzy dynamic systems and fuzzy linear programming problems even transportation problems, play an important role, on the other hand, the main and basic model of fuzzy linear programming problems is fuzzy linear systems.

In conclusion, fuzzy differential equations (as a special version of dynamic systems) [1–3] and fuzzy linear systems (as a basic model of fuzzy linear programming problems) [4], have an important role in this research. Recently several research has been done on investigating the advanced version of the uncertain information [2, 5–7] and moreover the above-mentioned basic models. Many research studies have been conducted to address the challenges of fuzzy systems [8–12].

One of the techniques for decision making is Data Envelopment Analysis (DEA), and many researchers have conducted research on this topic. Several recent papers have been cited to mention their research area [13–17]. Some authors have explored the topic in a different way: safety analysis and reliability [18–20].

In this chapter, we will first briefly review the fundamentals and basic models regarding the facility location problem in Sect. 2. Then, we will review the literature on healthcare location in Sect. 3. In Sect. 4, we will present the concept of efficiency and the fundamental models of data envelopment analysis, and finally, we will develop a model to determine the best place for establishing healthcare centers based on their efficiency. Section 6 will contain the conclusion.

2 Facility Location

The facility location problem (FLP) involves locating a number of facilities to serve a set of demands. There is a set of potential facility locations, and opening a facility at each location has an associated non-negative fixed cost and either limited or unlimited capacity of available supply. In a basic formulation, the facility location problem consists of a set of potential facility sites where a facility can be opened and a set of demand points that must be serviced. The goal is to select a subset of facilities to open, minimizing the sum of distances from each demand point to its nearest facility, plus the sum of opening costs of the facilities.

The location of facilities is critical in both industry and healthcare systems. Inappropriately choosing the number of locations may lead to customer dissatisfaction or excessive costs for the organization. Both of these outcomes will cause a lack of proper productivity, leading to a negative impact on the organization's performance, including financial indicators, credit, and brand.

In the field of healthcare, this problem becomes even more critical and acute. Inadequate or insufficient facilities can lead to increased mortality rates and the spread of complications and diseases. Therefore, location modeling of healthcare facilities is significant. In cases where there is a surplus of these centers, the issue of costs and completing the treatment staff also highlights another aspect of the problem's importance.

Table 1 A classification of discrete location problem

Discrete location problem	Covering-based problem	Set covering location problem
		Maximal covering location problem
		P-center location problem
	Median-based problem	P-median location problem
		Fixed charge-facility location problem
	Other problems	P-dispersion, maxisum dispersion, MNS location problem

In general, facility location models are classified into two categories: continuous and discrete. In continuous location models, it is assumed that demands are continuously distributed throughout an area, allowing facilities to be located anywhere in the area. On the other hand, discrete models focus on selecting the best location for a facility from a given set of potential sites while minimizing total cost and satisfying customer demand. Discrete models assume that demands can be limited to a finite number of discrete points. Therefore, a general map of location areas can be represented by several hundred or even several thousand points or nodes (such as census tracts or even census blocks). In other words, discrete location models assume that there is a finite number of candidate locations or nodes where facilities can be placed [21]. Table 1 shows how discrete models are classified.

The majority of healthcare facility location problems are based on discrete models. Therefore, in the following sections, we will focus on these types of models.

As previously mentioned, there is a vast amount of research in the field of facility location models. A general introduction to facility location modeling and summary of general location models can be found in [22–24]. Applications of facility location models to problems in the public sector can be found in [25, 26]. Moreover, Laporte et al. [27] show that facility location is one of the most widely used and diverse decision-making problems, which has gathered significant knowledge over time, both in terms of theoretical properties and modeling frameworks, along with solution techniques. Several other applications of the subject in the transportation problems have been done by Mahmoodirad et al. [4].

2.1 Covering-Based Problem

2.1.1 Set Covering Location Problem

Coverage is the main concept in set covering and maximal covering models [28, 29]. Using this concept, it is possible to verify if all demands within the system are being met by at least one facility. Based on the development of the concept of coverage distance, a zero-one mathematical model can be presented, which named set covering model [30]. In the set covering model, the aim is to select facilities that cover all demand nodes while minimizing costs [21, 31]. With a slight change in objective function, another model can be presented, the aim of which is to minimize the number of facilities instead of reducing the cost.

2.1.2 Maximal Covering Location Problem

The maximal covering location problem is a type of facility location problem that aims to maximize the coverage of demand by locating a given number of facilities strategically. The problem involves identifying potential facility locations, demand points, and their corresponding coverage radii. The problem also requires that each potential facility has a fixed cost associated with its opening and that each demand point has a weight representing its level of importance. The objective of this problem is to select a subset of potential facility locations to open such that the sum of weights covered by the selected facilities is maximized [32].

As opening facilities comes with a cost, there is a budget constraint that limits the total expenditure on facility launch. The objective of the maximal covering location problem is to find the set of facilities that maximizes the total weight of all covered demand points while adhering to this budget constraint [33]. It is worth noting that the maximal covering location problem is an NP-hard optimization problem. Various algorithms exist for solving this problem, including integer programming formulations and heuristic approaches like greedy algorithms, simulated annealing, and genetic algorithms. While these methods can provide reasonably good approximate solutions, finding the optimal solution is often infeasible for large instances of the problem [34, 35].

2.1.3 P-center Location Problem

The P-center location problem is a classical optimization problem that seeks to identify the optimal location of P facilities in order to minimize the maximum distance between each customer and their closest facility. The problem can be stated as follows:

Given a set of potential facility locations, a set of customers with known demand, and a distance or travel time matrix between each pair of customers and facilities, determine the optimal location of P facilities such that the maximum distance between any customer and their closest facility is minimized.

The P-center location problem finds its application in transportation and logistics planning, where it is essential to ensure that customers can access necessary goods or services within a certain distance or time limit. It is also useful in public service planning to determine the optimal locations for hospitals or fire stations to serve a given population. Solving the P-center location problem typically involves a mixed-integer linear programming (MILP) formulation, which can be solved using various algorithms like branch-and-bound and branch-and-cut methods. In addition, heuristic and meta-heuristic methods such as simulated annealing and genetic algorithms have proved effective in finding good solutions for large-scale instances of the problem [36–38].

2.2 *Median-Based Problem*

2.2.1 P-median Location Problem

The P-median location problem is a classic optimization problem in that involves the selection of P facilities to serve a set of customers, with the aim of minimizing the overall distance or cost of serving those customers. The problem can be stated as follows:

Given a set of N potential facility locations, a set of M customers with known demand, and a distance or travel time matrix between each pair of customers and facilities, determine the optimal selection of P facilities such that the total distance or cost of serving all customers is minimized [33].

The P-median location problem is similar to the P-center problem, but instead of minimizing the maximum distance between any customer and their closest facility, it seeks to minimize the overall distance or cost of serving all customers. The P-median problem is often used in transportation and logistics planning, where it is important to optimize the allocation of resources to minimize costs while ensuring efficient service to customers [39]. Solving the P-median location problem typically involves a mixed-integer linear programming (MILP) formulation, which can be solved using various algorithms, including branch-and-bound and branch-and-cut methods. Heuristic and meta-heuristic methods, like simulated annealing and genetic algorithms, can also be effective in finding good solutions for large-scale instances of the problem [40].

2.2.2 Fixed Charge-Facility Location Problem

The fixed charge-facility location problem involves selecting the optimal locations of facilities while taking into account their fixed costs. The problem can be stated as follows:

Given a set of potential facility locations, a set of customers with known demand, and a cost matrix for each customer-facility pair, determine the optimal selection of facilities to open such that the sum of the fixed costs associated with opening facilities and the variable costs associated with serving customers is minimized [41, 42].

The fixed charge-facility location problem differs from other facility location problems in that it considers the fixed costs associated with establishing a facility in addition to the variable costs associated with serving customers. This makes the problem more complex and challenging to solve, but also more realistic since the fixed costs associated with establishing a facility cannot be easily changed once a decision has been made [27].

Typically, the fixed-charge facility location problem requires a mixed-integer linear programming (MILP) formulation to be solved. There are several algorithms available for this task, such as branch-and-bound and branch-and-cut methods. Heuristic and meta-heuristic approaches, such as simulated annealing and genetic algorithms, can also work well to find good solutions for larger instances of the problem.

2.3 Other Problem

The problems that do not fall under the two main categories, which are covering-based and median-based problems, are categorized in the final category. As instance, the p-dispersion is a measure of the spread or dispersion of facilities across a region. The p-dispersion is a useful measure for evaluating the effectiveness of facility location strategies. A low p-dispersion indicates that facilities are well-distributed and easily accessible throughout the region, while a high p-dispersion indicates that some areas may be underserved or poorly connected to facilities [43, 44]. Laporte et al. [27] present a comprehensive overview of location problems, including Anti-covering Problems, Location Problems with Multiple Criteria, Location Logistics in Supply Chain Management and etc. among others.

3 Healthcare Facility Location

Healthcare facility location refers to the process of selecting optimal sites for healthcare facilities such as hospitals, clinics, and health centers. The objective of healthcare facility location is to ensure that healthcare services are accessible to the population they serve. This involves identifying the areas where there is a need for healthcare services, analyzing the existing healthcare infrastructure in those areas, and deciding on the most suitable locations for new healthcare facilities.

The process of healthcare facility location can involve various factors, such as population density, demographics, disease prevalence, transportation links, and availability of healthcare professionals. Decisions on healthcare facility location also need to take into account factors such as cost-effectiveness, capacity planning, and service quality.

Optimizing healthcare facility location can help to improve access to healthcare services for people living in underserved areas, reduce healthcare disparities, and improve health outcomes. Additionally, efficient healthcare facility location can increase the utilization of healthcare services, reduce healthcare costs, and improve overall healthcare system efficiency.

Accessibility, adaptability, and availability are three important considerations when it comes to choosing a location for a healthcare facility.

Accessibility: Healthcare facilities must be easily accessible to patients, especially those with mobility issues or disabilities. Consider the proximity of public transportation, parking facilities, and the overall ease of access to the facility. Additionally, accessibility also refers to the availability of the necessary medical equipment and technology needed to provide top-quality care [45–47].

Adaptability: Healthcare is an ever-changing industry, so it's important to choose a location that can adapt to new technologies, changes in regulations, and evolving patient needs. It's important that the establishment has the flexibility to adjust its size when necessary, and it's crucial to verify that the site can support any future expansion or progress [48–50].

Availability: Healthcare facilities must be able to provide services when patients need them. Consider the operating hours of the facility and whether they align with the needs of the community. Additionally, it is necessary to ensure that there is sufficient staff to meet patient demand and they have the necessary training and expertise to provide high-quality care [51, 52].

4 Data Envelopment Analysis

Data Envelopment Analysis (DEA) is a non-parametric method used to measure the efficiency of decision-making units (DMUs) with multiple inputs and outputs [53]. DEA is the most commonly used tool for efficiency evaluation by estimating the frontier. As a non-parametric method, DEA does not require any assumptions that are the basis of parametric methods. Its ability to evaluate the efficiency of a DMU relative to a group of DMUs that perform in a certain domain makes it superior.

For years, data envelopment analysis (DEA) has been a powerful tool used to evaluate the efficiency of Decision-Making Units (DMUs). Over the last four decades, many models, various methods and interesting interpretations have been introduced to DEA. Simultaneously with the development of theories, models, and techniques in DEA, a wide range of applications have been found for it [54]. The first and most basic model presented to evaluate the performance of units using this method is named CCR model and is as follows:

Suppose that there are n DMUs such that each $DMU_p(p = 1, \ldots, n)$ uses a vector of inputs $I_p = (I_{1p}, \ldots, I_{mp})$ to produce a vector of outputs $O_p = (o_{1p}, \ldots, o_{sp})$. It is also assumed that $I_p \geq 0, I_p \neq 0$ and $O_p \geq 0, O_p \neq 0$ for every $p = 1, \ldots, n$. The production possibility set (PPS) is defined as follows:

$$T = \{(I, O) \mid output\ O\ can\ be\ produced\ by\ input\ I\}$$

The set T is characterized by the five postulates [55]. According to these postulates T_c can be defined as follows [53, 55]:

$$T_c = \left\{ (I, O) | I \geq \sum_p I_p \lambda_p, O \leq \sum_p O_p \lambda_p, \lambda_p \geq 0, p = 1, \ldots, n \right\}$$

Using T_c, the CCR model is formulated. A $DMU_k (k \in \{1, \ldots, n\})$, is said to be CCR-efficient if it lies on the frontier of T_c. The efficiency score of $DMU_k \equiv (I_k, O_k)$ is obtained by solving the problem

$$\begin{aligned} &\max \ \varphi \\ &s.t. (I_k, \varphi O_k) \in T_c \end{aligned}$$

That will be in the following form in details:

$$\begin{aligned} &\max \varphi \\ &s.t. \sum_p I_p \lambda_p \leq I_k \\ &\sum_p O_p \lambda_p \geq \varphi O_k \\ &\lambda_p \geq 0, p = 1, \ldots, n \end{aligned}$$

This is the output oriented CCR model (Envelopment form). It can be proved that in the optimal solution of model $\varphi^* \geq 1$ .If $\varphi^* = 1$ then DMU_k is efficient; otherwise, if $\varphi^* > 1$ then DMU_k is inefficient (this means all outputs of DMU_k can be increased proportionally by the amount of $\varphi^* > 1$). The dual of above model is the multiplier form of CCR model (output oriented).

$$\begin{aligned} \min \quad & vI_k \\ s.t. \quad & uO_k = 1 \\ & uO_p - vI_p \leq 0 \quad p = 1, \ldots, n \\ & u \geq 0, v \geq 0, \end{aligned}$$

where $u = (u_1, \ldots, u_s)$ is the vector of output weights and $v = (v_1, \ldots, v_m)$ is the vector of input weights.

4.1 Ranking in DEA

One of the most important challenges in DEA is deciding which efficient unit is the best when there are more than one efficient ones, and this has led to numerous attempts to solve the problem. A possible solution is the AP model introduced by Andersen and Petersen [56], which involves excluding the unit being evaluated from the PPS in order to rank efficient units.

Since then, a number of models for ranking have been proposed. Adler et al. [57] presented a classification of these models, which includes cross-efficiency [58], super-efficiency [59], benchmarking [60], statistical-based models [61], and multi-criteria decision-making models [62–64]. Another classification was developed by Aldamak and Zolfaghari [65]. Meanwhile, Rezaeiani and Foroughi [66] categorized other ranking methods, such as those involving weight restrictions, a common set of weights, an inverted frontier, and reference-based approaches.

There are additional methods for ranking units that can be found in the literature. For instance, Gholam Abri et al. [67] proposed a method for ranking non-extreme efficient units. Liu and Wang [68] suggested using upper and lower bounds, and Rezaeiani and Foroughi [66] proposed using the reference frontier share. There is also a group of models that use norms for ranking such as Tchebycheff [69] and norm-1 [70]. Jahanshahloo et al. [71] presented a Monte-Carlo simulation for ranking units. Wang and Jian [72] introduced the concept of the most efficient DMU to find the best non-dominated unit, which has been further developed by Toloo [73]. Davoodi and Zhiani [74] introduced a technique for ranking efficient units based on their crowding distance, which considers the diversity and variety of units located on the efficient frontier. This approach draws from existing literature on multi-objective evolutionary optimization.

4.2 Application of DEA on Healthcare

The use of DEA in evaluating the efficiency of healthcare systems has a long history in literature [75, 76]. Due to its high flexibility in selecting and using factors affecting efficiency, its ability to detect inefficiency factors, and the possibility of providing practical suggestions to improve efficiency, data envelopment analysis has become one of the accepted methods in healthcare facilities [77, 78]. Most of these studies have been related to the evaluation of health services providers. Klimberg and Ratick [79] were the first to formulate a model that allows for the DEA efficiencies of all operating units to be calculated in one linear program and then combine that formulation with the uncapacitated and capacitated fixed charge facility location problem in a multi-objective framework.

4.3 Application of DEA on Location Problem

In recent years, many facility location/allocation models have been introduced to find optimal allocations based on different location criteria. Most of these models have been formulated in a mathematical programming framework. Recently, the concept of efficiency has been taken into consideration, and DEA models have been used in spatial evaluations. Klimberg and Ratick [79] introduced a model that combines the efficiency score of units with the capacitated (and uncapacitated) fixed charge facility location problem. Fang and Li [80] used a combination of DEA, goal programming, and multi-criteria decision analysis to determine efficient location-allocation. Additionally, Hong and Jeong [81] used a combination of data envelopment analysis and multi-objective models for efficient facility location-allocation decisions. Georgantzinos and Giannikos [82] introduced a modeling framework for incorporating DEA efficiency into set covering, packing, and partitioning formulations.

5 Healthcare Facility Location Using DEA

A few studies have utilized DEA for healthcare facility location. Segal et al. [83] employed basic DEA models to evaluate candidate towns for healthcare facility location planning, but they did not consider some of the significant factors in selecting the location.

Following the work of Klimberg and Ratick, Mitropoulos et al. [84] introduced an innovative method for using DEA in healthcare facility location evaluation. They considered efficiency as a new factor in spatial evaluation and applied its effect in the evaluation by combining it with a multi-objective program model. They evaluated healthcare facility locations to determine health providers' locations and service allocations, which included both new services distribution and existing services redistribution.

In this section, we aim to utilize data envelopment analysis models to find the best place for construction of healthcare facilities. To achieve this goal, we must initially define the conditions upon which the centers should be established.

Based on these assumptions, health centers should be selected in a manner that ensures they are located at the shortest distance from the population centers. Additionally, the variable costs of providing services should also be minimized in them. Moreover, the selection method should prioritize considering the coverage of the required demand. In general, the problem entails choosing a set of potential centers for building a healthcare facility that can meet the needs of multiple population centers.

When we use DEA for selection or allocation, the decision-making process will be based on efficiency. Unlike other Healthcare facility location models where the data is given to the problem without any orientation, in DEA, selected factors should be classified into two categories, input and output, so that the efficiency can be determined based on the best performance of the outputs to the inputs. In other words, although there is a similarity between the factors in conventional location models with the DEA model, in conventional location models, the decision factors are considered in the objective function or in constraints, but they will be employed based on the efficiency through DEA. In the following numerical example, based on the factors extracted from literature review, we will reach a set of factors that we will use for a typical healthcare facility location. Table 2 shows the input and output indicators for evaluating the construction of centers

Table 2 Input and output factors

Inputs	Outputs
The distance from the healthcare facility to the population centers	The rate of coverage provided by the facility
The fixed and variable costs of constructing the facility	The level of quality provided

Note that in other DEA models used for healthcare center location, each health center is considered as a DMU and evaluated individually based on its related input and output indicators, from which its efficiency score is obtained. The resulting efficiencies may be used in the second stage or combined with another objective function to evaluate the centers or locations.

In our presented method, we consider every possible facility location scenario (specifically, each potential location selection mode) as a decision-making unit. This approach allows us to consider all possible allocations simultaneously, leading to a more precise selection of the best location. To apply this idea, we first need to introduce the sets of demands and facility sites as:

$$\begin{aligned} &D: set\ of\ demand\ nodes \\ &S: \ set\ of\ candidates\ facility\ sites \end{aligned}$$

And the variables related to different allocation modes and assignments are defined as follows:

$$x_j = \begin{cases} 1\ if\ site\ j\ is\ selected\ (j \in S) \\ 0\ otherwise \end{cases}$$

$$y_{ij} = \begin{cases} 1 & \begin{array}{l} if\ demand\ node\ i\ (i \in D)\ can\ be\ covered \\ \ \ by\ a\ facility\ at\ candidate\ site\ j\ (j \in S) \end{array} \\ 0\ otherwise \end{cases}$$

It is clear that a set of n possible facility locations leads to at most 2^n possible solutions, each has a large number of assignments in terms of y_{ij}.

Other parameters are:

d_{ij}: *The distance of demand node i to the facility site (possible healthcare) j*

p_i: *The amount of demand node i*

ca_j: *The capacity of possible healthcare j*

q_j: *The quality of service at possible healthcare j*

c_j: *The fixed cost of building the healthcare j*

m_j: *The maintenance cost of possible healthcare j based on the service number.*

A typical DMU must be defined by its input–output vector. Considering that we are going to define each scenario (or method of selection and allocation) as a DMU and the fact that the scenarios are written based on variables x_j and y_{ij}, the general form of DMU_k is as follows (Table 3).

Table 3 Input and output formulation for a typical DMU

Inputs	Input 1:	$\sum_j(\sum_i d_{ij} y^k_{ij})x^k_j$
	Input 2:	$\sum_j c_j x^k_j + \sum_j(\sum_i p_i y^k_{ij})m_j x^k_j$
Outputs	Output 1:	$\sum_j(\sum_i p_i y^k_{ij})q_j x^k_j$
	Output 2:	$(\sum_j c_j x^k_j)/\sum_i p_i$

Unlike other DEA models where input and output data are clear and specific, here the data is expressed in a general formulaic format and their precise values are not specified as they depend on the value of x_j and y_{ij}. However, we can write the general mode of evaluating DMU_k in CCR output-oriented multiplier form:

$$Min z = v_1\left(\sum_j\left(\sum_i d_{ij} y^k_{ij}\right)x^k_j\right) + v_2\left(\sum_j c_j x^k_j + \sum_j\left(\sum_i p_i y^k_{ij}\right)m_j x^k_j\right)$$

$$s.t: \quad u_1\left(\sum_j\left(\sum_i p_i y^k_{ij}\right)q_j x^k_j\right) + u_2\left(\left(\sum_j c_j x^k_j\right)/\sum_i p_i\right)$$

$$- v_1\left(\sum_j\left(\sum_i d_{ij} y^k_{ij}\right)x^k_j\right)$$

$$- v_2\left(\sum_j c_j x^k_j + \sum_j\left(\sum_i p_i y^k_{ij}\right)m_j x^k_j\right) \le 0 \text{ Model(2)} \tag{1}$$

$$u_1\left(\sum_j\left(\sum_i p_i y^k_{ij}\right)q_j x^k_j\right) + u_2\left(\left(\sum_j c_j x^k_j\right)/\sum_i p_i\right) = 1 \tag{2}$$

$$\sum_i y^k_{ij} \le M x^k_j \forall j \tag{3}$$

$$\sum_j y^k_{ij} = 1 \forall i \tag{4}$$

$$u_1, u_2, v_1, v_2 \ge 0, \; y^k_{ij}, x^k_j \in \{0, 1\}$$

In this model, $v_1 and v_2$ show the weights of inputs as $u_1 and u_2$ indicate the weights of outputs respectively used in DEA model. Restrictions (1) and (2) are related to the DMUs. Equation (3) indicates that if a site is not selected, it will not respond to any demand where M is a big number. Equation (4) states that the needs of each population center should be answered by only one site. If we have the values of x_j and y_{ij}, the model will be linear in terms of variables(u_1, u_2, v_1, v_2). But as mentioned earlier, finding the values of x_j and its corresponding assignments (y_{ij}) is not simply possible. On the other hand, considering that we are going to determine the way of location based on the efficiency scores, we need to have all the information of the DMUs, which is not available. Therefore, we design the problem in such a way that the optimal search is performed simultaneously in the space of x_j and y_{ij} so that it leads to the formation of an efficient unit. The optimal solution of the model will definitely be equal to unity due to the unknown values of x_j. In other words, the model provides an answer that is on the efficient frontier. At the same time, it will also show the values of x_j and the way of the allocation of population centers to healthcare facilities by y_{ij}. It has been observed that in this case we have a mixed binary non-linear programming which is not as easy to be solved. Although the problem can be solved using the metaheuristic algorithms [85–88], here we present a method to solve this model based on a Lexicographic method on the distance factor.

5.1 Solving the Model Based on Distance Priority

Consider a scenario in which 4 sites are being evaluated to meet the healthcare (HC) needs of 5 population centers (PC). Table 4 provides relevant data for evaluation. Note that Table 4 does not directly exhibit the input and output indicators, rather they must be constructed based on the raw data provided. The data in the table represents the distance between the population centers and facility locations (FLs). The demand column indicates the number of potential clients (demands) for each PC. For each FL, the capacity is denoted as the accepted number (norm) of clients per month.

Setting up any FL involves two types of costs: fixed cost and variable cost. The fixed cost includes the expenses required for acquiring the land, building the structure, and equipping the center. On the other hand, the variable cost is calculated based on

Table 4 Data of example

		Facility location (site)				
		I	II	III	IV	Demand (Person)
Population center	1	2	5	10	5	1000
	2	3	14	7	4	2000
	3	6	2	1	2	1500
	4	5	6	0	4	2500
	5	3	1	11	3	3000
Capacity (Person)		3000	2000	2500	3500	
Manufacturing fixed cost		7000	5000	6000	6500	
Maintenance cost rate (Per demand)		1.2	1	0.9	1.1	
Quality of services		2	1.7	1.5	1.9	

the number of (potential) demands for each center and the maintenance cost rate. Additionally, the quality of service depends on factors such as the number of staff members, the experience of the staff, and the equipment available.

Since the distance factor has high priority, we have applied a Lexicographic method to find the optimal solution. It is clear that there are 15 ($= 2^4 - 1$) different scenarios for construction of FLs. We have removed the case where no FL is considered. We represent these scenarios by the form of (x_1, x_2, x_3, x_4), where each of its components is zero or one. For example, $(1, 0, 1, 1)$ means the first, third and fourth sited are selected and the second site is not.

According to the lexicographic method, the first step involves solving allocation problems using the distance data between population centers and sites (as provided in Table 4) to obtain the optimal allocation. In the second step, based on the results of the first step, the inputs and outputs of each DMU (scenario) are determined and their efficiency is evaluated. These steps will ultimately lead to the optimal selection of sites and the allocation of population centers to the selected sites.

In the first step, utilizing an improved assignment problem [89], we obtained the optimal allocation of FLs and PCs for each scenario. To achieve this, we solved 15 linear problems.

$$
\begin{aligned}
\min & \sum_i \sum_j d_{ij} y_{ij} \\
s.t. & \sum_j y_{ij} = 1 \quad i = 1, \ldots, P \\
& y_{ij} \in \{0, 1\}
\end{aligned}
$$

where d_{ij} is the distance between the ith PC and the jth site (Table 4). The optimal solution of the problems (the best assignment for each scenario) are shown in Table 5.

For example, for the scenario no. 14 (Selecting sites 2, 3 and 4) the best allocation is:

Population Center 1 $\rightarrow$ site 2
Population Center 2 $\rightarrow$ site 4
Population Center 3 $\rightarrow$ site 3
Population Center 4 $\rightarrow$ site 3
Population Center 5 $\rightarrow$ site 2

Now, considering each scenario as a decision making unit (DMU), we can calculate its inputs and outputs based on the above allocations (y_{ij}). The inputs are Total Distance (TD) and Total Cost (TC), while the outputs are Weighted Cover (WC) and Total Quality of Service (TQS). The Total Distance is calculated using the assignment model, while the Total Cost is determined by adding the fixed cost and variable cost. The variable cost is obtained by multiplying the Maintenance Cost Rate by the number of demands referred to each site. Weighted Cover is calculated by dividing the number of demand referrals to a particular center by the total number of demands

Table 5 Optimal solutions of model

No	Scenario	Assignments				Total distance
1	(1,0,0,0)	1	0	0	0	19
		1	0	0	0	
		1	0	0	0	
		1	0	0	0	
		1	0	0	0	
2	(0,1,0,0)	0	1	0	0	28
		0	1	0	0	
		0	1	0	0	
		0	1	0	0	
		0	1	0	0	
3	(0,0,1,0)	0	0	1	0	29
		0	0	1	0	
		0	0	1	0	
		0	0	1	0	
		0	0	1	0	
4	(0,0,0,1)	0	0	0	1	18
		0	0	0	1	
		0	0	0	1	
		0	0	0	1	
		0	0	0	1	
5	(1,1,0,0)	1	0	0	0	13
		1	0	0	0	
		0	1	0	0	
		1	0	0	0	
		0	1	0	0	
6	(1,0,1,0)	1	0	0	0	9
		1	0	0	0	
		0	0	1	0	
		0	0	1	0	
		1	0	0	0	
7	(1,0,0,1)	1	0	0	0	14
		1	0	0	0	
		0	0	0	1	
		0	0	0	1	
		1	0	0	0	
8	(0,1,1,0)	0	1	0	0	14
		0	0	1	0	

(continued)

Table 5 (continued)

No	Scenario	Assignments				Total distance
		0	0	1	0	
		0	0	1	0	
		0	1	0	0	
9	(0,1,0,1)	0	1	0	0	16
		0	0	0	1	
		0	1	0	0	
		0	0	0	1	
		0	1	0	0	
10	(0,0,1,1)	0	0	0	1	13
		0	0	0	1	
		0	0	1	0	
		0	0	1	0	
		0	0	0	1	
11	(1,1,1,0)	1	0	0	0	7
		1	0	0	0	
		0	0	1	0	
		0	0	1	0	
		0	1	0	0	
12	(1,1,0,1)	1	0	0	0	12
		1	0	0	0	
		0	1	0	0	
		0	0	0	1	
		0	1	0	0	
13	(1,0,1,1)	1	0	0	0	9
		1	0	0	0	
		0	0	1	0	
		0	0	1	0	
		1	0	0	0	
14	(0,1,1,1)	0	1	0	0	11
		0	0	0	1	
		0	0	1	0	
		0	0	1	0	
		0	1	0	0	
15	(1,1,1,1)	1	0	0	0	7
		1	0	0	0	
		0	0	1	0	
		0	0	1	0	
		0	1	0	0	

(=10,000). Finally, TQS is the product of the number of demand referrals to a particular center and the Quality of Service provided. To evaluate the efficiency of each DMU (scenario), we used Model (1), and the resulting values, along with the inputs and outputs of each unit, are listed in Table 6.

Table 6's efficiency column indicates that out of the 15 units, only 6 are efficient. To determine which efficient unit performs better, we utilized the AP ranking method [56]. The optimal solution of the AP model is presented in Table 7.

Therefore, scenario 11 is the most favorable, indicating that sites 1, 2, and 3 should be selected for healthcare facility locations. The optimal allocation of population centers to these sites is presented in Table 5, row 11.

Table 6 The data of inputs and outputs and the efficiency of scenarios

	DMU (Scenario)	Input		Output		CCR efficiency (Output oriented)
		TD	TC	WC	TQS	
1	(1,0,0,0)	19	19,000	0.3	20,000	1.029
2	(0,1,0,0)	28	15,000	0.2	17,000	1
3	(0,0,1,0)	29	15,000	0.25	15,000	1.098
4	(0,0,0,1)	18	17,500	0.35	19,000	1
5	(1,1,0,0)	13	23,100	0.5	18,650	1.252
6	(1,0,1,0)	9	23,650	0.55	17,750	1.055
7	(1,0,0,1)	14	25,100	0.65	26,100	1
8	(0,1,1,0)	14	20,400	0.45	15,800	1.274
9	(0,1,0,1)	16	21,950	0.55	17,900	1.173
10	(0,0,1,1)	13	22,700	0.6	17,400	1.187
11	(1,1,1,0)	7	28,200	0.75	17,100	1
12	(1,1,0,1)	12	29,350	0.85	18,400	1.258
13	(1,0,1,1)	9	23,800	0.9	18,000	1
14	(0,1,1,1)	11	27,300	0.8	16,600	1.269
15	(1,1,1,1)	7	28,200	1.1	17,100	1

Table 7 The result of ranking scenarios

No	DMU (Scenario)	Rank	AP (OO)
2	(0,1,0,0)	3	0.958
4	(0,0,0,1)	2	0.989
7	(1,0,0,1)	5	0.815
11	(1,1,1,0)	1	1
13	(1,0,1,1)	4	0.945
15	(1,1,1,1)	6	0.682

6 Conclusion

In this chapter, we have used the combination of facility location methods and data envelopment analysis to evaluate the sites and select the efficient ones to determine the best healthcare facility location. First, we presented a non-linear model, the solution of which leads to the simultaneous finding of the best site and the best allocation of population centers to each site. We also illustrated how to convert the model into linear models with the help of a lexicographic method via an example. In order to determine the best scenario among the efficient ones, a ranking method was used. However, other methods such as weight restrictions on input and output factors [90, 91] or using DEA network models [92] can also be used to increase the discrimination power of the model.

References

1. Abbasbandy, S., Viranloo, T.A.: Numerical solution of fuzzy differential equation. Math. Comput. Appl. **7**(1), 41–52 (2002)
2. Allahviranloo, T., Lotfi, F.H., Kiasari, M.K., Khezerloo, M.: On the fuzzy solution of LR fuzzy linear systems. Appl. Math. Model. **37**(3), 1170–1176 (2013)
3. Chelabi, M., Allahviranloo, T.: Concreted solutions to fuzzy linear fractional differential equations. Appl. Soft Comput. **44**, 108–116 (2016)
4. Mahmoodirad, A., Allahviranloo, T., Niroomand, S.: A new effective solution method for fully intuitionistic fuzzy transportation problem. Soft. Comput. **23**(12), 4521–4530 (2019)
5. Allahviranloo, T., Ezadi, S.: Z-Advanced numbers processes. Inf. Sci. **480**, 130–143 (2019)
6. Rahmani, A., Lotfi, F.H., Rostamy-Malkhalifeh, M., Allahviranloo, T.: A new method for defuzzification and ranking of fuzzy numbers based on the statistical beta distribution. Adv. Fuzzy Syst. **2016**, 1–8 (2016)
7. Moloudzadeh, S., Allahviranloo, T., Darabi, P.: A new method for solving an arbitrary fully fuzzy linear system. Soft. Comput. **17**(9), 1725–1731 (2013)
8. Abbasi, F., Allahviranloo, T.: Conception and implementation of a new Data-Driven Fuzzy Method for Reliability and Safety Analysis. New Math. Nat. Comput. **16**(02), 339–361 (2020). https://doi.org/10.1142/s1793005720500210
9. Allahviranloo, T., Abbasbandy, S., Rouhparvar, H.: The exact solutions of fuzzy wave-like equations with variable coefficients by a variational iteration method. Appl. Soft Comput. **11**(2), 2186–2192 (2011)
10. Allahviranloo, T., Gouyandeh, Z., Armand, A.: A full fuzzy method for solving differential equation based on Taylor expansion. J. Intell. Fuzzy Syst. **29**(3), 1039–1055 (2015)
11. Allahviranloo, T.A., Kermani, M.: Numerical methods for fuzzy linear partial differential equations under new definition for derivative. Iran. J. Fuzzy Syst. **7**(3), 33–50 (2010)
12. Allahviranloo, T.: Uncertain Information and Linear Systems, vol. 254 (2020). https://doi.org/10.1007/978-3-030-31324-1
13. Akram, M., Shahzadi, S., Shah, S.M.U., Allahviranloo, T.: A fully Fermatean fuzzy multi-objective transportation model using an extended DEA technique. Granular Comput. (2023). https://doi.org/10.1007/s41066-023-00399-6
14. Amirteimoori, A., Allahviranloo, T., Kordrostami, S., Bagheri, S.F.: Improving decision-making units in performance analysis methods: a data envelopment analysis approach. Math. Sci. (2023). https://doi.org/10.1007/s40096-023-00512-5

15. Amirteimoori, A., Allahviranloo, T., Zadmirzaei, M.: Scale elasticity and technical efficiency analysis in the European forest sector: a stochastic value-based approach. Eur. J. Forest Res. (2023). https://doi.org/10.1007/s10342-023-01589-2
16. Amirteimoori, A., Allahviranloo, T., Zadmirzaei, M., Hasanzadeh, F.: On the environmental performance analysis: a combined fuzzy data envelopment analysis and artificial intelligence algorithms. Expert Syst. Appl. **224**, 119953 (2023). https://doi.org/10.1016/j.eswa.2023.119953
17. Banker, R.D., Amirteimoori, A., Allahviranloo, T., Sinha, R.P.: Performance analysis and managerial ability in the general insurance market: a study of India and Iran. Inf. Technol. Manage. (2023). https://doi.org/10.1007/s10799-023-00405-y
18. Abbasi, F., Allahviranloo, T.: The fuzzy arithmetic operations of transmission average on Pseudo-Hexagonal fuzzy numbers and its application in fuzzy system reliability analysis. Fuzzy Inf. Eng. **13**(1), 58–78 (2021). https://doi.org/10.1080/16168658.2021.1915449
19. Abbasi, F., Allahviranloo, T.: Realistic solution of fuzzy critical path problems, case study: the airport's cargo ground operation systems. Granular Comput. **8**(3), 617–632 (2022). https://doi.org/10.1007/s41066-022-00347-w
20. Allahviranloo, T., Abbasi, F.: A new estimation of failure analysis in fuzzy environment, case study: the electrical model failure for the football stadium. New Math. Nat. Comput. **18**(03), 791–817 (2022). https://doi.org/10.1142/s1793005722500387
21. Daskin, M.S.: Network and Discrete Location: Models, Algorithms, and Applications. Wiley & Sons (2004)
22. Current, J., Daskin, M., Schilling, D.: Discrete network location models. In: Drezner, Z., Hamacher, H.W. (eds.) Facility Location: Applications and Theory. Springer, Berlin (2002)
23. Daskin, M., Hesse, S.M., ReVelle, C.S.: α-Reliable P-minimax regret: a new model for strategic facility location modeling. Locat. Sci. **5**, 227–246 (1997)
24. ReVelle, C.S., Eiselt, H.A.: Location analysis: a synthesis and survey. Eur. J. Oper. Res. **165**(1), 1–19 (2005)
25. Marianov, V., Serra, D.: Location problems in the public sector. In: Drezner, Z., Hamacher, H.W. (eds.) Facility Location: Applications and Theory. Springer, Berlin (2002)
26. Marianov, V., Serra, D.: Strategic facility location: a review. Eur. J. Oper. Res. **202**(2), 447–463 (2010)
27. Laporte, G., Nickel, S., Saldanha da Gama, F. (eds.): Location Science. Springer International Publishing (2019)
28. Balas, E., Xhonneux, L.: Integer programming formulations of set covering and vertex-covering problems. Manage. Sci. **24**(11), 1098–1106 (1978)
29. Pisinger, D.: Where are the hard set covering problems? Comput. Oper. Res. **32**(9), 2271–2284 (2005)
30. Zhang, W., Li, X., Hu, Q., Wu, Y.: A novel heuristic algorithm for the set covering problem. J. Intell. Manuf. **31**(4), 961–971 (2020)
31. Lim, J., Lee, D.H.: An effective set covering-based optimization model for computing reliable travel routes in public transportation networks. Transp. Res. Part C Emerg. Technol. **101**, 297–313 (2019)
32. Beasley, J.E.: Heuristics for the maximal covering location problem. Ann. Oper. Res. **6**(1), 319–329 (1987)
33. Mirchandani, P.B., Francis, R.L.: Discrete Location Theory, vol. 15. Wiley & Sons (1990)
34. Current, J.R., Schilling, D.A., Szmerekovsky, J.G.: The maximal covering location problem: a review. Eur. J. Oper. Res. **192**(3), 723–737 (2009)
35. Ghiani, G., Laporte, G., Musmanno, R.: Introduction to Logistics Systems Planning and Control, vol. 43. Wiley & Sons (2013)
36. Albareda-Sambola, M., Díaz, J.A., Fernández, E.: Lagrangean duals and exact solution to the capacitated p-center problem. Eur. J. Oper. Res. **201**(1), 71–81 (2010)
37. Mousavi, S.M., Akhavan Niaki, S.T., Mehdizadeh, E., Tavarroth, M.R.: The capacitated multi-facility location–allocation problem with probabilistic customer location and demand: two hybrid meta-heuristic algorithms. Int. J. Syst. Sci. **44**(10), 1897–1912 (2013)

38. Wang, Y., Liu, L., Zhang, A.: An effective algorithm for the capacitated p-center location problem. J. Clean. Prod. **259**, 120812 (2020)
39. Karatas, M., Yakıcı, E.: An iterative solution approach to a multi-objective facility location problem. Appl. Soft Comput. **62**, 272–287 (2018)
40. Basti, M., Sevkli, M.: An artificial bee colony algorithm for the p-median facility location problem. Int. J. Metaheuristics. **4**(1), 91–113 (2015)
41. Alumur, S.A., Nickel, S.: Facility location: a survey of applications and methods. Eur. J. Oper. Res. **211**(3), 329–341 (2012)
42. Bard, J.F., Tuncbilek, I.: Facility Location: Applications and Theory. Springer Science & Business Media (2008)
43. Huang, R., Kim, S., Menezes, M.B.: Facility location for large-scale emergencies. Ann. Oper. Res. **181**(1), 271–286 (2010)
44. Kuby, M.J.: Programming models for facility dispersion: the p-dispersion and maxisum dispersion problems. Geogr. Anal. **19**(4), 315–329 (1987)
45. Adenso-Díaz, B., Rodríguez, F.: A simple search heuristic for the MCLP: application to the location of ambulance bases in a rural region. OMEGA Int. J. Manage. Sci. **25**, 181–187 (1997)
46. Bruno, G., Cavola, M., Diglio, A., Piccolo, C.: Improving spatial accessibility to regional health systems through facility capacity management. Socio-Econ. Plan. Sci Elsevier **71**(C) (2020)
47. Sayadi, M.K., Mohammadi, M., Tavakkoli-Moghaddam, R.: A multi-objective robust model for locating emergency medical service stations with real-time uncertainty. Health Care Manage. Sci. **21**(2), 295–311 (2018)
48. Bashford, H.: Preparing for the future: using scenario planning for community-based waste management. Waste Manage. Res. **21**(6), 515–523 (2003)
49. Zhang, H., Zhang, K., Chen, Y., Ma, L.: Multi-objective two-level medical facility location problem and tabu search algorithm. Inf. Sci. **608**, 734–756 (2022)
50. Jia, M., Zhang, B., Chen, J.: A robust optimization model for multi-stage logistics network design under uncertainty. Int. J. Prod. Econ. **183**, 680–693 (2017)
51. Daskin, M., Stern, E.: A hierarchical objective set covering model for EMS vehicle deployment. Transp. Sci. **15**, 137–152 (1981)
52. Liu, S., Sun, L., Zhang, T., Zhang, X., Huang, J.: A bi-objective model for optimizing the location-routing problem of emergency material delivery in large-scale disasters. Transp. Res. Part E Logistics Transp. Rev. **126**, 176–195 (2019)
53. Charnes, A., Cooper, W.W., Rhodes, E.: Measuring the efficiency of decision-making units. Eur. J. Oper. Res. **2**(6), 429–444 (1978)
54. Liu, J.S., Lu, L.Y.Y., Lu, W., Lin, B.J.Y.: A survey of DEA applications. Omega **41**(5), 893–902 (2013)
55. Cooper, W.W., Seiford, L.M., Tone, K.: Data Envelopment Analysis: A Comprehensive Text with Models, Applications, References and DEA-Solver Software. Springer (2007)
56. Andersen, P., Petersen, N.C.: A procedure for ranking efficient units in data envelopment analysis. Manage. Sci. **39**(10), 1261–1264 (1993)
57. Adler, N., Friedman, L., Sinuany-Stern, Z.: Review of ranking methods in the data envelopment analysis context. Eur. J. Oper. Res. **140**(2), 249–265 (2002)
58. Sexton, T.R., Silkman, R.H., Hogan, A.J.: Data Envelopment Analysis: Critique and Extensions. Wiley & Sons, Inc. (1986)
59. Hashimoto, A.: A ranked voting system using a DEA/AR exclusion model: a note. Eur. J. Oper. Res. **97**(3), 600–604 (1997)
60. Torgersen, A.M., Forsund, F.R., Kittelsen, S.A.C.: Slack-adjusted efficiency measures and ranking of efficient units. J. Prod. Anal. **7**(4), 379–398 (1996)
61. Friedman, L., Sinuany-Stern, Z.: Combining ranking scales and selecting variables in the DEA context: the case of industrial branches. Comput. Oper. Res. **25**(9), 781–791 (1998)
62. Carrillo, M., Jorge, M.: A multiobjective DEA approach to ranking alternatives. Expert Syst. Appl. **50**, 130–139 (2016)
63. Hatami-Marbini, A., Toloo, M.: An extended multiple criteria data envelopment analysis model. Expert Syst. Appl. **73**, 201–219 (2017)

64. dos Santos Rubem, A.P., Soares de Mello, J.C.C., Meza, L.A.: A goal programming approach to solve the multiple criteria DEA model. Eur. J. Oper. Res. **260**(1), 134–139 (2017)
65. Aldamak, A.M., Zolfaghari, S.: Review of efficiency ranking methods in data envelopment analysis. Measurement **106**, 161–172 (2017)
66. Rezaeiani, M.J., Foroughi, A.A.: Ranking efficient decision-making units in data envelopment analysis based on reference frontier share. Eur. J. Oper. Res. **264**(2), 665–674 (2018)
67. Gholam Abri, A., Jahanshahloo, G.R., Hosseinzadeh Lotfi, F., Shoja, N., Fallah Jelodar, M.: A new method for ranking non-extreme efficient units in data envelopment analysis. Optim. Lett. **7**(2), 309–324 (2013)
68. Liu, W., Wang, Y.: Ranking DMUs by using the upper and lower bounds of the normalized efficiency in data envelopment analysis. Comput. Ind. Eng. **125**, 135–143 (2018)
69. Rezai Balf, F., Zhiani Rezai, H., Jahanshahloo, G.R., Hosseinzadeh Lotfi, F.: Ranking efficient DMUs using the Tchebycheff norm. Appl. Math. Model. **36**(1), 46–56 (2012)
70. Ziari, S.: An alternative transformation in ranking using l1-norm in data envelopment analysis. J. Ind. Eng. **12**, 401–405 (2016)
71. Jahanshahloo, G.R., Hosseinzadeh Lotfi, F., Zhiani Rezai, H., Rezai Balf, F.: Using Monte Carlo method for ranking efficient DMUs. Appl. Math. Comput. **162**(1), 371–379 (2005)
72. Wang, Y.M., Jiang, P.: Alternative mixed integer linear programming models for identifying the most efficient decision-making unit in data envelopment analysis. Comput. Ind. Eng. **62**(2), 546–553 (2012)
73. Toloo, M.: Alternative minimax model for finding the most efficient unit in data envelopment analysis. Comput. Ind. Eng. **81**, 186–194 (2015)
74. Davoodi, A., Zhiani, R.H.: Crowding distance development for ranking efficient units in DEA. J. Ind. Manage. Optim. **19**(8), 5902–5915 (2023)
75. Oikonomou, N., Tountas, Y., Mariolis, A., Souliotis, K., Athanasakis, K., Kyriopoulos, J.: Measuring the efficiency of the Greek rural primary health care using a restricted DEA model; the case of southern and western Greece. Health Care Manage. Sci. **19**(4) (2015)
76. Shwartz, M., Burgess, J.F., Jr., Zhu, J.: A DEA based composite measure of quality and its associated data uncertainty interval for health care provider profiling and pay-for-performance. Health Serv. Res. **51**(2), 489–502 (2016)
77. Makheti, A.J.: Technical efficiency in public health facilities in Meru County: DEA analysis. Health Econ. Outcome Res. **3**(4) (2017)
78. Stefko, R., Gavurova, B., Kocisova, K.: Healthcare efficiency assessment using DEA analysis in the Slovak Republic. Health Econ. Rev. **8**(6) (2018)
79. Klimberg, R., Ratick, S.: Modeling data envelopment analysis (DEA) efficient location/ allocation decisions. Comput. Oper. Res. **35**, 457–474 (2008)
80. Fang, L., Li, H.: Multi-criteria decision analysis for efficient location- allocation problem combining DEA and goal programming. RAIRO-Oper. Res. **49**, 753–772 (2015)
81. Hong, J., Jeong, K.: Combining data envelopment analysis and multi-objective model for the efficient facility location-allocation decision. J. Ind. Eng.Int. **15**, 315–331 (2018)
82. Georgantzinos, S.K., Giannikos, I.: A modeling framework for incorporating DEA efficiency into set covering, packing, and partitioning formulations. Int. Trans. Oper. Res. **24**(1), 213–235 (2017)
83. Segall, M., Lumb, R., Lall, V., Moreno, A.: Healthcare facility location: a DEA approach. Am. J. Manage. **17**(6), 54–65 (2017)
84. Mitropoulos, P., Mitropoulos, I., Giannikos, I.: Combining DEA with location analysis for the effective consolidation of services in the health sector. Comput. Oper. Res. **40**(9), 2241–2250 (2013)
85. Seyyedabbasi, A.: WOASCALF: a new hybrid whale optimization algorithm based on sine cosine algorithm and levy flight to solve global optimization problems. Adv. Eng. Softw. **173**, 103272 (2022). https://doi.org/10.1016/j.advengsoft.2022.103272
86. Seyyedabbasi, A.: A reinforcement learning-based metaheuristic algorithm for solving global optimization problems. Adv. Eng. Softw. **178**, 103411 (2023). https://doi.org/10.1016/j.advengsoft.2023.10341

87. Seyyedabbasi, A.: Binary sand cat swarm optimization algorithm for wrapper feature selection on biological data. Biomimetics **8**(3), 310 (2023)
88. Seyyedabbasi, A., Kiani, F., Allahviranloo, T., Fernandez-Gamiz, U., Noeiaghdam, S.: Optimal data transmission and pathfinding for WSN and decentralized IoT systems using I-GWO and Ex-GWO algorithms. Alex. Eng. J. **63**, 339–357 (2023)
89. Bazaraa, M.S., Jarvis, J.J., Sherali, H.D.: Linear Programming and Network Flows, 4th edn. Wiley & Sons.
90. Davoodi, A., Zhiani Rezai, H.: Improving production possibility set with production tradeoffs. Appl. Math. Model. **39**(8), 1966–1974 (2015)
91. Davoodi, A., Zhiani Rezai, H., Fallahnejad, R.: Congestion analysis in DEA inputs under weight restrictions. J. Oper. Res. Soc. **63**(8), 1089–1097 (2012)
92. Kao, C.: Network data envelopment analysis: a review. Eur. J. Oper. Res. **239**(1), 1–16 (2014)
93. Sarkis, J.: A comparative analysis of DEA as a discrete alternative multiple criteria decision tool. Eur. J. Oper. Res. **123**(3), 543–557 (2000)

Fuzzy Transportation Model for Resource Allocation in a Dental Hospital

Alize Yaprak Gul and Saliha Karadayi-Usta

Abstract The transportation models are of paramount importance as a powerful tool for health institutions with resource allocation abilities. Movement of patients, medical supplies, employees, and other individuals across various locations are all covered in this field of study to enhance efficiency and reduce costs. However, there are limited number of papers discussing nursing staff and bed capacity as a resource allocation problem within the scope of transportation models. Hence, the purpose of the study is to examine the transportation model with a fuzzy mixed integer linear programming (FMILP) approach to allocate the nursing staff and bed capacity as resources with a case study of dental hospital. Findings illustrate that the highest patient demand is observed in the last three months of the year, and there is a need to increase the capacity in that time period. Besides, the sensitivity analysis highlights that while volume of domestic patients' demand is relatively stable, the number of international patients varies greatly throughout the year and causes a change in total patient demand significantly. This chapter contributes to the literature by emphasizing the transportation models' wide range of utilization ability for the healthcare resource allocation problems. Indeed, the practitioners can benefit from this paper in order to handle its resources to allocate exact dates and operating rooms.

Keywords Transportation model · Healthcare · Dental · Nursing staff · Capacity planning · Resource allocation · Fuzzy mixed integer linear programming

---

A. Y. Gul · S. Karadayi-Usta (✉)
Industrial Engineering Department, Istinye University, Istanbul, Turkey
e-mail: saliha.usta@istinye.edu.tr

A. Y. Gul
Industrial Engineering Department, Istanbul Technical University, Istanbul, Turkey

T. Allahviranloo et al. (eds.), *Decision Making in Healthcare Systems*,
Studies in Systems, Decision and Control 513,
https://doi.org/10.1007/978-3-031-46735-6_7

1 Introduction and Motivation

A health system integrates the value network of "access to care", "care process", "administrative efficiency", "equity", and "health care outcomes" with the movement of people, materials, and wastes [1]. Moreover, the transportation model offers a powerful solution for health institutions seeking to improve resource allocation within health systems. By simulating the movement of patients, medical supplies, staff, and other individuals across various locations, including hospitals, clinics, healthcare facilities, pharmaceutical warehouses, and waste disposal facilities, health institutions can enhance efficiency and reduce costs [2]. Among the benefits it provides, minimizing travel time for patients and staff, ensuring accurate delivery of medical supplies, and optimizing staffing levels based on patient demand are available [3].

Transportation (i.e., delivery) model in health systems covers both people and materials' movement, assignment and allocation. The literature review of transportation models in health systems addresses the distribution model for COVID-19 vaccines [4], optimisation of COVID-19 vaccination process [5], distribution and transportation of emergency materials [2], evacuation support system for healthcare infrastructures [6], personal protective equipment [7], medical waste collection and transportation [8], RFID-enabled medical waste transportation system [9], distribution strategy to blood services [10], geographic information systems (GIS) in public health [11], inventory and transportation cost reduction in swine flu vaccination supply logistics [12]. There is a limited number of papers discussing nursing staff and bed capacity to plan and schedule as a resource allocation problem within the scope of transportation models.

Furthermore, the literature review clearly demonstrates that mathematical programming models are the preferred method for addressing people and material movement issues in health system transportation models (see Literature Review part). A gap exists in the literature of this research field in terms of providing applications of fuzzy logic.

Besides, since the health industry reports emphasize the importance of hospital beds and nursing staff [13], the motivation of this study grounds on this fact. Hence, the purpose of the study is to elaborate the transportation model with a fuzzy mixed integer linear programming (FMILP) approach to allocate the nursing staff and bed capacity as resources with a case study of dental hospital [14].

The reason behind why this methodology is selected is based on the fact that Fuzzy MILP optimization's incorporating ability of subjectivity and uncertainty in the mathematical models [15]. Since in this study, the demand, the number of admitted and transferred patients are uncertain and dependent on various factors, fuzzy sets are required in some part of the optimization procedure.

Findings illustrates that as a consequence of the optimal solution for the allocation of hospital beds and nursing staff, the highest patient demand is observed in the last three months of the year, and there is a need to extent the bed and nurse capacity accordingly (which is more profitable to not admit patients). The sensitivity analysis addresses that by changing the α value (the parameter associated with the degree of constraint violation), regarding the patient demand, volume of domestic patients is relatively stable, while the number of international patients varies greatly throughout the year. In other words, this situation generates a change in total patient demand significantly as a result of the international demand [16].

The following part of the paper covers the literature review; preliminaries of fuzzy sets; problem, formulation and proposed solution of FMILP; application; sensitivity analysis; discussion and concluding remarks.

2 Literature Review

Transportation models in health systems literature provides optimization problems including hospitals, production, and pollution/vehicle emission sides of a healthcare-transportation modeling [3].

A transportation model is a collection of mathematical connections used to depict individuals'/firms'/intermediaries' travel decisions. These options include how many trips to take, where to travel, and which mode to reach there. The transportation model can be used to optimize resource allocation in health systems by assisting health institutions to improve efficiency and save costs by simulating the flow of patients, medical supplies, staff and people between different locations such as hospitals, clinics, other healthcare facilities, pharmaceutical warehouses and waste disposal facilities [2]. Healthcare businesses may increase efficiency, mitigate costs, and ultimately deliver better patient care by using health-transportation models. It can, for example, assist to save patient and staff travel time, guarantee that medical supplies are delivered to the correct place at the right time, and optimize staffing levels depending on patient demand [3].

In addition, the distribution of ambulances is one use of the transportation model in health systems. The transportation model can assist health services in determining the best number and placement of ambulances to guarantee fast responses to crises by examining historical data on emergency calls and ambulance response times [17, 18].

The transportation model also refers to the "distribution model" [4], and considered as an important part of "urban modeling" [19] with different scenario-based good and services plan of transportation.

Optimization techniques are the most preferred tools to determine the routes with optimized resource allocations [10]. Mixed integer programming (MIP) is used with multi objective functions [4] like maximizing the rescue effect [2] or minimum shortage [10]. Moreover, forecasting scenario building process [19], participatory planning [11], clustering by coupling and text analysis [20], exposure assessment [6], fuzzy programming [21], genetic algorithm [4], and systematic review [19] are the other methodologies discussed.

In the mathematical programming models of healthcare-transportation models; vehicle emission, air pollution, consumption, corruption, air quality, carbon emission reduction and climate change issues are commonly addressed in the objective functions to minimize the effects to enable the environmental, social and financial sustainability [6, 22–24].

Besides, service/material production, inventory, cost-effectiveness, and urgency of demand are the issues to handle in line with the management of healthcare-transportation systems [12, 22]. In the COVID-19 pandemic period, vaccine hubs and supply chain infrastructure, emergency supplies and public health emergency are the special important topics for the literature [5, 7].

Medical wastes are significant in designing the transportation network of the health systems with vehicle routing problem solutions [8], or RFID-based transportation solutions [9], or GIS and machine learning solutions [5].

According to literature review on Scopus database with "transportation model" and "health" keywords searched in titles, abstracts and keywords, 63 document results are obtained on 29th June 2023. The number of publications is in increasing trend since 2012. Furthermore, United States, China, India and Turkey are the country of residence for the authors publishing most in this field of study. While 64% of these documents are articles, the remaining 24% of them are conference papers, 6% of them are book chapters, 3% of them are conference reviews, and 3% of them are reviews. Moreover, the disciplines addressing the field of study are engineering (19%), environmental science (16%), medicine (10%), computer science (9%), social sciences (8%), business, management, and accounting (6%), earth and planetary sciences (6%), decision sciences (5%), mathematics (5%), and others. Table 1 indicates the details of the field of this research.

As it can be clearly observed by the literature review regarding the transportation models of health systems, mathematical programming models are the ones mostly preferred with vehicle routing and material movement problems. There is a gap in literature in this field of research in terms of providing fuzzy logic applications.

The following section explains the preliminaries of triangular fuzzy numbers, basic operations, and ranking functions.

3 Preliminaries

This section presents the primary definitions on fuzzy sets, triangular fuzzy numbers (TFNs) and the basic concepts in fuzzy optimization models.

Definition 1 Let X be a non-empty set. A fuzzy set in X is an object $\tilde{A}$ of the form $\tilde{A} = \{(x, \mu_{\tilde{A}}(x)) \mid x \in X\}$, where $\mu_{\tilde{A}}(x)$ is the membership degree of x in set $\tilde{A}$, and is defined for the interval [0, 1], $\mu_{\tilde{A}}(x) \in [0, 1]$.

Definition 2 A triangular fuzzy number (TFN) is represented by the form $\tilde{A} = (a^l, a^m, a^u)$, where a^l, a^m, a^u denote the left threshold value, the midpoint, and the right threshold value of a TFN, respectively. The membership function of $\tilde{A}$ is then defined as follows:

Table 1 Literature review of transportation models in health systems

Publication	Focus	Methodology/ Problem	Findings
Kumar et al. [4]	Distribution model for COVID-19 vaccine	Mixed integer programming	Number of people vaccinated is maximized, the cost of transportation over the entire network is minimized
Mengüç et al. [5]	Optimization of COVID-19 vaccination process	Mathematical modelling, k-means algorithm	The vaccination procedure may be cut down from 108 to 44 days, representing a 40% improvement in vaccine administration pace
Zhou et al. [2]	Distribution and transportation of emergency materials	Genetic algorithm	The limited supply, transportation and delay costs have an adverse correlation
Yazdani et al. [6]	Evacuation support system for healthcare infrastructures	Framework of multiple mathematical models	As a complex system composed of multiple interactive and interdependent components, the evacuation framework is defined
Bala et al. [7]	Personal protective equipment	Linear programming	The proposed algorithm could be deployed when the healthcare supply chain is insufficient
Babaee Tirkolaee and Aydın [8]	Medical waste collection and transportation	Meta-goal programming, vehicle routing problem	The objective is achieved to minimize the total costs due to transportation, emissions-related pollution, outsourcing and use of vehicles
Liu et al. [9]	RFID-enabled medical waste transportation system	Conceptual model	RFID technology models might alleviate challenges in the medical waste transportation process and execute safe medical waste transportation management
Nurprihatin et al. [10]	Distribution strategy to blood services	Two-step stochastic optimization	It is ensured that the destination points are the only ones fastest to arrive, the capacitated vehicle routing is used to ensure that the routing is global optimum
Yasobant et al. [11]	Applications of geographic information systems (GIS) in public health	GIS, data analysis, pattern recognition	Increased use of GIS in public health practice, such as program design, implementation, and monitoring, as well as developing an evidence foundation for policymaking, would help minimize inequalities in health and deliver universal healthcare
Gupta [12]	Inventory and transportation cost reduction in swine flu vaccination supply logistics	Linear programming	The number of units that should be obtained from distribution centers to reduce the overall cost of acquiring the drug is determined, followed by the size of the order

$$\mu_{\tilde{A}}(x) = \left\{ \begin{array}{ll} \frac{x-a^l}{a^m-a^l} & a^l \le x \le a^m \\ \frac{a^u-x}{a^u-a^m} & a^m \le x \le a^u \\ 0 & a^l < 0, a^u > 0 \end{array} \right\} \quad (1)$$

Definition 3 [25] A TFN is said to be nonnegative if and only if $a^l \ge 0$. The collection of the nonnegative TFNs is denoted by $TF(\mathbb{R})^+$.

Definition 4 [26] Let $\tilde{A} = (a^l, a^m, a^u)$ and $\tilde{B} = (b^l, b^m, b^u)$ be two TFNs and $t \in \mathbb{R}^+$. The basic operations between two TFNs are defined as follows:

$$\tilde{A} \oplus \tilde{B} = (a^l + b^l, a^m + b^m, a^u + b^u)$$

$$\tilde{A} \ominus \tilde{B} = (a^l - b^u, a^m - b^m, a^u - b^l)$$

$$\tilde{A} \otimes \tilde{B} = (a^l b^l, a^m b^m, a^u b^u)$$

$$\frac{\tilde{A}}{\tilde{B}} = \left(\frac{a^l}{b^u}, \frac{a^m}{b^m}, \frac{a^u}{b^l}\right)$$

$$\frac{1}{\tilde{A}} = \left(\frac{1}{a^u}, \frac{1}{a^m}, \frac{1}{a^l}\right)$$

$$t\tilde{A} = (ta^l, ta^m, ta^u)$$

Definition 5 [25] Let $F(R)$ be the collection of TFNs. A ranking function of the TFNs is a function $\mathfrak{R}$ that maps each TFN defined over R to a real number, $\mathfrak{R} : F(R) \to R$. The ranking function for a TFN is given as:

$$Defuzz(\tilde{A}) = \mathfrak{R}\left(\tilde{A}\right) = \frac{a^l + 2a^m + a^u}{4} \quad (2)$$

Definition 6 Let $\tilde{A} = (a^l, a^m, a^u)$ and $\tilde{B} = (b^l, b^m, b^u)$ be two TFNs, then

1. If $\mathfrak{R}\left(\tilde{A}\right) > \mathfrak{R}\left(\tilde{B}\right)$, then $\tilde{A} > \tilde{B}$,
2. If $\mathfrak{R}\left(\tilde{A}\right) = \mathfrak{R}\left(\tilde{B}\right)$, then $\tilde{A} = \tilde{B}$,
3. If $\mathfrak{R}\left(\tilde{A}\right) < \mathfrak{R}\left(\tilde{B}\right)$, then $\tilde{A} < \tilde{B}$.

4 Fuzzy Mixed Integer Linear Programming Model

This section first outlines a resource allocation problem in a healthcare unit considering the planning of nursing staff and bed capacity. Then, the formulation of the fuzzy mixed integer linear programming (FMILP) model of the given problem is presented along with an approach from the literature to solve the FMILP model.

- **Problem description**

The presented model is developed based on the model proposed by Breuer et al. [27]. The model introduced in this study aims to determine the optimal bed capacity and planning of nurse staffing in a healthcare unit by minimizing the salary expense of the staff and the acquisition cost of hospital beds. The patients may request treatment by either a direct consultation or may be transferred from an external institution. Due to the profitability reasons, the unit may decline to give treatment to patients which are then called the non-admissions or non-admitted patients. Further, there are certain measures which the model should surpass such as the hospital beds have to be occupied by a predefined level, the nursing staff must ensure a certain minimum service level and a predefined minimum nurse-to-patient ratio must be sustained. The model also considers different types of patients and resources, namely the nurse personnel differentiated according to their qualification and hospital beds of different types. The healthcare unit is also allowed to borrow a certain amount of hospital bed in each period from other units. The model finds the optimal number of beds and nurses allocated in each period for each patient type, the maximum number of beds and nurses required during the modeling horizon and the number of non-admissions in each period.

- **Formulation of fuzzy model**

The above-described problem is modelled by a fuzzy mixed integer linear programming model to incorporate the uncertainty in the problem. The number of admitted and transferred patients is uncertain and dependent on various factors that are not in the focus of this study. To capture the demand uncertainty in healthcare, widely utilized methods are stochastic optimization [10, 28, 29], robust optimization [30], possibilistic optimization [31], data envelopment analysis [32] and simulation-based optimization [31] approaches among others. We use fuzzy sets to represent the demand volume to account for the lack of information and its uncertain nature. Further the predefined performance measures are represented by fuzzy numbers granting the model flexibility to some extent [33]. The costs associated with the resources are assumed to be definite and fixed. Table 2 shows the set of indices, parameters, and decision variables of the FMILP model.

The model is constructed as follows:

$$\text{Minimize } \tilde{\text{w}} \approx \sum_k c_k^b B_k + \sum_i \sum_j \sum_k c_k^s s_{ijk}$$

Table 2 Notation for the model

Notation	Description	Type
Index sets		
i	Index for months, $i = 1, 2, .., m$	Integer
j	Index for patient types, $j = 1, 2, .., n$	Integer
k	Index for resource types, $k = 1, 2, .., l$	Integer
Decision variables		
b_{ijk}	Number of beds of type k used in month i for patient type j	Integer
s_{ijk}	Number of nursing personnel of type k assigned in month i for patient type j	Integer
B_k	Maximum number of beds of type k used	Integer
S_k	Maximum number of nursing personnel of type k assigned	Integer
t_{ij}^{-}	Number of non-admissions in month i for patient type j	Integer
Parameters		
$\tilde{z}_{ij}$	Number of incoming patients in month i for patient type j	Fuzzy
$\tilde{t}_{ij}^{+}$	Number of patients transferred from external institutions in month i for patient type j	Fuzzy
c_k^b	Purchasing cost of a bed of type k	Real
c_k^s	Monthly salary of a nursing personnel of type k	Real
c_j^{-}	Cost incurred from each non-admission of patient type j	Real
c_j^{+}	Income generated from each treated patient of patient type j	Real
$\tilde{\alpha}^{OC}$	Maximum acceptable level of resource occupancy	Fuzzy
$\tilde{\alpha}_j^{NPR}$	Minimum acceptable level of nurse-to-patient ratio for patient type j	Fuzzy
$\tilde{\alpha}^{SL}$	Minimum acceptable service level	Fuzzy

$$+\sum_i \sum_j \left(c_j^{-} t_{ij}^{-}\right) - \sum_i \sum_j c_j^{+}\left(\Re(\tilde{z}_{ij} \oplus \tilde{t}_{ij}^{+}) - t_{ij}^{-}\right) \tag{3}$$

subject to

$$\Re(\tilde{z}_{ij} \oplus \tilde{t}_{ij}^{+}) - t_{ij}^{-} \tilde{\leq} \Re(\tilde{\alpha}^{OC}) \sum_k b_{ijk}, i = 1, 2, \ldots, m, j = 1, 2, \ldots, n \tag{4}$$

$$\Re(\tilde{\alpha}_j^{NPR})\left(\Re(\tilde{z}_{ij} \oplus \tilde{t}_{ij}^{+}) - t_{ij}^{-}\right) \leq \sum_k s_{ijk}, i = 1, 2, \ldots, m, j = 1, 2, \ldots, n \tag{5}$$

$$\Re(\tilde{\alpha}^{SL} \otimes \left(\tilde{z}_{ij} \oplus \tilde{t}_{ij}^{+}\right)) \tilde{\leq} \sum_k b_{ijk}, i = 1, 2, \ldots, m, j = 1, 2, \ldots, n \tag{6}$$

$$\Re(\tilde{\alpha}^{NPR} \otimes \tilde{\alpha}^{SL} \otimes \left(\tilde{z}_{ij} \oplus \tilde{t}_{ij}^{+}\right)) \leq \sum_k s_{ijk}, i = 1, 2, \ldots, m, j = 1, 2, \ldots, n \tag{7}$$

$$\sum_j b_{ijk} \le B_k, i = 1, 2, \ldots, m, k = 1, 2, \ldots, l \tag{8}$$

$$\sum_j s_{ijk} \le S_k, i = 1, 2, \ldots, m, k = 1, 2, \ldots, l \tag{9}$$

$$b_{ijk}, s_{ijk}, t_{ij}^-, B_k, S_k \in \mathbb{Z}^+ \tag{10}$$

$$c_k^b, c_k^s, c_j^-, c_j^+ \ge 0 \tag{11}$$

$$\tilde{z}_{ij}, \tilde{t}_{ij}^+, \tilde{\alpha}^{NPR}, \tilde{\alpha}^{SL}, \tilde{\alpha}^{OC} \; are\ nonnegative\ triangular\ fuzzy\ numbers \tag{12}$$

The presented model determines the number of beds b_{ijk} and nursing personnel s_{ijk} of type $k, k = 1, 2, .., l$ assigned for month i, $i = 1, 2, .., m$ for the patient type $j, j = 1, 2, .., n$. Additionally, the maximum number of beds B_k and personnel S_k contracted and the number of non-admissions t_{ij}^- in month i for patient type j are determined.

Equation 3 gives the total cost of the healthcare unit that consists of the sum of costs incurred from bed acquisition, non-admissions and nurse salary expenses deducted by the profits earned by the treatment of patients. Equation 4 signifies the constraint that in each month the number of treated patients must be below the maximum number of beds available for patient type while satisfying the predefined maximum occupancy threshold. Equation 5 guarantees that in each month and for each patient type the minimum requirement for nursing staff is satisfied for the given minimum nurse-to-patient ratio. The available hospital beds must be sufficient so that the minimum service level is attained which is determined by the incoming patients only, as indicated by Eq. 6. The constraints on the available number of hospital beds in each period given in Eqs. (4) and (6) can be relaxed since the unit may borrow beds from other units and extend the available capacity which indicates that these constraints can be violated to a predetermined degree. Therefore, Eqs. (4) and (6) are modelled as fuzzy constraints by $\tilde{\le}$. Equation 7 gives the available nursing personnel that satisfies both the minimum nurse-to-patient ratio and minimum service level for the incoming patients to the unit. Finally, the maximum number of beds and nursing personnel required during the interested period is determined by Eqs. 8 and 9, respectively.

- **Solution of the proposed fuzzy model**

This section presents an approach to solve the FMILP model through its transformation into a deterministic mixed integer linear programming (MILP) model. The proposed FMILP model incorporates both the uncertain and incomplete information in data and the fuzzy constraints. The model is aligned with the fuzzy linear programming (FLP) model studied by Cadenas and Verdegay [34] and Peidro et al. [35] and follows the solution approach presented in these studies.

The solution approach in Cadenas and Verdegay [34] consists of two stages; first, the fuzzy constraints are transformed based on the decomposition theorem for fuzzy sets, and second, the fuzzy constraint set is substituted by a convex fuzzy set to obtain a comparison among fuzzy numbers. For this purpose, either a linear ranking or a nonlinear ranking function is applicable, which is given in Definition 5. Definition 6 shows the relationship associated with the ranking function between two fuzzy numbers.

The general FLP model is given as follows:

$$Maximize\, w = \sum_j \tilde{c}_j x_j$$

subject to

$$\sum_j \tilde{a}_{ij} x_j \tilde{\leq} \tilde{b}_i, i = 1, \ldots, m, j = 1, \ldots, n, x_j \geq 0 \tag{13}$$

where

$\tilde{c}_j$, $\tilde{a}_{ij}$, $\tilde{b}_i$ denote the fuzzy cost, the fuzzy technological constant and the fuzzy right-hand side coefficient related to the resource availability.

To solve the FLP in (13), let $\varrho\left(\tilde{a}_i x, \tilde{b}_i\right) : F(R) \times F(R) \rightarrow F(R)$ be the function and $\mathfrak{R}$ be the linear ranking function such that

$$\varrho\left(\tilde{a}_i x, \tilde{b}_i\right) = \left\{ \begin{array}{cc} \tilde{\rho}_i, & \tilde{a}_i x \leq_{\mathfrak{R}} \tilde{b}_i \\ \tilde{\rho}_i \ominus \tilde{a}_i x \oplus \tilde{b}_i, & \tilde{b}_i \leq_{\mathfrak{R}} \tilde{a}_i x \leq_{\mathfrak{R}} \tilde{b}_i \oplus \tilde{\rho}_i \\ 0, & \tilde{a}_i x \leq_{\mathfrak{R}} \tilde{b}_i \oplus \tilde{\rho}_i \end{array} \right\}$$

where ϱ represents a function that is related to the fuzzy constraint $\sum_j \tilde{a}_{ij} x_j \tilde{\leq} \tilde{b}_i$ incorporating the maximum fuzzy violation $\tilde{\rho}_i$ permitted in the respective fuzzy constraint and $\tilde{\rho}_i$ satisfies $\tilde{\rho}_i \in F(R)$ while its support is included in R^+.

The membership function of the fuzzy ith constraint $\mu^i : F(R) \rightarrow [0, 1]$ is then derived by constructing the ratio of defuzzified $\varrho\left(\tilde{a}_i x, \tilde{b}_i\right)$ and defuzzified maximum violation $\tilde{\rho}_i$ where the ranking function $\mathfrak{R}$ is used for defuzzification [36] and the following equation is obtained:

$$\mu^i\left(\tilde{a}_i x, \tilde{b}_i\right) = \frac{\mathfrak{R}\left(\varrho\left(\tilde{a}_i x, \tilde{b}_i\right)\right)}{\mathfrak{R}(\tilde{\rho}_i)} \tag{14}$$

By the application of Eq. (14) to Eq. (13) and the utilization of the decomposition theorem [37, 38], we find:

$$\mu^i\left(\tilde{a}_i x, \tilde{b}_i\right) \geq \alpha \Leftrightarrow \frac{\Re\left(\varrho\left(\tilde{a}_i x, \tilde{b}_i\right)\right)}{\Re(\tilde{\rho}_i)} \geq \alpha$$
$$\Leftrightarrow \frac{\Re\left(\tilde{\rho}_i \ominus \tilde{a}_i x \oplus \tilde{b}_i\right)}{\Re(\tilde{\rho}_i)} \geq \alpha \Leftrightarrow \Re(\tilde{\rho}_i) - \Re(\tilde{a}_i x) + \Re\left(\tilde{b}_i\right) \geq \Re(\tilde{\rho}_i)\alpha$$
$$\Leftrightarrow \Re(\tilde{a}_i x) \leq \Re\left(\tilde{b}_i \oplus \tilde{\rho}_i(1-\alpha)\right) \Leftrightarrow \tilde{a}_i x \leq_{\Re} \tilde{b}_i + \tilde{\rho}_i(1-\alpha) \tag{15}$$

Thus, an equivalent model to (13) is obtained as follows:

$$Maximize\, w = \sum_j \tilde{c}_j x_j$$

subject to

$$\sum_j \tilde{a}_{ij} x_j \leq_{\Re} \tilde{b}_i + \tilde{\rho}_i(1-\alpha), i = 1, \ldots, m, j = 1, \ldots, n, x_j \geq 0, \alpha \in [0, 1] \tag{16}$$

where α is a parameter taking a value between 0 and 1 that is associated with the violation permitted in the fuzzy constraint and is determined by the problem-owner.

Now, the fuzzy numbers in (16) should be defuzzified by either using different ranking methods functions in constraints and the objective function or by using different ranking methods in constraints and α-cuts in the objective function [39]. Here we use the ranking function for triangular fuzzy numbers given in Eq. (2) for the transformation of both the objective function and constraints and obtained:

$$Maximize\, w = \sum_j \left(\frac{c_j^l + 2c_j^m + c_j^u}{4}\right) x_j$$

subject to

$$\sum_j \left(\frac{a_{ij}^l + 2a_{ij}^m + a_{ij}^u}{4}\right) x_j \leq \left(\frac{b_i^l + 2b_i^m + b_i^u}{4}\right) + \left(\frac{\rho_i^l + 2\rho_i^m + \rho_i^u}{4}\right)(1-\alpha),$$
$$i = 1, \ldots, m, j = 1, \ldots, n, x_j \geq 0, \alpha \in [0, 1] \tag{17}$$

where the triangular fuzzy numbers are denoted by the superscripts *l, m, u* for the application of ranking function. Utilizing the discussed approach, the FMILP model given in Eqs. (3)–(12) is transformed into a deterministic MILP model.

Thus, the proposed approach consists of the following steps:

Step 1 Let the decision makers submit the fuzzy mixed integer linear programming model where the fuzzy elements are represented by triangular fuzzy numbers.

Step 2 The fuzzy constraints are transformed by incorporating the constraint violation as given in Eqs. (14) and (15). The standard constraints do not require any modifications.

Step 3 The ranking function for triangular fuzzy numbers is determined as given in Eq. (2).

Step 4 An equivalent deterministic linear programming model is constructed by applying the ranking function for the fuzzy values and is solved by using a standard method to derive the optimal solution.

- **Deterministic model**

According to the approach of Cadenas and Verdegay [34] for the classical fuzzy linear programming, first the fuzzy constraints should be transformed using the decomposition theorem. In our model, the constraints on the available number of hospital beds in each period in Eqs. (4) and (6) are fuzzy constraints and must be adjusted as given in Eq. (15) by including the possible violation of the constraint. Then the fuzzy numbers in the model are defuzzified by the ranking function $\mathfrak{R}$. The index in parameter p_t denotes the index of the fuzzy constraint. The following deterministic model is then obtained:

$$\text{Minimize w} = \sum_k c_k^b B_k + \sum_i \sum_j \sum_k c_k^s s_{ijk} + \sum_i \sum_j \left(c_j^- t_{ij}^-\right) - \sum_i \sum_j c_j^+ \left(\left(\frac{z_{ij}^l + 2z_{ij}^m + z_{ij}^u}{4}\right) + \left(\frac{\left(t_{ij}^+\right)^l + 2\left(t_{ij}^+\right)^m + \left(t_{ij}^+\right)^u}{4}\right) - t_{ij}^- \right) \tag{18}$$

subject to

$$\left(\frac{z_{ij}^l + 2z_{ij}^m + z_{ij}^u}{4}\right) + \left(\frac{\left(t_{ij}^+\right)^l + 2\left(t_{ij}^+\right)^m + \left(t_{ij}^+\right)^u}{4}\right) - t_{ij}^- \leq \left(\frac{\left(\alpha^{OC}\right)^l + 2\left(\alpha^{OC}\right)^m + \left(\alpha^{OC}\right)^u}{4}\right) \sum_k b_{ijk} + \left(\frac{p_t^l + 2p_t^m + p_t^u}{4}\right)(1 - \alpha), i = 1, 2, .., m, j = 1, 2, .., n \tag{19}$$

$$\left(\frac{\left(\alpha_j^{NPR}\right)^l + 2\left(\alpha_j^{NPR}\right)^m + \left(\alpha_j^{NPR}\right)^u}{4}\right)$$

$$\left(\left(\frac{z_{ij}^{l}+2z_{ij}^{m}+z_{ij}^{u}}{4}\right)+\left(\frac{\left(t_{ij}^{+}\right)^{l}+2\left(t_{ij}^{+}\right)^{m}+\left(t_{ij}^{+}\right)^{u}}{4}\right)-t_{ij}^{-}\right)$$

$$\leq \sum_{k} s_{ijk}, i=1,2,..,m, j=1,2,..,n \tag{20}$$

$$\left(\frac{(\alpha^{SL})^{l}+2(\alpha^{SL})^{m}+(\alpha^{SL})^{u}}{4}\right)$$

$$\left(\left(\frac{z_{ij}^{l}+2z_{ij}^{m}+z_{ij}^{u}}{4}\right)+\left(\frac{\left(t_{ij}^{+}\right)^{l}+2\left(t_{ij}^{+}\right)^{m}+\left(t_{ij}^{+}\right)^{u}}{4}\right)\right)\leq \sum_{k} b_{ijk}$$

$$+\left(\frac{p_{t}^{l}+2p_{t}^{m}+p_{t}^{u}}{4}\right)(1-\alpha), i=1,2,..,m, j=1,2,..,n \tag{21}$$

$$\left(\frac{\left(\alpha_{j}^{NPR}\right)^{l}+2\left(\alpha_{j}^{NPR}\right)^{m}+\left(\alpha_{j}^{NPR}\right)^{u}}{4}\right)\left(\frac{(\alpha^{SL})^{l}+2(\alpha^{SL})^{m}+(\alpha^{SL})^{u}}{4}\right)$$

$$\left(\left(\frac{z_{ij}^{l}+2z_{ij}^{m}+z_{ij}^{u}}{4}\right)+\left(\frac{\left(t_{ij}^{+}\right)^{l}+2\left(t_{ij}^{+}\right)^{m}+\left(t_{ij}^{+}\right)^{u}}{4}\right)\right)\leq \sum_{k} s_{ijk},$$

$$i=1,2,..,m, j=1,2,..,n \tag{22}$$

$$\sum_{j} b_{ijk} \leq B_{k}, i=1,2,..,m, k=1,2,..,l \tag{23}$$

$$\sum_{j} s_{ijk} \leq S_{k}, i=1,2,..,m, k=1,2,..,l \tag{24}$$

$$b_{ijk}, s_{ijk}, t_{ij}^{-}, c_{k}^{b}, c_{k}^{s}, c_{j}^{-}, c_{j}^{+}, B_{k}, S_{k} \in \mathbb{Z}^{+} \tag{25}$$

$$\alpha \in [0,1] \tag{26}$$

where $\tilde{\rho}_i$ denotes the allowed violation in the ith constraint in terms of resource quantities and α presents the parameter associated with the degree of constraint violation $(1-\alpha)$, where $\alpha = 1$ signifies no violation is allowed and $\alpha = 0$ indicates that a complete relaxation is allowed in the fuzzy constraints.

5 Application

This section presents the application of FMILP model using for the data of a dental hospital that is adopted from the case study in [40]. The data on incoming patients and transfers from external sources for the period 2020–2022 are examined to predict the patient demand for the year 2023 which is given in Table 3. The incoming patients represent the domestic patients, whereas the transferred patients are the international patients applying for a dental treatment.

Further, the parameter values used in the model are shown in Table 4 along with the description and source of information. The occupation types for nurses are selected as Dental Assistants ($k = 1$) and Dental Hygienists ($k = 2$), whose mean annual salary are estimated to be 44,710 and 84,860 US dollars, respectively according to the U.S. [41]. The monthly mean salaries of these occupations are calculated based on this information. The parameter values of opportunity cost of non-admissions and profit per treatment have been assumed hypothetically. Further the service-related parameters from the model of [27] have been converted to triangular fuzzy numbers for the FMILP model.

The solution of model given in Eqs. (18)–(26) has been implemented in GAMS software and Table 5 presents the obtained optimal solution with a total profit of 2316721.26 US dollars in one-year period. The highest patient demand is observed in the last three months, for which the bed and nurse capacity have been adjusted accordingly, where also it has become more profitable to not admit patients in October and December.

Table 3 Predicted fuzzy patient demand for each month

Month	Incoming patients $\tilde{z}_{ij}$	Transferred patients $\tilde{t}^{+}_{ij}$
January	(77,108,231)	(22,35,111)
February	(78,81,203)	(20,40,68)
March	(95,153,248)	(33,84,110)
April	(90,182,209)	(30,72,90)
May	(72,192,206)	(21,71,83)
June	(52,142,190)	(15,59,68)
July	(73,190,237)	(21,85,86)
August	(98,176,221)	(31,57,71)
September	(67,165,220)	(24,75,79)
October	(131,188,220)	(26,81,95)
November	(119,181,222)	(30,85,96)
December	(136,198,257)	(36,87,90)

Table 4 Parameter values

	$j = 1, k = 1$	$j = 1, k = 2$	Description
c_k^b(in US dollars)	20,000	30,000	Includes all the costs associated with the acquisition of a hospital bed, taken from [27]
c_k^s(in US dollars)	3725.83	7071.67	Monthly salary of the nursing staff calculated from the mean annual salary information for 2022 by U.S. Bureau of Labor Statistics
c_j^-(in US dollars)	5000		Opportunity cost of each non admitted patient, assumed hypothetically
c_j^+(in US dollars)	4000		Profit earned per each treated patient, assumed hypothetically
$\tilde{\rho}_1$	(9, 10, 11)		Maximum number of beds which can be used if allowed for constraint relaxation, assumed hypothetically
$\tilde{\alpha}^{OC}$	(1, 1, 1)		Occupancy level, taken from [27] and converted to fuzzy number
$\tilde{\alpha}_j^{NPR}$	(0.26, 0.33, 0.4)		Nurse-to-patient ratio, taken from [27] and converted to fuzzy number
$\tilde{\alpha}^{SL}$	(0.26, 0.33, 0.4)		Service level, taken from [27] and converted to fuzzy number
α	0.3		Parameter associated with the degree of constraint violation

Table 5 Results of the FMILP model

Month	b_{ijk}	s_{ijk}	t_{ij}^-
January	175	60	0
February	146	51	0
March	233	80	0
April	225	77	0
May	220	75	0
June	175	60	0
July	235	80	0
August	215	74	0
September	211	72	0
October	243	83	3
November	243	83	0
December	243	83	23
Max. number of beds and nursing personnel required	243	83	–

6 Sensitivity Analysis

A one-at-a-time sensitivity analysis is conducted to observe the change in bed allocation to each month with respect to the change in degree of constraint violation $(1 - \alpha)$. The number of beds per month are collected for different values of parameter of degree of constraint violation $\alpha \in [0, 1]$ varied by the increment of 0.1 and presented in Table 6. For $\alpha = 0$, the complete violation of fuzzy constraints is allowed, where it incorporates the maximum relaxation in the constraint yielding the usage of the highest possible number of beds and thus the highest profit for the healthcare unit. Contrarily, for $\alpha = 1$, no relaxation is allowed, and the lowest possible profit is obtained while keeping all other variables constant.

Figure 1 illustrates the bed capacity for each month under the variation of α value. It can be clearly observed that regarding the patient demand given in Table 2 that the volume of domestic patients is relatively stable, and the number of international patients varies greatly throughout the year. This indicates that the change in total patient demand is significantly affected by the change in international demand volume. High demand has been observed in March, April May, July, October, November, and December. In months March, April and May, the number of international patients increases due to school vacation and Easter holidays and high demand in July is explicable by the expanded tourism since tourists seek to get treatment during their vacation. The period from October to December coincides with Christmas holiday, where the highest demand for treatment in the dental unit has been observed. In months October and December, patients have been rejected for the treatment indicating that it has been more profitable to not admit instead of accordingly extending the capacity. It could be recommended that the unit might consider collaborating with another healthcare unit or lease the required space and bed capacity for the high demand seasons.

7 Concluding Remarks

The employment of the transportation model presents a robust solution for health institutions that aim to optimize resource allocation within healthcare systems. Simulating the movement of patients, medical supplies, staff, and other individuals across a range of locations, such as hospitals, clinics, healthcare facilities, pharmaceutical warehouses, and waste disposal facilities, can help health institutions enhance efficiency and reduce costs. Among the advantages it provides: It is possible to minimize travel time for patients and staff, ensure accurate delivery of medical supplies, and optimize staffing levels based on patient demand with available solutions. In health systems, the transportation model covers the assignment, allocation, and movement of both people and materials. Despite this, there exist a limited number of papers that delve into the matter of nursing staff and bed capacity as a resource allocation problem within the transportation model framework.

Table 6 Bed capacity allocation with respect to the parameter α

	α										
Month	0.0	0.1	0.2	0.3	0.4	0.5	0.6	0.7	0.8	0.9	1.0
January	172	173	174	175	176	177	178	179	180	181	182
February	143	144	145	146	147	148	149	150	151	152	153
March	230	231	232	233	234	235	236	237	238	239	240
April	222	223	224	225	226	227	228	229	230	231	232
May	217	218	219	220	221	222	223	224	225	226	227
June	172	173	174	175	176	177	178	179	180	181	182
July	232	233	234	235	236	237	238	239	240	241	242
August	212	213	214	215	216	217	218	219	220	221	222
September	208	209	210	211	212	213	214	215	216	217	218
October	240	241	242	243	244	245	246	247	248	249	250
November	240	241	242	243	244	245	246	247	248	249	250
December	240	241	242	243	244	245	246	247	248	249	250
Total profit	2,376,721	2,356,721	2,336,721	2,316,721	2,296,721	2,276,721	2,256,721	2,236,721	2,216,721	2,196,721	2,176,721

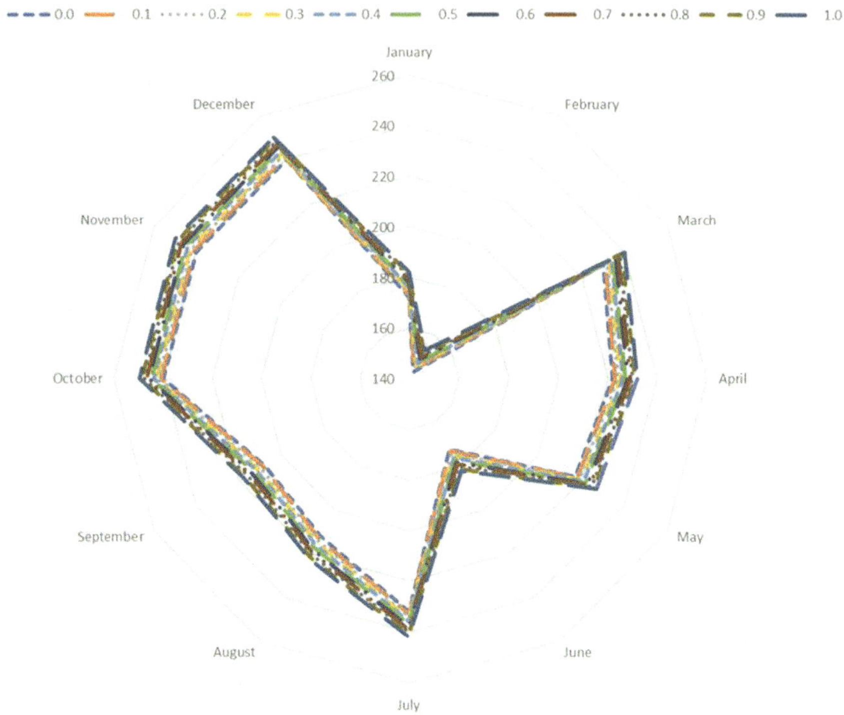

Fig. 1 Result of the sensitivity analysis

Henceforth, the purpose of the study is to expound on the transportation model through the utilization of a fuzzy mixed integer linear programming (FMILP) approach to allocate nursing staff and bed capacity as resources, using a dental hospital's case study. The rationale for selecting this methodology is rooted in the Fuzzy MILP optimization capacity to incorporate subjectivity and uncertainty into the mathematical model. In view of the fact that the demand, number of admitted and transferred patients are subject to uncertainty and reliant on multiple factors in this study, the utilization of fuzzy sets is necessary in some parts of the optimization procedure.

According to the findings, the highest patient demand is observed in the last three months of the year as a result of the optimal solution for the allocation of hospital beds and nursing staff, and there is a need to increase bed and nurse capacity accordingly (which is more profitable to not admit patients).

The sensitivity analysis examines this case study by modifying the α value in terms of patient demand. The number of domestic patients is rather steady throughout the year; however, the number of international patients changes substantially. In other words, as a result of foreign demand, this circumstance causes a major shift in total patient demand.

This chapter adds to the literature by highlighting the wide range of application abilities of transportation models for healthcare resource allocation issues. Practitioners may gain from this work in order to manage its resources in order to assign specific dates and operating rooms.

The limitation of this study grounds on the case study by having only one dental hospitals' data of a particular country. However, the model can be easily adapted to the different scenarios and institutions. Although this study's findings are not generic for the whole literature, the mathematical model is highly generic for the wide range of use in several fields of studies.

Further research opportunities are available by enhancing the data gathered from different health systems. Besides, recently introduced fuzzy sets such as picture fuzzy sets, neutrosophic sets, Fermatean sets can be used to extend this proposed approach in future studies.

References

1. Vankar, P.: Health care system: health outcomes ranking of select countries worldwide 2021. Statista (2022)
2. Zhou, C.-Y., Zhang, S.-Z., Sun, Y.: Research on the distribution and transportation of emergency materials under public health emergencies. In: International Conference on Smart Transportation and City Engineering, p. 12460 (2022)
3. Younkin, S.G., Fremont, H.C., Patz, J.A.: The health-oriented transportation model: estimating the health benefits of active transportation. J. Transp. Health **22** (2021)
4. Kumar, A., Amin, M.A.S., Tarakci, H., Prybutok, V.: Distribution and transportation model for COVID-19 vaccine. Int. J. Enterp. Netw. Manage. **14**(1–2), 78–98 (2023)
5. Mengüç, K., Aydin, N., Ulu, M.: Optimisation of COVID-19 vaccination process using GIS, machine learning, and the multi-layered transportation model. Int. J. Prod. Res. (2023)
6. Yazdani, M., Mojtahedi, M., Loosemore, M., Sanderson, D.: A modelling framework to design an evacuation support system for healthcare infrastructures in response to major flood events. Prog. Disaster Sci. **13** (2022)
7. Bala, R., Lee, C., Pallant, B., Srinivasan, M., Lurie, D., Jacob, R., Bhagchandani, N., Ranney, M., He, S.: Algorithmic matching of personal protective equipment donations with healthcare facilities during the COVID-19 pandemic. Digital Med. **4**(1) (2021)
8. Babaee Tirkolaee, E., Aydın, N.S.: A sustainable medical waste collection and transportation model for pandemics. Waste Manage. Res. **39**(1_suppl), 34–44 (2021)
9. Liu, H., Yao, Z., Chang, F., Meyer, S.: An RFID-based medical waste transportation management system: assessment of a new model on a hospital in China. Fresenius Environ. Bull. **29**(2), 773–784 (2020)
10. Nurprihatin, F., Elnathan, R., Rumawan, R.E., Regina, T.: A distribution strategy using a two-step optimisation to maximize blood services considering stochastic travel times. In: 1st International Conference of Construction, Infrastructure, and Materials, ICCIM 2019, vol. 650, no. 1. Scopus (2019)
11. Yasobant, S., Vora, K.S., Upadhyay, A.: Geographic information system applications in public health: advancing health research. In: Healthcare Policy and Reform: Concepts, Methodologies, Tools, and Applications, vol. 2, pp. 538–561 (2018)
12. Gupta, K.: Inventory and transportation cost minimization in the delivery logistics of swine flu vaccine. Yugoslav J. Oper. Res. **27**(4), 481–497 (2017)
13. Michas, F.: Hospital bed density select countries 2020. Statista (2022)

14. Belien, J.: Exact and heuristic methodologies for scheduling in hospitals: problems, formulations and algorithms. 4OR **5**(2), 157–160 (2007)
15. Migo-Sumagang, M.V., Tan, R.R., Tapia, J.F.D., Aviso, K.B.: Fuzzy mixed-integer linear and quadratic programming models for planning negative emissions technologies portfolios with synergistic interactions. Cleaner Eng. Technol. **9**, 100507 (2022)
16. Baker, K.B.: Workforce allocation in cyclical scheduling problems: a survey. J. Oper. Res. Soc. **27**(1), 155–167 (1976)
17. Knyazkov, K., Derevitsky, I., Mednikov, L., Yakovlev, A.: Evaluation of dynamic ambulance routing for the transportation of patients with acute coronary syndrome in Saint-Petersburg. Proc. Comput. Sci. **66**, 419–428 (2015)
18. Li, M., Vanberkel, P., Carter, A.: A review on ambulance offload delay literature. Health Care Manage. Sci. **22** (2019)
19. Perveen, S., Yigitcanlar, T., Kamruzzaman, M., Hayes, J.: Evaluating transport externalities of urban growth: a critical review of scenario-based planning methods. Int. J. Environ. Sci. Technol. **14**(3), 663–678 (2017)
20. Prasetyadi, A., Trianggoro, C., Rezaldi, M.Y., Nugroho, B.: The autonomous vehicle models to minimize the impact of pandemic. In: International Conference on Computer, Control, Informatics and Its Applications, pp. 122–125 (2021)
21. Sivakumar, G., Hari Ganesh, A.: Application of fuzzy multi objective linear programming in the efficient treatment of communicable diseases. Glob. J. Pure Appl. Math. **11**(3), 1363–1377 (2015)
22. Bhattacharya, P.P., Bhattacharya, K., De, S.K.: A study on pollution sensitive sponge iron-based production transportation model under fuzzy environment. Decision Making Appl. Manage. Eng. **5**(1), 225–245 (2022)
23. Liu, C., He, Z., Lu, X.: Optimisation analysis of carbon emission reduction from crop straw collection and transportation under the sustainable development goals. Nongye Gongcheng Xuebao/Trans. Chin. Soc. Agric. Eng. **38**(10), 239–248 (2022)
24. Shekarrizfard, M., Valois, M.-F., Goldberg, M.S., Crouse, D., Ross, N., Parent, M.-E., Yasmin, S., Hatzopoulou, M.: Investigating the role of transportation models in epidemiologic studies of traffic related air pollution and health effects. Environ. Res. **140**, 282–291 (2015)
25. Arya, R., Singh, P., Kumari, S., Obaidat, M.S.: An approach for solving fully fuzzy multi-objective linear fractional optimisation problems. Soft. Comput. **24**(12), 9105–9119 (2020)
26. Kannan, D., de Sousa Jabbour, A.B.L., Jabbour, C.J.C.: Selecting green suppliers based on GSCM practices: Using Fuzzy TOPSIS applied to a Brazilian electronics company. Eur. J. Oper. Res. **233**(2), 432–447 (2014)
27. Breuer, D.J., Kapadia, S., Lahrichi, N., Benneyan, J.C.: Joint robust optimisation of bed capacity, nurse staffing, and care access under uncertainty. Ann. Oper. Res. **312**(2), 673–689 (2022)
28. Olya, M.H., Badri, H., Teimoori, S., Yang, K.: An integrated deep learning and stochastic optimization approach for resource management in team-based healthcare systems. Expert Syst. Appl. (2022)
29. Pei, Z., Yuan, Y., Yu, T., Li, N.: Dynamic allocation of medical resources during the outbreak of epidemics. IEEE Trans. Autom. Sci. Eng. **19**(2), 663–676 (2022)
30. Ash, C., Diallo, C., Venkatadri, U., VanBerkel, P.: Distributionally robust optimization of a Canadian healthcare supply chain to enhance resilience during the COVID-19 pandemic. Comput. Ind. Eng. **168** (2022)
31. Goli, A., Ala, A., Mirjalili, S.: A robust possibilistic programming framework for designing an organ transplant supply chain under uncertainty. Ann. Oper. Res. (2022)
32. Wu, J.S.: Healthcare service efficiency: an empirical study on healthcare capacity in various counties and cities in Taiwan. Healthcare (Switzerland) **11**(11) (2023)
33. Banker, R.D., Amirteimoori, A., Allahviranloo, T., Sinha, R.P.: Performance analysis and managerial ability in the general insurance market: a study of India and Iran. Inf. Technol. Manage. (2023). https://doi.org/10.1007/s10799-023-00405-y

34. Cadenas, J.M., Verdegay, J.L.: Using fuzzy numbers in linear programming. IEEE Trans. Syst. Man Cybern. B Cybern. **27**(6), 1016–1022 (1997). https://doi.org/10.1109/3477.650062
35. Peidro, D., Mula, J., Poler, R., Verdegay J.: Fuzzy optimization for supply chain planning under supply, demand and process uncertainties. Fuzzy Sets Syst. **160**, 2640–2657 (2009). https://doi.org/10.1016/j.fss.2009.02.021
36. Rahmani, A., Lotfi, F.H., Rostamy-Malkhalifeh, M., Allahviranloo, T.: A new method for defuzzification and ranking of fuzzy numbers based on the statistical beta distribution. Adv. Fuzzy Syst. **2016**, 1–8 (2016)
37. Cadenas, J.M.: Design and implementation of an interactive system to solve fuzzy optimisations problems. Ph.D. Dissertation, Universidad de Granada, Spain
38. Negoita, C.V., Ralescu, D.A.: Application of Fuzzy Sets to System Analysis. Interdisciplinary Systems Research, Birkhäuser Verlag, Stuttgart (1975)
39. Cadenas, J.M., Verdegay, J.L.: Métodos Y Modelos De Programación Lineal Borrosa. In: Alonso-Ayuso, A., Cerdá, E., Escudero, L.F., Sala, R. (eds.) Optimización Bajo Incertidumbre, pp. 77–98. Tirant Lo Blanch, Madrid (2004)
40. Isikli, E., SerdarAsan, S., Karadayi-Usta, S.: Predicting the Medical Tourism Demand of Turkey, pp. 119–132 (2020)
41. Bureau of Labor Statistics.: Occupational employment and wages (2022)

Locating Problems for Medical Centers and Emergency Services

Mansour Soufi

Abstract The select location of Medical Centers and Emergency Services is regarding as the case study in this chapter.

This chapter has presented the integration of intuitionistic fuzzy preference relation and fuzzy PROMETHEE method for selecting the most desirable facility location. This work aimed to propose the use of a multi-criteria decision support for the prioritization location of static facilities. Selecting the wrong location for a new facility will increase the cost of decision makers and even in some cases it is irrecoverable, so any decision method which is less deviation would be more appropriate. The multi-criteria decision analysis is one of the evident areas of important points in integrated planning of the location problems. The model is presented based on the employment of four methodologies, F-Delphi, F-AHP, F-LLSM and F-PROMETHEE. This chapter solves a factor rating system facility location allocation problem defined as follows:

In F-Delphi area

- Selection of location criteria for evaluating potential locations for hypermarket centers.
- The decision makers use their knowledge, prior experience with the hypermarket conditions of the city and the presence of sustainable freight regulations in the city to identify candidate locations for implementing hyper market center.

In F-AHP area

- Provide fuzzy total pairwise comparisons matrix of criteria.

In F-LLSM area

- Using F-LLSM and LINGO software to calculate weights of criteria.

M. Soufi (✉)
Department of Industrial Management, Rasht Branch, Islamic Azad University, Rasht, Iran
e-mail: msoufi45@gmail.com

T. Allahviranloo et al. (eds.), *Decision Making in Healthcare Systems*,
Studies in Systems, Decision and Control 513,
https://doi.org/10.1007/978-3-031-46735-6_8

In F-PROMETHEE area

- Provide: Fuzzy aggregated decision matrix; fuzzy Preference matrix for all criteria; total Preference matrix; flow calculation for pre-ordering alternatives and the net flow. Finally, defuzzification and ranking of alternatives must be done. According to Table 17, prioritization of proposed location is calculated as follows: ***location3 > location4 > location5 > location6 > location1 > location2.***

Keywords Factor rating system · Facility location allocation problem · Medical centers and emergency services · F-MCDM · F-Delphi · FAHP · F-LLSM · F-PROMETHEE

1 Introduction and Motivation

The success of organizations depends on their ability to make the right strategic decisions. Choosing the location of facilities is one of these strategic decisions, which is a costly and difficult activity for organizations. Facility location or facility location problem is an important strategic decision for an organization. One of the key features of the conversion process (production system) is the efficiency with which products (services) are delivered to customers. This fact will include determining the location of the facility. Choosing a location is a key decision because a lot of investment is made in building the location. Changing locations frequently is not recommended or possible. Therefore, the inappropriate location of the facility may lead to a waste of all the investments made in the building and equipment [44]. Before choosing a location for a facility, long-term forecasts should be made by anticipating the future needs of the organization. The location of the facility should be based on the organization's development plan and policy, diversification plan for products (goods, services and ideas), changing market conditions, changing sources of raw materials and many other factors that affect the choice of location. The purpose of location study is to find the optimal location that has the greatest advantage for the organization [43]. While others must be credited for earlier work (e.g., Richard Cantillon, Etienne Bono de Condillac, David Hume, Sir James Stewart, and David Ricardo), prior to the publication of Johann Heinrich von Tonen's first volume of Der Isolierte. Staat in 1826, when we can say that the theory of place really began. In fact, the eminent regional scholar Walter Izard has called von Tonen the father of place theorists. Von Tonen notes in Der Isolierte Staat that the cost of transporting goods consumes some of Ricardo's economic rent. He points out that since these transportation costs and of course economic rents are different in goods, different uses and intensity of land use will increase the distance from the market. However, this argument has been criticized because Johann Heinrich von Tonen oversimplified the issue with his assumptions of, for example, isolated states or individual cities [27]. This chapter proposes an intuitive fuzzy multi-criteria decision-making method with a combination of the pair matrix "Fuzzy Hierarchical Analysis Process" (FAHP) and expert opinion weighting with "Fuzzy Logarithmic Least Squares Method" (F-LLSM). After that, the fuzzy priority ranking organizational method for enrichment evaluation (FPROMETHEE) is used to rank the options. Hu [28] combined fuzzy set theory and developed the fuzzy PROMETHEE method, which is more flexible. The following steps are required to run the method:

Step1: Determine alternatives, criteria and decision makers;
Step2: Define linguistic values and their corresponding fuzzy number;
Step3: Aggregate the decision-maker's estimation;
Step4: Compute the average fuzzy weight and construct the fuzzy decision matrix;
Step5: Construct the fuzzy preference function;
Step6: Define the multi-criteria preference index to decide the valued out ranking relation;
Step7: Calculate the flow to preorder the alternatives.

In this chapter, the first three steps run with F-Delphi method for gathering expert's opinion about criteria's values for each location and F-AHP to determine the composed matrix of paired comparisons. The fourth step is performed with F-LLSM in which the criteria weights are determined. Next steps run with F-PROMETHEE that during which, the weights of alternatives determined then by the Excel are prioritized. The LLSM is a very natural method, and for an AHP with complete information, the solution of LLSM is equivalent to that of the geometric mean method. This of course gives a positive solution, because exponential values obtained by the inverse transformation of logarithm are always positive [30]. Geldermann et al. proposed an adaptation of the PROMETHEE method using operations with fuzzy numbers. The weights of the criteria are treated as linguistic variables, represented as triangle fuzzy numbers. In the context of plant location or the facilities location problem in which this paper is included, the performance of alternatives (Location) in each of the criteria can be obtained only at rough. Thus, the use of fuzzy numbers in the evaluation of each alternative is very adequate and important, since its usage allows a closer look at the reality of the problem, obtaining a more realistic ranking. On the other hand, the impact of alternatives on criteria provided by decision makers is usually difficult to be precisely expressed by the crisp data in the facility location selection [16]. An intuitionistic fuzzy set is characterized by three parameters: Membership function, non-membership function and hesitation margin namely, which is a flexible way to deal with uncertainty, while a fuzzy set is only characterized by membership function.

Recent research points out that most mathematical models like dynamic systems and also linear systems get involved with real-world problems. Since their related information has different forms like certainty and uncertainty, the uncertain version of these models does have more importance in the applications. In health problems, two types of mathematical models; fuzzy dynamic systems and fuzzy linear programming problems even transportation problems, play an important role, on the other hand, the main and basic model of fuzzy linear programming problems is fuzzy linear systems.

In conclusion, fuzzy differential equations (as a special version of dynamic systems) [1, 9, 18], and fuzzy linear systems (as a basic model of fuzzy linear programming problems) [32], have an important role in this research. Recently several research has been done on investigating the advanced version of the uncertain information [8, 9, 34, 38], and moreover the above-mentioned basic models.

One of the techniques for decision making is Data Envelopment Analysis (DEA), and many researchers have conducted research on this topic. Several recent papers have been cited to mention their research area [5, 15–13]. Some authors have explored the topic in a different way: safety analysis and reliability [2, 3, 7].

2 Literature Review

Various models can be used to locate health care and related services centers based on the considered criteria. Among these models, we can mention:

(a) Neural network models: These models can predict the best possible locations for health care and related services centers by using different data such as demographic, spatial and health information, traffic, and so on.
(b) Multi-criteria decision-making models: By considering various criteria such as population, disease prevalence in different regions, the need for health services, cost, etc., these models propose the best possible locations for health care and related services centers.
(c) Bayesian network models: By using population, spatial, and health data, these models predict the best possible locations for health care and related services centers.
(d) GIS application models: By using spatial and geographical data, these models propose the best possible locations for health care and related services centers [10].

As there are various criteria for locating health care and related services centers, the use of combined models that consider multiple criteria simultaneously is recommended due to their higher accuracy in predicting the best possible locations. In these models, different criteria such as distance to existing centers, population, disease prevalence in different regions, the need for health services, cost, etc., are taken into account, and as a result, a better prediction of the best possible locations for health care and related services centers is achieved. Therefore, in this chapter, we will explain how to locate a new health care and related services center based on health criteria using combined models [42].

The first concern of managers of any institution is the appropriate and optimal conversion of existing capital resources at the appropriate time and place. Therefore, in today's economic conditions, deciding how and where to invest will be a complicated and risky matter. Choosing a suitable location for the establishment of service and production units has been the focus of managers of organizations and researchers. The choice of location itself has a great impact on the unit costs of production or services, as well as the possibility of access to production resources, including transportation facilities, raw materials, and labor. Additionally, due to the distance from markets and access to customers, it will have an undeniable effect on the income of these organizations. This matter, especially in the case of service organizations that mainly have face-to-face communication with the final consumers of their services, means the corners of marketing strategies. Uneven and suboptimal distribution of service and treatment centers has been mentioned as one of the important factors in the lack of development of health culture. At the level of the cities of each country, it is possible to provide adequate coverage to the problem. In some places, the number of service and treatment centers is high, while in other areas, the number of these centers is limited and faces the problem of inadequate service coverage. Abundance indicators should be considered in choosing the best place for services. Some of these indicators are personnel costs, population density, age, access to suppliers, environmental issues, and social considerations, etc., which change according to the conditions. A number of the above variables, along with many other indicators, can be included in the selection of a suitable place for the establishment of various facilities, including service and treatment centers. However, they have not been identified. Therefore, managers' decisions in dealing with the location category of service and treatment centers are mostly accompanied by some kind of confusion and based on coincidences and personal perceptions [33].

Many models have been developed for making decisions based on simple and quick perceptions in order to choose the best option among the available options. However, many of these models seem to be inefficient when considering the complex and unstructured context of today's decision-making issues. In fact, most of the existing decision-making models are limited to summarizing the indicators that can be considered when choosing the best option from among the available options. Therefore, it seems necessary to use multi-criteria decision-making methods. The spatial problem is usually a multi-criteria decision-making problem that involves the following conditions:

a. There are m candidates to choose from for the selection of a place.
b. There are n decision-making attributes that should be considered when choosing a location, and usually, these criteria behave inversely. Thus, an increase in one index can lead to a decrease in another.
c. The opinions and evaluations of a group of decision-makers should be taken into account when selecting a place. Moreover, due to the varying levels of experience, knowledge, and influence among the members of this decision-making group, the importance and weight of each decision-maker's viewpoint differ from the others. This must be considered [21].

Studies on personnel employment and planning in hospitals and other health institutions are still among the important studies today. Provide timely and good quality care to sick individuals. When making these choices, it is important to note that most hospitals are obliged to have 24-h staff in their nursing and emergency units. There are also many pressures to reduce the costs of health care. Health care providers should control the cost. An element that has a significant impact on cost is the staff [22].

Due to the advancement of information and communication technology and the shift towards remote activities during the multi-year period of the COVID-19 pandemic, as well as the emergence of operational management paradigms and the expansion of supply chains in the service sector, location perspectives have also undergone significant transformations.

Yu et al. [47] focused their literature review on the closed-loop supply chain network design problem, which involves location decisions for facilities considering both forward and reverse logistics. It covers various models, algorithms, and recent research advancements in this area. Fernández et al. [23] In a literature review, they focused on location allocation models for supply chain network design, discussing different models, solution methods, and recent developments in this field. Aksen and Klose [6] provided a comprehensive synthesis and review of location analysis, covering both classic and recent developments in the field, including facility location, coverage models, network design, and more. Current and Min [19] in a review paper on the global facility location literature, a discussion of state-of-the-art models, solution methods, and future research directions focused on providing insight into current developments and potential areas for further exploration. In summary, recent studies on the location of healthcare facilities and medical emergencies have been presented in Table 1.

3 Location

We need to select a suitable location for facility deployment for three reasons:

I. When a new organization starts operating

When choosing a location for a new organization for the first time, cost savings are very important, but the long-term business goals should also be considered. The following are factors that should be taken into account when selecting a location for a new organization:

(a) Identifying the region: regional objectives, along with various long-term considerations regarding marketing, technology, internal strengths and weaknesses, resources available in the region, the business environment, governmental and legal environment, social environment, and geographical environment should be considered.
(b) Selecting a location within the region: after choosing the appropriate region, the next step is to select the best location from a series of accessible locations. The choice of location depends less on the organization's long-term strategies. Evaluating various locations solves facility-related cost issues. The problem of choosing a location within a region can be analyzed dimensionally through a non-behavioral cost model approach, which will be explained below.

Table 1 Literature review about using MCDM techniques for Location problems

Author	Year	Method	Subject
Acar and Kizilay [4]	2021	Literature review	Location-allocation models for healthcare facility planning: a systematic literature review
Kumar et al. [30]	2020	Meta-heuristic techniques	A review on healthcare facility location and resource allocation using meta-heuristic techniques
Mosadeghrad and Esfahanipour [35]	2020	Literature review	An overview of location-allocation models and methods in the healthcare facility planning literature
Yazdani and Asgharizadeh [45]	2020	MCDM	A sustainable healthcare facility location model under uncertainty: a case study of the Kerman province, Iran
Goia and Gupta	2020	Hybrid MCDM	A decision support system for healthcare facility location selection using a hybrid multi-criteria decision-making approach
Bostel and Karimi [17]	2019	Literature review	Facility location in healthcare: a comprehensive review
Shabanpour et al. [41]	2019	MCDM	A hybrid location-allocation model for healthcare facility planning in a green supply chain under uncertainty
Zarrinpoor et al. [48]	2019	Fuzzy MODM	An integrated fuzzy multi-objective facility location and network design model for healthcare delivery systems: a case study
Li and Huang [31]	2019	Fuzzy MCDM	Fuzzy-based facility location selection for healthcare waste disposal under sustainability and environmental risks
Yousefi-Babadi et al. [46]	2019	Hybrid MCDM	A hybrid MCDM model for sustainable healthcare facility location selection considering uncertainty and interdependent criteria
Gupta and Misra [25]	2018	Fuzzy AHP—TOPSIS	Decision-making in healthcare facility location selection using fuzzy AHP and fuzzy TOPSIS
Hadi-Vencheh et al. [26]	2017	MODM	Sustainable healthcare facility location: a dynamic multi-objective approach

(continued)

Table 1 (continued)

Author	Year	Method	Subject
Karakaya and Ekici	2017	Fuzzy MCDM	A fuzzy multi-criteria decision-making approach for healthcare facility location selection
Hansen and Peeters [27]	2017	Literature review	Fifty years of location analysis: a review
Banaeian and Mobini [15]	2016	Fuzzy MCDM	Fuzzy multi-criteria decision-making approaches for facility location selection: a review
Khan et al. [29]	2015	Literature review	A systematic literature review of facility location decisions: a focus on healthcare facility location
Çelik [20]	2014	Fuzzy MCDM	A fuzzy multi-criteria decision-making approach for the selection of healthcare facility locations
Ashtiani and Gholamian [14]	2013	Fuzzy AHP—TOPSIS	A hybrid fuzzy AHP-TOPSIS framework for assessment of hospital location selection: a case study
Govindan et al. [24]	2013	Fuzzy MCDM	A fuzzy multi criteria approach for measuring sustainability performance of a supplier based on triple bottom line approach

(c) Dimensional analysis: if all costs are tangible, comparing and selecting a location is easy. The location with the lowest cost is selected. In most cases, intangible costs are defined relatively, not absolutely. Since both tangible and intangible costs must be considered when choosing a location, we need dimensional analysis. Dimensional analysis involves calculating relative values (cost share) for each of the cost items in both locations. For each share, a suitable coefficient has been assigned according to their power, and multiplying these variables will provide a comprehensible measure of the relative value of both locations.

Different costs, $C_{1m}, C_{2m}, \ldots, C_{zm}$, are associated with location m for z units, and different costs, $C_{1n}, C_{2n}, \ldots, C_{zn}$, are associated with location n for z units. Additionally, $w_1, w_2, \ldots, w_z$ are coefficients assigned to each cost item. Thus, the relative value of location M and N is calculated as follows:

$$(C_{1m}/C_{1n})^{w_1} \times (C_{2m}/C_{2n})^{w_2} \times \cdots \times (C_{zm}/C_{zn})^{w_z}$$

If the result is greater than one, location N is preferred, and vice versa.

When a new office is launched, the decision of its location is crucial as it directly impacts financial factors, employment, and distribution patterns. In the long term, the office location can even have benefits for the organization, but changing the location can cause disruptions in production and also result in relocation and transfer costs. Additionally, it can disrupt the normal business of the organization. Therefore, when starting a business or industry, different locations for establishing both light and heavy central buildings should be considered, and after proper analysis, the best possible location should be selected. The location of warehouses and other facilities is equally important in the organization's performance. An organization that is currently operating is always looking for new locations to expand its business, open new branches, or relocate its current facilities. When demand for a product (goods, services or ideas) increase, it leads to many decision-making processes:

- Should we expand our current facilities and capacity?
- Should we look for new locations for new facilities?
- Should we shut down current facilities in order to make the most out of new locations?

II. Location selection for current organization

In this regard, a service organization must have a coordinated multi-branch strategy. This means having additional locations for branches in the same current location or elsewhere under the following conditions:

1. Branches provide separate products.
2. The service organization serves a particular market area.
3. Branches are separated based on the process or stages of service delivery.
4. Branches emphasize flexibility.

Various operational strategies in the above conditions can be as follows:

(a) Separate branches produce distinct products: Each branch covers a separate region. This strategy is necessary when technological needs and input resources for service delivery are different, specialized, or distinct. For example, providing a high-quality and precise service should not be alongside other services that require less precision and quality. As much as possible, opposing factors such as high-end and old equipment, specialized and non-specialized staff, sensitive and non-sensitive processes, should not be located under one roof or managed side by side. Such arrangements can create confusion about management policies. Exclusive products may be needed in highly competitive markets. It may be necessary to utilize specific resources in a particular area. The more these opposing factors are separate in terms of management and physical location, the easier it is to plan, control, and utilize them.

(b) A branch serves a particular area in the market: Here, each branch offers almost all of the company's insurance products. This strategy is useful when proximity to market resources and technology is dominant. This strategy requires significant coordination at the headquarters.

(c) Branches are separate based on the service process or stages: Each process or stage of insurance services requires separate and different equipment, capacity, specialized workforce, technology, and management policies. Since a company's products are a source of nourishment for other companies, this strategy requires high coordination at the headquarters, which is expected to understand the needs and technological aspects of all companies.

Companies emphasize on flexibility: this strategy requires high coordination among branches to be able to address changing needs simultaneously and ensure optimal utilization of facilities and resources. Continuous changes in long-term strategy are not recommended for the sake of temporary performance improvements. The main question for the location problem is whether there is a location where the company can remain competitive in the long run. The following are ways for an organization to expand its capacity:

- Expansion of facilities in the current location: as long as it does not compromise the overall management and business plan of the organization such as philosophy, goals, strategy, and capabilities, it is acceptable. For example, developing a factory should not jeopardize quality, delay time, and customer service.
- Transfer of facilities (shutting down current facilities): This is a risky step known as "relocation and migration." Changing and relocating a location should only be done if there are compelling reasons for it. These reasons can include fundamental changes in technology, resources, availability, etc. All of these factors can apply to production organizations that may have different goals, priorities, and strategies than service organizations.

III. Due to globalization

As a result of globalization, multinational companies are establishing their organizations in different countries, while those countries are also considering expanding their businesses to other countries. Regarding global locations, there is also a domain for virtual proximity and virtual services.

(a) Virtual proximity

With advances in telecommunications technology, a company can be virtually close to its customers. A software services company conducts most of its activities through information or communication channels. Many companies use the information superhighway for a large number of their business transactions. However, logistics is an important factor in decision-making for location, whether within or outside the country. Markets must be accessible and customers must be in contact with the organization. As a result, being present in the customers' country is necessary.

(b) Virtual organization

Today, many domestic and foreign companies, through strong legal contracts in the services or production sector, usually outsource part of their business process to other companies. As a result, an organization can use its partner company's facilities instead of its own operations. This means that the location can belong to another organization and the organization itself can only exist legally on the internet.

3.1 Location Models

Location models are used to determine the best location for a facility, such as a warehouse, distribution center, or manufacturing plant, based on various criteria such as transportation costs, labor costs, and market access. There are several types of location models, including the p-median model, which involves determining the best location for p facilities to minimize total transportation costs; the location set covering model, which involves selecting a minimum number of locations to meet a certain level of demand; and the capacitated facility location model, which takes into account the capacity constraints of facilities. These models can help businesses make informed decisions about where to locate their facilities to optimize efficiency and profitability.

There are various models available to help identify an ideal location, some of the most common ones are as follows.

4 Factor Evaluation Method

- The process of selecting a new facility location includes the following steps:
- Identify the important location factors.
- Estimate each factor's relative importance, with a higher estimation rate indicating a more important factor.
- Determine the rate for each location based on its value for each factor.
- Calculate the score for each location by multiplying the rated factors.
- Add up the calculated results for each factor and choose the location with the highest total score.

4.1 Factor Rating Method

In this method, the factors have been weighted based on their importance, and the score for each location is calculated using a matrix with weighted coefficients. The location with the highest score is chosen as the suitable location.

4.2 Distance-Loading Method

Assuming there are m healthcare centers located at points $P_1(a_1, b_1)$, $P_2(a_2, b_2)$, ..., $P_m(a_m, b_m)$ we want to determine the location for a new center. The coordinates for the new center, which will be constructed, are considered as $X = (x, y)$. The objective is to minimize the total transportation cost. Assuming that w_i is the cost of transportation for each unit of distance between the $i - t_h$ existing center and the new center x, and $d(x, P_i)$ is the distance between the location of the new center (x) and the $i - t_h$ existing center, the mathematical model of the problem is defined as follows:

$$Min\ F(x) = \sum_{i=1}^{m} w_i .\ d(x\ ,\ p_i)$$

The distance-loading method is a mathematical model used to evaluate a location based on its proximity factors. The goal is to choose a location that minimizes the loads that enter and exit the location. The distance between two points is defined by assigning scores to the coordinates on the map. Another approach is to use time instead of location.

Assume that a new healthcare and service center is going to be established in city A, which will receive shipments from various suppliers, one of which is located in city B. What will be the distance between the two facilities? If the shipments are transported by truck, the distance will depend on the highway and road system that they pass through. There are software programs available that can calculate the distance between two locations in a country. However, for the distance-loading method, usually the calculation is done through Euclidean or straight-line distance. Euclidean distance is the shortest distance or shortest path between two locations. The distance between location A and B is the length of the hypotenuse of the triangle or as shown below: d(AB) represents the distance between points A and B. X_A is the coordinates of point A, X_B is the coordinates of point B, Y_A is the coordinates of point A, and Y_A is the coordinates of point B.

$$d_{AB} = Sqrt((X_A - X_B)^2 + (Y_A - Y_B)^2)$$

The distance traveled along the path X is the absolute difference in the X coordinates. Adding this value to the absolute difference in the Y coordinates gives the following formula:

$$D_{AB} = |X_A - X_B| + |Y_A - Y_B|$$

$$Min\ F(x) = \sum_{i=1}^{m} w_i .\ d(x\ ,\ p_i) = \sum_{i=1}^{m} w_i[|x - a_i| + |y - b_i|]$$

$$= \sum_{i=1}^{m} w_i |x - a_i| + \sum_{i=1}^{m} w_i |y - b_i| = F_1(x) + F_2(x)$$

If both f and g are minimized separately, then in fact, the whole F(x) has been minimized.

$$Min \sum w_i |x - a_i| \Rightarrow x*$$

$$Min \sum w_i |y - b_i| \Rightarrow y*$$

This type of function (absolute value) has several properties:

- The point x* falls on one of the xi's and y* falls on one of the yi's.
- The point x* is a point where half of the transportation occurs to the right and half occurs to the left, and y* is a point where half of the movements occur above it and half occur below it.
- Due to the presence of the absolute value, these functions are necessarily convex, so the slope of the function is positive in some places and negative in others, and precisely where the slope changes sign, the optimal point is located.
- The optimal point lies on one of the corners of the piecewise linear function. (since it is a linear function).

4.3 Gravity Center

The center of gravity, more than anything, focuses on cost concentration considerations. This method can be used to help managers balance costs. The center of gravity method considers the location of the factory and markets, the volume of goods, transportation and relocation costs to find the best location for an average warehouse. The center of gravity is a location that reduces the distance between the warehouse and the source and distribution points. Here, the distance is multiplied by the number of tons that are supplied or consumed. The first step is to place the location on a coordinate system. This can be easily done by placing grid lines on a regular map. The center of gravity is calculated using the following formula:

$$C_X = \frac{\sum D_{ix}.\, W_i}{\sum W_i}, \qquad C_Y = \frac{\sum D_{iy}.\, W_i}{\sum W_i}$$

Here, C_x represents the coordinates of the center of gravity, C_y represents the y-coordinate of the center of gravity, D_{ix} represents the x-coordinate of point i, and D_{iy} represents the y-coordinate of point i.

I. The break-even point analysis

The Break-Even Point (BEP) analysis occurs when the total revenue equals the total costs at a particular point in the operation. The BEP analysis is the point at which the revenues precisely equal the costs. It is the point where the output volume generates neither profit nor loss.

II. Cost savings in location

An ideal location is a place that has the lowest fixed and variable costs for each unit. Among the various costs that are effective in location cost savings, we can mention land, buildings, equipment, labor, and raw materials. Other factors such as social behavior, community facilities, and the region also affect the choice of the best location.

5 The Location of Healthcare and Related Service Centers

The location of health-related centers and services is of great importance. These centers include hospitals, clinics, pharmacies, research centers, and so on. In choosing a suitable location for these centers, factors such as access to transportation facilities, access to the target population, and basic infrastructure should be considered.

The primary factor in locating healthcare centers is access to them. It should be examined whether the healthcare center is located within the geographical area of the target population or not. It should also be checked whether the route to the healthcare center has any transportation difficulties or not. For example, in urban areas, the distance between healthcare and service centers with various transportation facilities is less, but in rural areas, the distances are greater and special means of transportation should be used.

Another factor that should be considered in locating health-related centers and services is basic infrastructure. These infrastructures include water, electricity, gas, water and sewage treatment systems, etc. These infrastructures are necessary for the operation of the required healthcare centers and services and should be taken into account.

Finally, the third factor that should be considered in locating healthcare centers is the ability to coordinate with other related centers and services.

5.1 Location Selection of Healthcare and Service Centers Using MADM Methods

Location selection of healthcare and related service centers can be a complex decision-making process that requires considering multiple criteria. In such cases, Multi-Attributes Decision Making (MADM) techniques can be used to facilitate the decision-making process.

In Chap. 5, several MADM techniques were introduced and this chapter, additional MADM techniques are explained for the location selection of healthcare and related service centers. By using MADM techniques, decision-makers can evaluate different location alternatives based on several criteria, such as accessibility, proximity to the target population, availability of basic infrastructure, coordination with other related services, and more. These techniques can help decision-makers to prioritize different criteria and select the best location based on their objectives and preferences.

6 Fuzzy PROMETHEE

The PROMETHEE method, which stands for "Preference Ranking Organization Method for Enrichment Evaluations," is classified under the category of option ranking techniques. The first versions of PROMETHEE, PROMETHEE 1 (incomplete ranking) and PROMETHEE 2 (complete ranking), were introduced by Brans and his colleagues in 1982, and a few years later, they also proposed PROMETHEE 3 (ranking based on distance) and PROMETHEE 4 (continuous case). Subsequently, other versions of this technique were developed, including PROMETHEE 5 (multi-criteria decision-making with divided constraints) and PROMETHEE 6 (human brain representation). So far, it has had successful applications in various fields. The fuzzy PROMETHEE method, which combines fuzzy logic and the PROMETHEE method has greater flexibility [39]. The steps of this method are as follows:

Step 1: Constructing the decision matrix.

(a) Identifying alternatives (m), criteria (c), and decision makers (n).
(b) Defining linguistic and fuzzy numerical values for them. To do this, we can use the proposed linguistic variables by Chen and Huang, which are expressed as triangular fuzzy numbers.
(c) Aggregating decision maker's estimates: The weighted average of each criterion's superiority is defined as (Table 2):

$$\tilde{w}_j = \frac{1}{n}\left[\sum_{e=1}^{n} \tilde{w}_j^e\right] = \frac{1}{n}\left[\tilde{w}_j^1(+)\tilde{w}_j^2(+)...(+)\tilde{w}_j^n\right]$$

The evaluated value of alternative i under criterion j is equal to:

$$\tilde{x}_{ij} = \frac{1}{n}\left[\sum_{e=1}^{n} \tilde{x}_{ij}^e\right] = \frac{1}{n}\left[\tilde{x}_{ij}^1(+)\tilde{x}_{ij}^2(+)\cdots(+)\tilde{x}_{ij}^n\right]$$

Since a weight is specified for each decision maker, instead of n in the denominator of the fraction in the above formula, the sum of decision makers' weights is used, and these weights are also applied in the numerator of the fraction. In other words,

Table 2 Linguistic variable

Linguistic scale	Triangular fuzzy numbers
VL (Very low)	0, 0.5, 2
L (Low)	1, 2, 3
ML (Moderately low)	2, 3.5, 5
M (Middle)	4, 5, 6
MH (Moderately high)	5, 6.5, 8
H (High)	7, 8, 9
VH (Very high)	8, 8.5, 10

a fuzzy weighted average is calculated. Accordingly, the fuzzy decision matrix is formed as follows:

$$\tilde{D} = \left[\tilde{x}_{ij}\right]_{m\times k} = \begin{array}{|c|c|c|c|c|} \hline & C_1 & C_2 & \dots & C_k \\ \hline A_1 & \tilde{x}_{11} & \tilde{x}_{12} & \dots & x_{1k} \\ \hline A_2 & \tilde{x}_{21} & \tilde{x}_{22} & \dots & x_{2k} \\ \hline \dots & \dots & \dots & \dots & \dots \\ \hline A_m & \tilde{x}_{m1} & \tilde{x}_{m2} & \dots & x_{mk} \\ \hline \end{array}$$

This indicates the evaluated value of alternative i under criterion j.

$$\tilde{x}_{ij} = (l_{ij}, m_{ij}, u_{ij})$$

Step 2: Construct Pairwise Comparison Matrix.

In this step, you need to construct a pairwise comparison matrix. The matrix should be square and each element represents your evaluation of the priority of one item over another. To construct this matrix, you can use one of the following methods:

1. Divide-into-Two method: In this method, you need to choose two items from your list and evaluate the priority of one over the other. Then, choose two more items and repeat the process. As you progress, you will automatically obtain a square matrix of all pairwise priorities.
2. Direct-determination method: In this method, you choose a number between 1 and 9 for each pair of items and determine their priority accordingly. For example, if you want to evaluate the priority between the first and second item and decide that the first item should have a higher priority, you can assign a value of 9 as their priority.

After completing this step, you will have a square matrix with dimensions equal to the number of items you want to evaluate (Table 3).

$$\tilde{P}_{ij}^{Ck} = (pl_{ij}^{ck}, pm_{ij}^{ck}, pu_{ij}^{ck}),\ k = 1, 2, 3, 4.$$

To calculate X, we proceed as follows:
If $\tilde{A} = (a_1, a_2, a_3)$ and $\tilde{B} = (b_1, b_2, b_3)$ Then $\tilde{P}_{AB} = (pl_{AB}, pm_{AB}, pu_{AB})$

$$pl_{AB} = \begin{cases} 0 & \frac{a_1, a_2, a_3}{3} \leq \frac{b_1, b_2, b_3}{3} \\ a_1 - b_3 & otherwise. \end{cases}$$

$$pm_{AB} = \begin{cases} 0 & \frac{a_1, a_2, a_3}{3} \leq \frac{b_1, b_2, b_3}{3} \\ a_2 - b_2 & otherwise. \end{cases}$$

$$pu_{AB} = \begin{cases} 0 & \frac{a_1, a_2, a_3}{3} \leq \frac{b_1, b_2, b_3}{3} \\ a_3 - b_1 & otherwise. \end{cases}$$

Step 3: Constructing a Preference Matrix and Multi-Criteria Preference List (Table 4).

The Preference Matrix is presented below $[\pi(a, b)]$:

Step 4: Calculating $\tilde{\phi}+$ Fuzzy PROMETHEE 1 and $\tilde{\phi}-$ Fuzzy PROMETHEE 2

$$\tilde{\phi}^+ = \sum_{j=1}^{m} \sum_{k=1}^{n} \tilde{p}_j^{ck} \tilde{w}_k, \quad \tilde{\phi}^- = \sum_{i=1}^{m} \sum_{k=1}^{n} \tilde{p}_i^{ck} \tilde{w}_k$$

Table 3 An example of a pairwise comparison matrix for the first criterion

C_1	A_1	A_2	A_3	A_4	A_5
A_1	$\tilde{P}_{11}^{C_1}$	$\tilde{P}_{12}^{C_1}$	$\tilde{P}_{13}^{C_1}$	$\tilde{P}_{14}^{C_1}$	$\tilde{P}_{15}^{C_1}$
A_2	$\tilde{P}_{21}^{C_1}$	$\tilde{P}_{22}^{C_1}$	$\tilde{P}_{23}^{C_1}$	$\tilde{P}_{24}^{C_1}$	$\tilde{P}_{25}^{C_1}$
A_3	$\tilde{P}_{31}^{C_1}$	$\tilde{P}_{32}^{C_1}$	$\tilde{P}_{33}^{C_1}$	$\tilde{P}_{34}^{C_1}$	$\tilde{P}_{35}^{C_1}$
A_4	$\tilde{P}_{41}^{C_1}$	$\tilde{P}_{42}^{C_1}$	$\tilde{P}_{43}^{C_1}$	$\tilde{P}_{44}^{C_1}$	$\tilde{P}_{45}^{C_1}$
A_5	$\tilde{P}_{41}^{C_1}$	$\tilde{P}_{52}^{C_1}$	$\tilde{P}_{53}^{C_1}$	$\tilde{P}_{54}^{C_1}$	$\tilde{P}_{55}^{C_1}$

Table 4 Constructing a preference matrix

π	A_1	A_2	A_3	A_4	A_5
A_1	$\sum_{k=1}^{n} \tilde{p}_{11}^{ck} \tilde{w}_k$	…	…	…	$\sum_{k=1}^{n} \tilde{p}_{51}^{ck} \tilde{w}_k$
A_2	$\sum_{k=1}^{n} \tilde{p}_{21}^{ck} \tilde{w}_k$	…	…	…	$\sum_{k=1}^{n} \tilde{p}_{52}^{ck} \tilde{w}_k$
A_3		$\sum_{k=1}^{n} \tilde{p}_{32}^{ck} \tilde{w}_k$			$\sum_{k=1}^{n} \tilde{p}_{53}^{ck} \tilde{w}_k$
A_4	…	…	…	…	$\sum_{k=1}^{n} \tilde{p}_{54}^{ck} \tilde{w}_k$
A_5	$\sum_{k=1}^{n} \tilde{p}_{51}^{ck} \tilde{w}_k$	…	…	…	$\sum_{k=1}^{n} \tilde{p}_{54}^{ck} \tilde{w}_k$

$\tilde{\phi}^{+}(a)$ represents the total preference of option "a" relative to the other options. The larger the value of $\tilde{\phi}^{+}(a)$, the better alternative "A" is. Additionally, $\tilde{\phi}^{-}(a)$ is the total preference of option "A" over the other options, and the smaller this value, the better alternative "A" is (Table 5).

Step 5: Calculating Net Cash Flow.

$\tilde{\phi}$ is calculated as the difference between $\tilde{\phi}+$ and $\tilde{\phi}-$.

$$\tilde{\phi}_1 = (\tilde{\phi}_1+) - (\tilde{\phi}_1-)$$

Step 6: Given that the output of step 5 is in the form of fuzzy numbers, to determine the rank of each alternative, the fuzzy numbers must be defuzzification. Defuzzification is one of the simplest methods that can be obtained using the $\frac{l+4m+u}{6}$ equation. In this study, a part of Chang's developmental analysis method is used. Therefore, the degree of magnitude $\tilde{M}_2 = (l_2, m_2, u_2) \geq \tilde{M}_1 = (l_1, m_1, u_1)$ is defined as follows:

$$V(\tilde{M}_2 \geq \tilde{M}_1) = \sup\left[\min(\tilde{M}_1(x), \tilde{M}_2(y))\right]$$

Which can be expressed as follows:

$$V(\tilde{M}_2 \geq \tilde{M}_1) = hgt(\tilde{M}_2 \cap \tilde{M}_1) = \tilde{M}_2(d) = \begin{cases} 1 & if\ m_2 \geq m_1, \\ 0 & if\ l_1 \geq u_2, \\ \frac{l_1 - u_2}{(m_2 - u_2) - (m_1 - l_1)} & otherwise. \end{cases}$$

Then, the degree of possible conformity is calculated based on the following equation:

$$V(\tilde{M} \geq \tilde{M}_1, \tilde{M}_2, ..., \tilde{M}_k) = \min V((\tilde{M} \geq \tilde{M}_i), i = 1, 2, ..., k,$$

Table 5 Calculation of $\tilde{\phi}+$ and $\tilde{\phi}-$

π	A_1	A_2	A_3	A_4	A_5	$\tilde{\phi}+$
A_1	$\sum_{k=1}^{n} \tilde{p}_{11}^{ck} \tilde{w}_k$	…	…	…	$\sum_{k=1}^{n} \tilde{p}_{15}^{ck} \tilde{w}_k$	$\tilde{\phi}_1^+ = \sum_{j=1}^{m} \sum_{k=1}^{n} \tilde{p}_{1j}^{ck} \tilde{w}_k$
A_2	$\sum_{k=1}^{n} \tilde{p}_{21}^{ck} \tilde{w}_k$			…	$\sum_{k=1}^{n} \tilde{p}_{25}^{ck} \tilde{w}_k$	…
A_3	…			…	$\sum_{k=1}^{n} \tilde{p}_{35}^{ck} \tilde{w}_k$	…
A_4	…			…	$\sum_{k=1}^{n} \tilde{p}_{45}^{ck} \tilde{w}_k$	…
A_5	$\sum_{k=1}^{n} \tilde{p}_{51}^{ck} \tilde{w}_k$	…	…	…	$\sum_{k=1}^{n} \tilde{p}_{55}^{ck} \tilde{w}_k$	…
$\tilde{\phi}-$	$\tilde{\phi}_1^- = \sum_{i=1}^{m} \sum_{k=1}^{n} \tilde{p}_{i1}^{ck} \tilde{w}_k$	…	…	…	…	

And finally, the weight or rank of each alternative is obtained using the following equation [36]:

$$W = (\min V(s_1 \geq s_k), \min V(s_2 \geq s_k), \ldots, \min V(s_n \geq s_k)T,$$

6.1 Fuzzy Hierarchical Analysis Process

Fuzzy hierarchical analysis process is one of the most well-known multi-criteria decision-making techniques introduced by Saaty. When faced with multiple options and criteria in decision-making, this method can be useful. Although experts rely on their competencies and mental abilities to conduct comparisons, it should be noted that the traditional hierarchical analysis process does not fully reflect the human thinking style. In other words, the use of fuzzy sets has a better compatibility with human verbal descriptions and sometimes ambiguous expressions, and therefore, it is better to use fuzzy sets (employing fuzzy numbers) for long-term prediction and decision-making in the real world. In 1983, two Dutch researchers named Lahdelma and Pedrycz proposed a method for fuzzy hierarchical analysis process based on the logarithmic least squares method. The complexity of the steps in this method prevented it from being widely used. In 1996, another method called "developmental analysis method" was introduced by Chang. The numbers used in this method are fuzzy triangular numbers [40].

Concepts and definitions of the Fuzzy Hierarchical Analysis Process, based on the Development Analysis Method, are as follows:

- Fuzzy Set Theory: A mathematical concept that deals with sets that have degrees of membership between 0 and 1, allowing for a more flexible and nuanced approach to data analysis.
- Fuzzy Number: A number in which the degree of membership in a set is described by a membership function.
- Fuzzy Linguistic Variable: A variable whose values are described using linguistic terms, rather than numerical values.
- Fuzzy Linguistic Scale: A scale that uses linguistic terms to describe the degree of importance or preference of a variable.
- Fuzzy Hierarchical Analysis Process: A decision-making process that involves breaking down a complex problem into a hierarchy of sub-problems and evaluating the importance of each sub-problem using fuzzy linguistic variables and scales.
- Development Analysis Method: A specific approach to the fuzzy hierarchical analysis process that uses triangular fuzzy numbers and a set of linguistic variables to describe the degree of importance of each sub-problem.

In the Analytic Hierarchy Process (AHP) method, for each row of the pairwise comparison matrix, the value, which is a triangular number itself, is calculated using Eq. (4).

$$S_k = \sum_{j=1}^{n} M_{kj} * \left[\sum_{i=1}^{m} \sum_{j=1}^{n} M_{ij} \right]^{-1}$$

In equation, K represents the row number, and i and j represent the options and indices, respectively.

In the developmental analysis approach, after calculating the SKs, their degree of superiority over each other should be determined. Generally, if M_1 and M_2 are two fuzzy triangular numbers, the degree of superiority of M_1 over M_2, denoted by $V(M_1 \geq M_2)$, is defined as the following equation:

$$\begin{cases} V(M_1 \geq M_2) = 1 & if\ m_1 \geq m_2 \\ V(M_1 \geq M_2) = hgt(M_1 \cap M_2) & otherwise \end{cases}$$

We also have:

$$hgt(M_1 \cap M_2) = \frac{u_1 - l_2}{(u_1 - l_2) + (m_2 - m_1)}$$

The greater magnitude of a fuzzy triangular number compared to K other fuzzy triangular numbers can also be obtained from the following equation:

$$V(M_1 \geq M_2, \ldots, M_K) = V(M_1 \geq M_2), \ldots, V(M_1 \geq M_K)$$

The following formula is used to calculate the weight of criteria in a pairwise comparison matrix:

$$W'(x_i) = Min\{V(S_i \geq S_k)\}, \quad k = 1, 2, \ldots, n, \ k \neq i.$$

Therefore, the vector of weights for criteria will be as follows:

$$W'(x_i) = \left[W'(c_1), W'(c_2), \ldots, W'(c_n) \right]^T$$

This is the same as the vector of normalized weights in the fuzzy analytic hierarchy process.

Using the following equation, the abnormal results obtained from the above equation become normal. The normalized results obtained from the following equation are denoted as "W", while observing the grammatical rules of English.

$$W_i = \frac{w'_1}{\sum w'_i}$$

6.2 *Fuzzy Logarithmic Least Square Method (FLLSM)*

The Fuzzy Least Squares Method is a computational method in which the parameters of a fuzzy system are calculated precisely using fuzzy logic principles and error minimization optimization. In this method, the theory of fuzzy sets is used to investigate the relationships between inputs and outputs. By defining fuzzy membership functions for input and output variables, the parameters of the fuzzy system can be optimized using optimization algorithms.

The aim of this method is to optimize the parameters of the fuzzy system with the least possible error. This method is suitable for complex and unconventional problems where traditional methods cannot provide a final solution due to their lack of accuracy and efficiency [39].

The Analytic Hierarchy Process (AHP) logic is based on the assumption that the pairwise comparison scale and the pairwise comparison matrix are compatible. If the pairwise comparison matrix is completely consistent, it can be written as:

$a_{ik} \times a_{kj} = a_{ij}$ Then:$a_{ij} = \frac{w_i}{w_j}$, a_{ij}, $w_j - w_i = e = 0$.

In operational research, assuming complete compatibility seems to be an ideal hypothetical assumption in practical environments. Therefore, we are seeking the minimum error (e). In the method of least squares, we know that MIN error occurs for the sum of errors squared, i.e., for the second moment coefficient.

$$Min\ e = \sum_{i=1}^{n}\sum_{j=1}^{n}(a_{ij},\ w_j - w_i)^2$$

$$s.t.\ \sum_{i=1}^{n} w_i = 1,\ w_i \geq 0,\ i = 1, 2, \ldots, n.$$

According to the method of least squares in logarithmic form, MIN error occurs as follows:

$$Min\ e = \sum_{i=1}^{n}\sum_{j=1}^{n}(Loga_{ij} - \log\left(\frac{w_i}{wj}\right))^2$$

$$s.t.\ \sum_{i=1}^{n} w_i = 1,\ w_i \geq 0,\ i = 1, 2, \ldots, n.$$

There are two types of methods for extracting weights from pairwise fuzzy comparisons in operations research. The first type of method involves weights that are obtained as real numbers, such as the FPP method and the LFPP method. The second type of method involves weights that are extracted as fuzzy numbers, including the LAMBDA-Max method, the fuzzy ideal method, and the fuzzy logarithmic least squares method.

The fuzzy logarithmic least squares method is capable of extracting weights from a group pairwise comparison matrix (Table 6) by solving the following nonlinear programming problem:

$$\begin{cases} Min\ \ J = \sum_{i=1}^{n}\sum_{\substack{j=1\\ j\neq i}}^{n}\sum_{k=1}^{e_{ij}} \begin{pmatrix} (Ln\ w_i^L - Ln\ w_i^U - Ln\ a_{ijk}^L)^2 \\ +(Ln\ w_i^M - Ln\ w_i^M - Ln\ a_{ijk}^M)^2 \\ +(Ln\ w_i^U - Ln\ w_i^L - Ln\ a_{ijk}^U)^2 \end{pmatrix} \\ Subject\ to: \begin{Bmatrix} w_i^L + \sum_{j=1, j\neq i}^{n} w_j^U \geq 1, \\ w_i^U + \sum_{j=1, j\neq i}^{n} w_j^L \leq 1, \\ \sum_{i=1}^{n} w_i^M \geq 1, \\ \sum_{i=1}^{n} (w_i^L + w_i^U) \geq 2, \\ w_i^U \geq w_i^M \geq w_i^L \geq 0, i = 1, 2, .., n \end{Bmatrix} \end{cases}$$

The limitations imposed in the fuzzy method as opposed to the non-fuzzy method are aimed at normalizing the output fuzzy weights of the model.

Table 6 Fuzzy pairwise group comparison

Criteria	Criteria 1	Criteria 2	…	Criteria n
Criteria 1	(1, 1, 1)	$\begin{Bmatrix} (l_{121}, m_{121}, u_{121}) \\ (l_{12e_{12}}, m_{12e_{12}}, u_{12e_{12}}) \end{Bmatrix}$	…	$\begin{Bmatrix} (l_{1n1}, m_{1n1}, u_{1n1}) \\ (l_{1ne_{1n}}, m_{1ne_{1n}}, u_{1ne_{1n}}) \end{Bmatrix}$
Criteria 2	$\begin{Bmatrix} (l_{211}, m_{211}, u_{211}) \\ (l_{21e_{21}}, m_{21e_{21}}, u_{21e_{21}}) \end{Bmatrix}$	(1, 1, 1)	…	$\begin{Bmatrix} (l_{2n1}, m_{2n1}, u_{2n1}) \\ (l_{2ne_{1n}}, m_{2ne_{1n}}, u_{2ne_{1n}}) \end{Bmatrix}$
…	…	…	…	…
Criteria n	$\begin{Bmatrix} (l_{n11}, m_{n11}, u_{n11}) \\ (l_{n1e_{n1}}, m_{n1e_{n1}}, u_{n1e_{n1}}) \end{Bmatrix}$	$\begin{Bmatrix} (l_{n21}, m_{n21}, u_{n21}) \\ (l_{n2e_{n2}}, m_{n2e_{n2}}, u_{n2e_{n2}}) \end{Bmatrix}$	…	(1, 1, 1)

$$\begin{cases} Min\ J = \sum_{i=1}^{6} \sum_{\substack{j=1 \\ j \neq i}}^{6} \sum_{k=1}^{5} \begin{pmatrix} (Ln\, w_i^L - Ln\, w_i^U - Ln\, a_{ijk}^L)^2 + (Ln\, w_i^M - Ln\, w_i^M - Ln\, a_{ijk}^M)^2 \\ +(Ln\, w_i^U - Ln\, w_i^L - Ln\, a_{ijk}^U)^2 \end{pmatrix} \\ Subject\ to: \begin{Bmatrix} w_i^L + \sum_{j=1, j\neq i}^{n} w_j^U \geq 1, \\ w_i^U + \sum_{j=1, j\neq i}^{n} w_j^L \leq 1, \\ \sum_{i=1}^{n} w_i^M \geq 1, \\ \sum_{i=1}^{n} (w_i^L + w_i^U) \geq 2, \\ w_i^U \geq w_i^M \geq w_i^L \geq 0, i = 1, 2, .., 6 \end{Bmatrix} \end{cases}$$

For the above pairwise comparison matrix, there exists a triangular fuzzy normalized weighted matrix.

$$\tilde{W} = (\tilde{w}_1, ..., \tilde{w}_n)^T = ((w_1^L, w_1^M, w_1^U), ..., (w_n^L, w_n^M, w_n^U))^T$$

$$\tilde{a}_{ijk} = (l_{ijk}, m_{ijk}, u_{ijk}) \approx \tilde{w}_i/\tilde{w}_j \approx (w_i^L/w_j^U, w_i^M/w_j^M, w_i^U/w_j^L),$$
$$i, j = 1, ..., n; \quad i \neq j, \quad k = 1, ..., \delta_{ij}.$$

One can use the logarithm of the least squares method to determine the fuzzy weight vector ˜W of the fuzzy model.

$$Min\ J = \sum_{i=1}^{n} \sum_{\substack{j=1 \\ j\neq i}}^{n} \sum_{k=1}^{\delta_{ij}} \begin{pmatrix} (Ln\ w_i^L - Ln\ w_i^U - Ln\ a_{ijk}^L)^2 \\ +(Ln\ w_i^M - Ln\ w_i^M - Ln\ a_{ijk}^M)^2 \\ +(Ln\ w_i^U - Ln\ w_i^L - Ln\ a_{ijk}^U)^2 \end{pmatrix}$$

Let $\frac{\partial J}{\partial w_i^L} = 0, \frac{\partial J}{\partial w_i^M} = 0, \frac{\partial J}{\partial w_i^U} = 0$ for $i = 1, 2, ..., n$. It follows that

$$\frac{\partial J}{\partial w_i^L} = \frac{2}{\partial w_i^L} \sum_{\substack{j=1 \\ j \neq i}}^{n} \sum_{k=1}^{\delta_{ij}} \left(Ln\, w_i^L - Ln\, w_i^U - Ln\, a_{ijk}^L\right)$$

$$= \frac{2}{\partial w_i^L}\left[(Ln\, w_i^L)\sum_{\substack{j=1\\ j\neq i}}^{n}\delta_{ij} - \sum_{\substack{j=1\\ j\neq i}}^{n}\delta_{ij}\left(Ln\, w_i^U\right) - \sum_{\substack{j=1\\ j\neq i}}^{n}\sum_{k=1}^{\delta_{ij}}\left(Ln\, a_{ijk}^L\right)\right],$$

$i = 1, \ldots, n.$

$$\frac{\partial J}{\partial w_i^M} = \frac{2}{\partial w_i^M}\sum_{\substack{j=1\\ j\neq i}}^{n}\sum_{k=1}^{\delta_{ij}}\left(Ln\, w_i^M - Ln\, w_i^M - Ln\, a_{ijk}^M\right)$$

$$= \frac{2}{\partial w_i^M}\left[(Ln\, w_i^M)\sum_{\substack{j=1\\ j\neq i}}^{n}\delta_{ij} - \sum_{\substack{j=1\\ j\neq i}}^{n}\delta_{ij}\left(Ln\, w_i^M\right) - \sum_{\substack{j=1\\ j\neq i}}^{n}\sum_{k=1}^{\delta_{ij}}\left(Ln\, a_{ijk}^M\right)\right],$$

$i = 1, \ldots, n.$

$$\frac{\partial J}{\partial w_i^U} = \frac{2}{\partial w_i^U}\sum_{\substack{j=1\\ j\neq i}}^{n}\sum_{k=1}^{\delta_{ij}}\left(Ln\, w_i^U - Ln\, w_i^L - Ln\, a_{ijk}^U\right)$$

$$= \frac{2}{\partial w_i^U}\left[(Ln\, w_i^U)\sum_{\substack{j=1\\ j\neq i}}^{n}\delta_{ij} - \sum_{\substack{j=1\\ j\neq i}}^{n}\delta_{ij}\left(Ln\, w_i^L\right) - \sum_{\substack{j=1\\ j\neq i}}^{n}\sum_{k=1}^{\delta_{ij}}\left(Ln\, a_{ijk}^U\right)\right],$$

$i = 1, \ldots, n.$

The above can be rewritten as follows for determining the fuzzy weight vector ˜W of the fuzzy model using the logarithm of the least squares method:

$$l_i\left(\sum_{j=1, j\neq i}^{n}\delta_{ij}\right) - \sum_{j=1, j\neq i}^{n}\delta_{ij}u_j = \sum_{j=1, j\neq i}^{n}\sum_{k=1}^{\delta_{ij}}\left(Ln\, a_{ijk}^L\right), \quad i = 1, \ldots, n.$$

$$m_i\left(\sum_{j=1, j\neq i}^{n}\delta_{ij}\right) - \sum_{j=1, j\neq i}^{n}\delta_{ij}m_j = \sum_{j=1, j\neq i}^{n}\sum_{k=1}^{\delta_{ij}}\left(Ln\, a_{ijk}^M\right), \quad i = 1, \ldots, n.$$

$$u_i\left(\sum_{j=1,j\neq i}^{n}\delta_{ij}\right)-\sum_{j=1,j\neq i}^{n}\delta_{ij}l_j=\sum_{j=1,j\neq i}^{n}\sum_{k=1}^{\delta_{ij}}\left(Ln\,a_{ijk}^{U}\right),\quad i=1,\ldots,n.$$

where $l_i = \ln w_i^l$, $m_i = \ln w_i^m$, and $u_i = \ln w_i^u$. Considering the reciprocal nature of the judgment elements in the above equations, some sections are equal to zero and therefore linearly dependent. This also applies to the following equation:

$$m_i\left(\sum_{j=1,j\neq i}^{n}\delta_{ij}\right)-\sum_{j=1,j\neq i}^{n}\delta_{ij}m_j=\sum_{j=1,j\neq i}^{n}\sum_{k=1}^{\delta_{ij}}\left(Ln\,a_{ijk}^{M}\right),\quad i=1,\ldots,n.$$

$$u_i\left(\sum_{j=1,j\neq i}^{n}\delta_{ij}\right)-\sum_{j=1,j\neq i}^{n}\delta_{ij}l_j=\sum_{j=1,j\neq i}^{n}\sum_{k=1}^{\delta_{ij}}\left(Ln\,a_{ijk}^{U}\right),\quad i=1,\ldots,n.$$

Finding the three numbers (I, M, U) subject to the condition of a power between one and infinity in the solutions of the first and third equations is hidden in the previous step and can be normalized using the following method:

$$\tilde{w}_i \approx (\exp(l_i+p_1), \exp(m_i+p_2), \exp(u_i+p_1)),\quad i=1,\ldots,n$$

After normalization, which was done using the above formula, we substitute the numbers into the following equation:

$$\tilde{w}_i \approx \left(\frac{\exp(l_i)}{\sum_{i=1}^{n}\exp(u_i)}, \frac{\exp(m_i)}{\sum_{i=1}^{n}\exp(m_i)}, \frac{\exp(u_i)}{\sum_{i=1}^{n}\exp(l_i)}\right),\quad i=1,\ldots,n.$$

Finally, by using the following formula, we obtain the normalized weights:

$$\tilde{w}_{Ai} \approx \sum_{j=1}^{m}\tilde{w}_j \otimes \tilde{w}_{ij} \approx \left(\sum_{j=1}^{m} w_i^L w_{ij}^L, \sum_{j=1}^{m} w_i^M w_{ij}^M, \sum_{j=1}^{m} w_i^U w_{ij}^U\right),\quad i=1,\ldots,n$$

Thus, the final weights of the indices are calculated [37].

6.3 *Location Selection of a Healthcare Center and Its Related Health Services Among Several Proposed Locations*

To accomplish this task, we need to consider some criteria for decision-making (Table 7).

A survey was conducted among 15 experts to determine the important criteria, but for the pairwise comparison matrix, five experts were selected, including two

Table 7 Criteria for location selection

Criterion	Definition
Accessibility (C_1)	Access to public transportation (taxi and bus)
Safety (C_2)	Safety of the location from accidents, theft, and vandalism
Proximity to the bank (C_3)	For performing tasks that require physical presence at the bank
Proximity to customers (C_4)	Distance of customers to the location
Parking (C_5)	Proximity of public parking to the location or the possibility of parking near the location

Table 8 Relationship between linguistic variables and fuzzy rankings

Linguistic variables	Fuzzy rankings		
VL	0	0	0.2
L	0.1	0.2	0.3
ML	0.2	0.3	0.5
M	0.4	0.5	0.6
MH	0.5	0.65	0.8
H	0.7	0.8	0.9
VH	0.8	1	1

managers of healthcare and service centers who had more work experience. After identifying the decision-makers, the linguistic variables in Table 8 were used to obtain the decision matrix for each decision-maker. Tables 9 and 10 are provided as an example for the first decision-maker. A scale of 0–10 was used to fuzzy the rankings of the criteria and options.

After writing the code for calculating weights based on the logarithmic least squares method and entering it into the Lingua software, the results are summarized for five expert decision-makers in Table 11 (Table 12).

Table 9 The linguistic variables of decision maker (1)

Location	Accessibility	Safety	Proximity to the bank	Proximity to customers	Parking
1	L	VL	L	M	M
2	ML	MH	VL	L	L
3	H	VH	H	M	M
4	H	M	MH	L	VL
5	M	MH	M	L	VL
6	H	MH	H	L	VL

Table 10 Converting linguistic variables to fuzzy numbers for decision-making (1)

Location	Criteria														
	Accessibility			Safety			Proximity to the bank			Proximity to customers			Parking		
1	0.1	0.2	0.3	0	0	0.2	0.1	0.2	0.3	0.4	0.5	0.6	0.4	0.5	0.6
2	0.2	0.35	0.5	0.5	0.65	0.8	0	0	0.2	0.1	0.2	0.3	0.1	0.2	0.3
3	0.7	0.8	0.9	0.8	0.9	1	0.7	0.8	0.9	0.4	0.5	0.6	0.4	0.5	0.6
4	0.7	0.8	0.9	0.4	0.5	0.6	0.5	0.65	0.8	0.1	0.2	0.3	0	0	0.2
5	0.4	0.5	0.6	0.5	0.65	0.8	0.4	0.5	0.6	0.1	0.2	0.3	0	0	0.2
6	0.7	0.8	0.9	0.2	0.35	0.5	0.7	0.8	0.9	0.1	0.2	0.3	0	0	0.2

A small part of the code is provided below as an example:

$$
\begin{aligned}
Min = {} & ((\log(w_{11}) - \log(w_{23}) - \log(1))^2) + ((\log(w_{12}) - \log(w_{22}) - \log(2))^2) \\
& + ((\log(w_{13}) - \log(w_{21}) - \log(3))^2) + ((\log(w_{11}) - \log(w_{23}) - \log(1))^2) \\
& + ((\log(w_{11}) - \log(w_{22}) - \log(1))^2) + ((\log(w_{13}) - \log(w_{21}) - \log(1))^2) \\
& + ((\log(w_{11}) - \log(w_{23}) - \log(1))^2) + ((\log(w_{12}) - \log(w_{22}) - \log(1))^2) \\
& + ((\log(w_{13}) - \log(w_{21}) - \log(1))^2) + ((\log(w_{11}) - \log(w_{23}) - \log(0.33))^2) \\
& + ((\log(w_{12}) - \log(w_{22}) - \log(0.5))^2) + ((\log(w_{13}) - \log(w_{21}) - \log(1))^2) \\
& + ((\log(w_{11}) - \log(w_{23}) - \log(0.33))^2) + ((\log(w_{12}) - \log(w_{22}) - \log(0.5))^2) \\
& + ((\log(w_{13}) - \log(w_{21}) - \log(1))^2) + ((\log(w_{11}) - \log(w_{33}) - \log(3))^2) \\
& + ((\log(w_{12}) - \log(w_{32}) - \log(4))^2) + ((\log(w_{13}) - \log(w_{31}) - \log(5))^2) + \cdots
\end{aligned}
$$

Step 2: Constructing the Preference Matrix and Multi-Criteria Preference List.

In this step, based on the fuzzy preference function, we construct a pairwise comparison matrix for each criterion separately (Tables 13, 14, 15, 16 and 17). For each criterion (C_j), a squared preference matrix (P_i) is formed where alternatives are compared pairwise (P_{ij}) based on criterion C_j.

In each preference matrix (P_i), the diagonal elements are set to 1 since an alternative is equal to itself. The upper triangular elements ($P_{ij}, i < j$) represent the preference degree of alternative i over alternative j based on criterion C_j, while the lower triangular elements ($P_{ij}, i > j$) represent the preference degree of alternative j over alternative i based on criterion C_j. Since the preference function is fuzzy, the values in the preference matrix are not crisp but rather represent the degree of preference.

Once all preference matrices are constructed, we can form a multi-criteria preference list by aggregating the preferences across all criteria. There are different methods for aggregating the preferences, such as weighted summation, weighted product, and others. The choice of the aggregation method depends on the decision-maker's preferences and the decision context.

Table 11 Fuzzy weights of criteria using FLLSM for experts

Criteria	Accessibility			Safety			Proximity to the bank			Proximity to customers			Parking		
Weight	W_{11}	W_{12}	W_{13}	W_{21}	W_{22}	W_{23}	W_{31}	W_{32}	W_{33}	W_{41}	W_{42}	W_{43}	W_{51}	W_{52}	W_{53}
DM1	0.09	0.17	0.30	0.29	0.42	0.54	0.47	0.58	0.70	0.47	0.59	0.72	0.63	0.72	0.83
DM2	0.08	0.14	0.30	0.30	0.42	0.55	0.47	0.58	0.68	0.41	0.54	0.66	0.45	0.52	0.65
DM3	0.07	0.13	0.30	0.32	0.44	0.56	0.49	0.59	0.70	0.46	0.58	0.70	0.38	0.45	0.58
DM4	0.05	0.09	0.26	0.28	0.40	0.51	0.45	0.55	0.65	0.39	0.51	0.64	0.43	0.50	0.63
DM5	0.06	0.11	0.27	0.26	0.37	0.49	0.46	0.56	0.67	0.44	0.57	0.70	0.52	0.60	0.72

Table 12 Formation of the comprehensive decision matrix

Criteria	Accessibility			Safety			Proximity to the bank			Proximity to customers			Parking		
1	0.58	0.68	0.78	0.20	0.28	0.40	0.26	0.34	0.46	0.46	0.58	0.70	0.42	0.53	0.64
2	0.24	0.38	0.52	0.38	0.49	0.64	0.06	0.11	0.28	0.18	0.29	0.40	0.34	0.44	0.54
3	0.72	0.82	0.92	0.66	0.77	0.88	0.66	0.77	0.88	0.40	0.50	0.60	0.50	0.61	0.72
4	0.42	0.51	0.64	0.34	0.44	0.54	0.38	0.50	0.62	0.46	0.58	0.70	0.28	0.36	0.52
5	0.40	0.50	0.60	0.42	0.56	0.70	0.48	0.59	0.70	0.26	0.38	0.50	0.36	0.43	0.58
6	0.40	0.53	0.66	0.30	0.44	0.58	0.50	0.61	0.72	0.30	0.41	0.52	0.24	0.30	0.44
Weight	0.07	0.13	0.29	0.29	0.41	0.53	0.47	0.57	0.68	0.43	0.56	0.68	0.48	0.56	0.68

Table 13 Fuzzy preference matrix for the measure of easy access to public transportation

Accessibility	A_1			A_2			A_3			A_4			A_5			A_6		
A_1	0	0	0	−0.20	0.26	0.15	0	0	0	0	0	0	0.07	0.13	0.33	−0.19	0.04	0.27
A_2	0	0	0	0	0	0	0	0	0	0	0	0	0	0	0	0	0	0
A_3	−0.02	0.18	0.38	−0.02	0.45	0.69	0	0	0	−0.07	0.15	0.53	0.12	0.32	0.52	0	0.22	0.45
A_4	0.32	0.08	−0.15	0.39	0.17	0.03	0	0	0	0	0	0	−0.03	0.17	0.39	−0.15	0.08	0.32
A_5	0	0	0	−0.33	0.13	0.37	0	0	0	0	0	0	0	0	0	0	0	0
A_6	0	0	0	−0.27	0.22	0.49	0	0	0	0	0	0	−0.13	0.09	0.32	0	0	0

Table 14 Fuzzy preference matrix for safety measure

Safety	A_1			A_2			A_3			A_4			A_5			A_6		
A_1	0	0	0	0	0	0	0	0	0	0	0	0	0	0	0	0	0	0
A_2	−0.06	0.17	0.04	0	0	0	0	0	0	0	0	0	0	0	0	0	0	0
A_3	0.37	0.60	0.78	0.37	0.43	0.64	0	0	0	0.17	0.38	0.59	−0.03	0.22	0.47	0.15	0.41	0.65
A_4	−0.01	0.22	0.39	−0.01	0.05	0.25	0	0	0	0	0	0	0	0	0	−0.22	0.03	0.26
A_5	0.12	0.36	0.06	0.12	0.22	0.46	0	0	0	−0.08	0.17	0.41	0	0	0	−0.10	0.20	0.47
A_6	−0.07	0.19	0.41	−0.07	0.02	0.27	0	0	0	0	0	0	0	0	0	0	0	0

Table 15 Fuzzy preference matrix for the measure of proximity to the operating bank

Proximity to the bank	A_1			A_2			A_3			A_4			A_5			A_6		
A_1	0	0	0	0	0	0	0	0	0	0	0	0	0	0	0	0	0	0
A_2	−0.36	0.08	0.12	0	0	0	0	0	0	0	0	0	0	0	0	0	0	0
A_3	0.48	0.60	0.77	0.19	0.37	0.46	0	0	0	0.15	0.18	0.69	−0.15	0.06	0.14	0.08	0.04	0.16
A_4	−0.09	0.12	0.19	−0.11	0.25	0.36	0	0	0	0	0	0	0	0	0	−0.22	0.23	0.36
A_5	0.18	0.36	0.46	0.17	0.34	0.65	0	0	0	−0.18	0.27	0.37	0	0	0	−0.29	0.34	0.57
A_6	−0.34	0.38	0.52	−0.05	0.02	0.07	0	0	0	0	0	0	0	0	0	0	0	0

Table 16 Fuzzy preference matrix for the customer proximity criterion to the office

Proximity to customers	A_1			A_2			A_3			A_4			A_5			A_6		
A_1	0	0	0	−0.24	0.27	0.50	0.17	0.05	0.27	0	0	0	−0.08	0.16	0.40	−0.04	0.19	0.42
A_2	0	0	0	0	0	0	0	0	0	0	0	0	0	0	0	0	0	0
A_3	0	0	0	0.27	0.22	0.43	0	0	0	0	0	0	−0.11	0.11	0.33	−0.07	0.14	0.35
A_4	−0.23	0.01	0.24	0.23	0.28	0.50	−0.16	0.05	0.27	0	0	0	−0.07	0.17	0.40	−0.03	0.19	0.42
A_5	0	0	0	0.40	0.11	0.34	0	0	0	0	0	0	0	0	0	−0.20	0.03	0.26
A_6	0	0	0	−0.42	0.08	0.30	0	0	0	0	0	0	0	0	0	0	0	0

Table 17 Fuzzy preference matrix for the parking criterion

Parking	A_1			A_2			A_3			A_4			A_5			A_6		
A_1	0	0	0	−0.21	0.07	0.28	0	0	0	−0.11	0.51	0.32	−0.08	0.18	0.37	0.01	0.27	0.34
A_2	0	0	0	0	0	0	0	0	0	−0.18	0.08	0.24	−0.15	0.11	0.29	−0.05	0.19	0.35
A_3	−0.14	0.07	0.28	−0.14	0.13	0.35	0	0	0	−0.04	0.22	0.39	−0.01	0.25	0.43	0.08	0.33	0.50
A_4	0	0	0	0	0	0	0	0	0	0	0	0	−0.19	0.03	0.26	−0.10	0.11	0.32
A_5	0	0	0	0	0	0	0	0	0	0	0	0	0	0	0	−0.14	0.08	0.30
A_6	0	0	0	0	0	0	0	0	0	0	0	0	0	0	0	0	0	0

Step 3: Formation of the Overall Preference Matrix (π).

In this step, you should create the overall preference matrix (π) by using the fuzzy preference matrices of different criteria and their respective weights. To do so, you need to consider the weight of each criterion first, multiply each fuzzy preference matrix by its weight, and then sum up the results. Finally, you can calculate the overall preference matrix (π) using the following formula:

$$\pi = W_1 \times F_1 + W_2 \times F_2 + \cdots + W_n \times F_n$$

In this formula, π represents the overall preference matrix, while W_1 to W_n are the weights assigned to each criterion and F_1 to F_n are the fuzzy preference matrices corresponding to each criterion (Table 18).

Step 4: Calculation of Fuzzy Flows [$\tilde{\phi}+$ (Phase 1) and $\tilde{\phi}-$ (Phase 2)] for Pre-Ranking Alternatives.

In step 4, you need to calculate the fuzzy flows $\tilde{\phi}+$ and $\tilde{\phi}-$ for pre-ranking the alternatives. These flows are obtained from the previous step (step 3). To calculate the fuzzy flow $\tilde{\phi}+$, you need to use the overall preference matrix.

(π) and calculate the flow $\tilde{\phi}+$ using the following formula:

$$\tilde{\phi}+ = \pi \times A$$

In this formula, A is the normalization matrix obtained by dividing each column of the overall preference matrix by the sum of values in that column. To calculate the fuzzy flow $\tilde{\phi}-$, you need to use the normalization matrix A and calculate the flow M using the following formula:

$$\tilde{\phi}- = A \times \pi$$

In this formula, π is the overall preference matrix obtained in step 3, using these fuzzy flows, you can pre-rank the alternatives and choose the best one (Table 19).

Step 5: Calculating the net flow $\tilde{\phi}$.

In step 5, you need to calculate the net flow for each alternative. The net flow consists of two parts: the fuzzy flow and the weight associated with each criterion. The fuzzy flow ($\tilde{\phi}+$ or $\tilde{\phi}-$) in each row is multiplied by the weight associated with that criterion, and the sum of these products is the net flow for that alternative. To calculate the net flow for each alternative, you first need to calculate the weight associated with each criterion. For this, you use the relative weight matrix obtained in step 2. Then, for each alternative, the fuzzy flow $\tilde{\phi}+$ or $\tilde{\phi}-$ (depending on the previous stage) is multiplied in each row, and the sum of these products is the fuzzy flow net for that criterion. This operation is performed for all criteria, and the sum of the fuzzy net flows for the alternative is the final net flow for that alternative.

Table 18 The overall preference matrix

π	A_1			A_2			A_3			A_4			A_5			A_6	
A_1	0	0	0	−0.31	0.33	0.90	−0.07	0.03	0.18	−0.05	0.08	0.22	−0.08	0.21	0.62	−0.02	0.26
A_2	−0.02	0.07	0.21	0	0	0	0	0	0	−0.08	0.04	0.17	−0.07	0.06	0.19	−0.02	0.11
A_3	0.18	0.61	1.20	0.06	0.84	1.67	0	0	0	0.05	0.46	1.02	0.05	0.46	1.21	0.01	0.53
A_4	−0.11	0.24	0.76	−0.11	0.46	1.21	0.07	0.03	0.18	0	0	0	−0.12	0.13	0.56	−0.13	0.19
A_5	0.07	0.33	0.65	−0.13	0.44	1.16	0	0	0	−0.11	0.10	0.41	0	0	0	−0.18	0.14
A_6	0.07	0.31	0.63	−0.13	0.42	1.15	0	0	0	−0.03	0.09	0.26	−0.06	0.08	0.31	0	0

Table 19 Calculation of Fuzzy Flows $\tilde{\phi}+$ and $\tilde{\phi}-$

$\tilde{\phi}^{+}(a)$			$\tilde{\phi}^{-}(a)$		
−0.54	0.91	2.58	0.20	1.56	3.45
−0.20	0.28	0.81	−0.61	2.49	6.09
0.25	2.89	6.37	−0.14	0.06	0.37
−0.54	1.06	3.45	−0.22	0.78	2.08
−0.34	1.01	2.85	−0.38	0.94	2.91
−0.14	0.91	2.35	−0.36	1.23	3.52

Table 20 Calculating the net flow

$\tilde{\phi}(a)$		
−4	−0/66	2/38
−6/29	−2/21	1/43
−0/12	2/84	6/51
−2/62	0/28	3/67
−3/25	0/07	3/23
−3/66	−0/32	2/71

Finally, by calculating the net flow for all alternatives, you can choose the best alternative. The net flow is calculated using the following formula (Table 20):

$$\tilde{\phi}_1 = (\tilde{\phi}_1+) - (\tilde{\phi}_1-)$$

Step 6: Defuzzification and Ranking of Alternatives

Given that the output of step 5 is in the form of fuzzy numbers, in order to determine the ranking of each alternative, fuzzy numbers must be converted to crisp numbers. Defuzzification is one of the simplest methods that can be obtained using the $\frac{l+4m+u}{6}$ relationship. In this study, part of the Chang's development analysis method has been used. Then, to determine the degree of possibility of each option, we select the minimum number of each column. To determine the weights of the options, we divide each element of the possibility degree row by the sum of the possibility degree row (Table 21).

Therefore, ***location3* > *location4* > *location5* > *location6* > *location1* > *location2.***

Table 21 Defuzzification and ranking of alternatives

A_6	A_5	A_4	A_3	A_2	A_1	
1	1	1	1	0.78	1	A_1
1	1	1	1	1	1	A_2
0.47	0.55	0.60	1	0.23	0.42	A_3
0.90	0.96	1	1	0.62	0.84	A_4
0.94	1	1	1	0.67	0.89	A_5
1	1	1	1	0.73	0.95	A_6
0.47	0.55	0.60	1	0.23	0.42	Possibility degree
0.14	0.17	0.18	0.31	0.07	0.13	Weight
4	3	2	1	6	5	Rank

References

1. Abbasbandy, S., Viranloo, T.A.: Numerical solution of fuzzy differential equation. Math. Comput. Appl. **7**(1), 41–52 (2002). https://doi.org/10.3390/mca7010041
2. Abbasi, F., Allahviranloo, T.: The fuzzy arithmetic operations of transmission average on Pseudo-Hexagonal fuzzy numbers and its application in fuzzy system reliability analysis. Fuzzy Inf. Eng. **13**(1), 58–78 (2021). https://doi.org/10.1080/16168658.2021.1915449
3. Abbasi, F., Allahviranloo, T.: Realistic solution of fuzzy critical path problems, case study: the airport's cargo ground operation systems. Granular Comput. **8**(3), 617–632 (2022). https://doi.org/10.1007/s41066-022-00347-w
4. Acar, Y., Kizilay, M.: Location-allocation models for healthcare facility planning: a systematic literature review. Ann. Oper. Res. 1–35 (2021)
5. Akram, M., Shahzadi, S., Shah, S.M.U., Allahviranloo, T.: A fully Fermatean fuzzy multi-objective transportation model using an extended DEA technique. Granular Comput. (2023). https://doi.org/10.1007/s41066-023-00399-6
6. Aksen, D., Klose, A.: Location analysis: a synthesis and survey. Eur. J. Oper. Res. **272**(2), 326–350 (2019)
7. Allahviranloo, T., Abbasi, F.: A new estimation of failure analysis in fuzzy environment, case study: the electrical model failure for the football stadium. New Math. Nat. Comput. **18**(03), 791–817 (2022). https://doi.org/10.1142/s1793005722500387
8. Allahviranloo, T., Ezadi, S.: Z-Advanced numbers processes. Inf. Sci. **480**, 130–143 (2019). https://doi.org/10.1016/j.ins.2018.12.012
9. Allahviranloo, T., Lotfi, F.H., Kiasari, M.K., Khezerloo, M.: On the fuzzy solution of LR fuzzy linear systems. Appl. Math. Model. **37**(3), 1170–1176 (2013). https://doi.org/10.1016/j.apm.2012.03.037
10. Amini, M., Saidi-Mehrabad, M., Mehrabi, A., Kazemi, Z.: Facility location in healthcare: a comprehensive review. Comput. Ind. Eng. **139**, 105650 (2020)
11. Amirteimoori, A., Allahviranloo, T., Kordrostami, S., Bagheri, S.F.: Improving decision-making units in performance analysis methods: a data envelopment analysis approach. Math. Sci. (2023). https://doi.org/10.1007/s40096-023-00512-5
12. Amirteimoori, A., Allahviranloo, T., Zadmirzaei, M.: Scale elasticity and technical efficiency analysis in the European forest sector: a stochastic value-based approach. Eur. J. Forest Res. (2023). https://doi.org/10.1007/s10342-023-01589-2
13. Amirteimoori, A., Allahviranloo, T., Zadmirzaei, M., Hasanzadeh, F.: On the environmental performance analysis: a combined fuzzy data envelopment analysis and artificial intelligence algorithms. Expert Syst. Appl. **224**, 119953 (2023). https://doi.org/10.1016/j.eswa.2023.119953

14. Ashtiani, B., Gholamian, M.R.: A hybrid fuzzy AHP-TOPSIS framework for assessment of hospital location selection: a case study. Health Care Manage. Sci. **16**(2), 150–164 (2013)
15. Banaeian, N., Mobini, M.: Fuzzy multi-criteria decision-making approaches for facility location selection: a review. Comput. Ind. Eng. **94**, 196–215 (2016)
16. Boran, F.E.: An integrated intuitionistic multi criteria decision making method for facility location selection. Math. Comput. Appl. **16**(2), 487–496 (2011)
17. Bostel, N., Karimi, B.: Facility location in healthcare: a comprehensive review. Ann. Oper. Res. **280**(1–2), 485–519 (2019)
18. Chehlabi, M., Allahviranloo, T.: Concreted solutions to fuzzy linear fractional differential equations. Appl. Soft Comput. **44**, 108–116 (2016). https://doi.org/10.1016/j.asoc.2016.03.011
19. Current, J.R., Min, H.: A review of the global facility location literature: state-of-the-art and future research directions. Eur. J. Oper. Res. **269**(2), 401–412 (2018)
20. Çelik, M.: A fuzzy multi-criteria decision-making approach for the selection of healthcare facility locations. J. Healthc. Eng. **5**(2), 219–238 (2014)
21. Daneshvar, S., Rezaei-Malek, M.: Sustainable healthcare facility location selection using fuzzy TOPSIS and VIKOR approaches. J. Clean. Prod. **280**, 124493 (2021)
22. Farrokhzad, M., Vahdani, B., Sadjadi, S.J.: A novel healthcare facility location-allocation model for supporting sustainable healthcare services. J. Clean. Prod. **208**, 1410–1428 (2019)
23. Fernández, E., Pelegrín, B., Pérez, G.: Location–allocation models for supply chain network design: a literature review. Eur. J. Ind. Eng. **14**(2), 209–252 (2020)
24. Govindan, K., Khodaverdi, R., Jafarian, A.: A fuzzy multi criteria approach for measuring sustainability performance of a supplier based on triple bottom line approach. J. Clean. Prod. **47**, 345–354 (2013)
25. Gupta, S., Misra, R.B.: Decision-making in healthcare facility location selection using fuzzy AHP and fuzzy TOPSIS. J. Model. Manage. **13**(3), 776–797 (2018)
26. Hadi-Vencheh, A., Chakhar, S., Torabi, S.A., Tavana, M.: Sustainable healthcare facility location: a dynamic multi-objective approach. Eur. J. Oper. Res. **259**(2), 626–640 (2017)
27. Hansen, P., Peeters, D.: Fifty years of location analysis: a review. Eur. J. Oper. Res. **262**(1), 1–35 (2017)
28. Hu, C.: Applying fuzzy multi criteria decision making for evaluating ERP system development methods and implementation strategies. Institute of Information Management, IShou University (2006)
29. Khan, M.A., Zain, S., Rehman, S.U.: A systematic literature review of facility location decisions: a focus on healthcare facility location. Eur. J. Oper. Res. **241**(2), 273–285 (2015)
30. Kumar, S., Kaur, R., Sangwan, K.S.: A review on healthcare facility location and resource allocation using meta-heuristic techniques. Comput. Mater. Continua **63**(3), 1593–1610 (2020)
31. Li, M.X., Huang, G.H.: Fuzzy-based facility location selection for healthcare waste disposal under sustainability and environmental risks. J. Clean. Prod. **229**, 1024–1035 (2019)
32. Mahmoodirad, A., Allahviranloo, T., Niroomand, S.: A new effective solution method for fully intuitionistic fuzzy transportation problem. Soft. Comput. **23**(12), 4521–4530 (2019). https://doi.org/10.1007/s00500-018-3115-z
33. Mohammadi, M., Dehnavi-Arani, A.: Location-allocation of healthcare centers considering the preferences of the served population and government. Comput. Ind. Eng. **149**, 106891 (2020)
34. Moloudzadeh, S., Allahviranloo, T., Darabi, P.: A new method for solving an arbitrary fully fuzzy linear system. Soft. Comput. **17**(9), 1725–1731 (2013). https://doi.org/10.1007/s00500-013-0986-x
35. Mosadeghrad, A.M., Esfahanipour, A.: An overview of location-allocation models and methods in the healthcare facility planning literature. Health Syst. **9**(4), 280–297 (2020)
36. Movahedi, M., Homayounfar, M., Fadaei, M., Soufi, M.: Ranking tehran stock exchange industries using a combined FCM-ELECTRE III-LA method. **14**(3), 173–188 (2022)
37. Movahedi, M., Homayounfar, M., Fadaei, M., Soufi, M.: Developing a hybrid model for comparative analysis of financial data clustering algorithms. J. Dec. Operat. Res. **8**(2), 507–526 (2023). https://doi.org/10.22105/dmor.2022.296982.1453

38. Rahmani, A., Lotfi, F.H., Rostamy-Malkhalifeh, M., Allahviranloo, T.: A new method for defuzzification and ranking of fuzzy numbers based on the statistical beta distribution. Adv. Fuzzy Syst. **2016**, 1–8 (2016). https://doi.org/10.1155/2016/6945184
39. Safari, H., Soufi, M.: Select a hypermarket location based on fuzzy multi criteria decision making (F-MCDM) techniques (Hybrid of F-Delphi, F-AHP, F-LLSM and F-PROMTHEE). Kuwait Chap. Arab. J. Bus. Manage. Rev. **4**(1), 76–95 (2014)
40. Safari, H., Soufi, M.: Prioritize barriers of e-factories in Iran's industries with hybrid multi criteria decision. Indian J. Fundam. Appl. Life Sci. **5**(1), 1329–1344 (2015)
41. Shabanpour, H., Baboli, A., Zavadskas, E.K.: A hybrid location-allocation model for healthcare facility planning in a green supply chain under uncertainty. Sustainability **11**(13), 3713 (2019)
42. Shahmoradi, B., Pourahmad, S., Kazemi, Z.: A systematic review of healthcare facility location models. Health Care Manage. Sci. **21**(1), 1–18 (2018)
43. Soufi, M.: Factory Management and Layout Planning. Farhang-e-Ilia Ltd. (2010)
44. Wong, I.L., Chan, T.M., Wong, Y.L.: Location-allocation models in healthcare: a systematic literature review. Eur. J. Oper. Res. **264**(1), 1–35 (2018)
45. Yazdani, M., Asgharizadeh, E.: A sustainable healthcare facility location model under uncertainty: a case study of the Kerman province, Iran. Int. J. Environ. Res. Public Health **17**(14), 5244 (2020)
46. Yousefi-Babadi, A., Torabi, S.A., Amin, S.H.: A hybrid MCDM model for sustainable healthcare facility location selection considering uncertainty and interdependent criteria. Ann. Oper. Res. **283**(1–2), 1307–1343 (2019)
47. Yu, G., Huang, G.Q., Zhou, Z.: Closed-loop supply chain network design: a review. Eur. J. Oper. Res. **294**(1), 1–18 (2021)
48. Zarrinpoor, N., Sadjadi, S.J., Tavakkoli-Moghaddam, R., Vahdani, B.: An integrated fuzzy multi-objective facility location and network design model for healthcare delivery systems: a case study. Health Care Manage. Sci. **22**(2), 223–241 (2019)

Budgeting in Healthcare

S. Khajavi, M. Etemedy Jooriaby, and E. Kermani

Abstract This chapter provides a comprehensive analysis of budgeting processes in healthcare organizations as not-for-profit entities. It emphasizes the significance of financial elements such as the reinvestment rate, financing rate, present value (PV), and future value (FV) in effective budgeting. The chapter introduces the Total Net Present Value (TNPV) concept, which includes both financial Net Present Value (NPV) and Net Present Social Value (NPSV). The TNPV emphasizes the importance of project proposals to achieve a balance between financial viability and social value. The manuscript stresses the importance of transparency and accountability when creating a budget. This budget serves as a guide for obtaining donors' trust and helps make decisions for an organization. It explains the different parts of a budget, including the various revenue sources, allocation of expenditures, and direct and indirect costs. The manuscript also distinguishes between operating budgets, which show projected annual income and expenditures, and capital budgets, which cover projects with long-term effects and substantial costs. Aligning budgeting with strategic planning is emphasized as a means to help achieve organizational goals.

Keywords Budgeting · Healthcare · Signal processing · Public sector · Financial management Innovation

S. Khajavi (✉)
Faculty of Commerce and Finance, University of Tehran, Tehran, Iran
e-mail: skhajavi@ut.ac.ir

M. Etemedy Jooriaby
Department of Accounting, Bandar Anzali Branch, Islamic Azad University, Bandar Anzali, Iran

E. Kermani
Department of Accounting, Dariun Branch, Islamic Azad University, Dariun, Iran

T. Allahviranloo et al. (eds.), *Decision Making in Healthcare Systems*,
Studies in Systems, Decision and Control 513,
https://doi.org/10.1007/978-3-031-46735-6_9

1 Introduction

Two factors make the provision of medical services different from other services. First, many healthcare providers are organized as nonprofit firms. Second, payment for services is usually made by insurance companies, not by the patients receiving the services.

In today's healthcare environment where financial realities play an important role in health care decision-making, it is very important for managers at all levels to understand the basic financial concepts of healthcare services and how to use these concepts to increase the organization's financial welfare.

The main subcategories of the healthcare field include the following:

- Medical services: the service area consists of medical service providers, including medical clinics, hospitals, nursing homes, home medical service agencies, and hospice service providers.
- Health Insurance: Insurance services that make most of the payments to health care providers include government programs, commercial insurers, and self-insurers.
- Medical equipment and supplies: this subcategory includes manufacturers of diagnostic equipment such as X-ray machines; durable medical equipment such as wheelchairs; and disposable medical supplies, such as disposable surgical instruments and hypodermic syringes.
- Pharmaceuticals and Biotechnology: This subcategory produces and markets drugs and other therapeutic products.
- Other: This broad category includes organizations such as consulting firms that advise hospitals on strategy and operations, educational institutions that train health care providers and managers, government agencies that direct various subsets of health care, and private agencies that they offer a wide range of services [21].

One of the techniques for decision making is Data Envelopment Analysis (DEA), and many researchers have conducted research on this topic. Several recent papers have been cited to mention their research area [4, 6–8]. Some authors have explored the topic in a different way: safety analysis and reliability [2, 3, 5].

2 Moving from Focusing on Financial Accounting to Financial Management

Finance affairs used in healthcare organizations consists of two areas: accounting and financial management (in many environments, accounting and financial management are separate disciplines). Accounting is related to the recording of financial and economic events that reflect the performance, resources and financing of an organization. The purpose of accounting is to prepare and provide useful information about the performance and financial condition of an organization, both internally and externally, to interested parties.

While accounting provides a logical means of measuring a business's financial performance and evaluating operations, financial management provides the theory, concepts, and tools necessary to help managers make better financial decisions. Of course, the line between accounting and financial management is ambiguous. Certain aspects of accounting involve decision-making, and the application of many financial management theories and concepts requires accounting data.

The primary role of financial affairs in healthcare organizations, as in all businesses, is to plan, acquire, and use resources to maximize organizational efficiency and value. The two broad areas of finance, accounting and financial management, have separate functions in larger organizations, although the accounting function is usually conducted under the direction of the organization's chief financial officer and is therefore included in the general category of finance.

In general, financial activities include the following:

Planning and budgeting: First of all, the financing of medical services includes evaluating the financial effectiveness of current operations and planning for the future. Budget plays an important role in this process.

- Financial Reporting: For various reasons, recording and reporting the results of operations and current financial condition is very important for businesses. This is done by a set of financial statements.
- Capital investment decisions: Although capital investments are usually made by top management, managers at all levels should be concerned with the investment decision process. Decisions resulting from this process, called capital budgeting decisions, focus on the acquisition of land, buildings, and equipment. These items are the primary means by which businesses implement strategic plans and thus play a key role in the financial future of an organization.
- Financing Decisions: All organizations must raise capital to purchase assets necessary to support operations. Such decisions include choosing between domestic and foreign funds, the use of debt versus equity capital, the use of long-term versus short-term debt, and the use of lease capital versus conventional financing. Although senior managers typically make financing decisions, these decisions have implications for managers at all levels.
- Revenue cycle and current account management: Revenue cycle management includes invoicing, invoices, and receivables, while current account management includes the organization's short-term assets, such as cash and inventories, and short-term liabilities, such as accounts payable and debts. Such functions and accounts must be properly managed to ensure operational effectiveness and reduce costs. In general, managers at all levels are involved to some extent in the revenue cycle and current account management.
- Contract Management: In today's health care environment, health care organizations must negotiate contracts with national health organizations and insurance companies and monitor them after they are signed. Finance staff usually have

primary responsibility for these tasks, but managers at all levels are involved in these activities and must be aware of their impact on operational decisions.
- Financial risk management: Many financial transactions that are carried out to support the operation of a business can themselves increase the risk of the business. Therefore, an important financial activity is financial risk control.

These specific financial activities can be summarized in four categories: expenses, cash, capital and control. Measuring and minimizing costs is critical to the financial success of any business. Cash has the role of "lubricant" that makes the wheels of a business run smoothly and without it, the business would grind to a halt. Capital represents funds used to acquire land, buildings, and equipment. Without capital, businesses do not have the physical resources needed to provide goods and services. Finally, a business must have adequate control mechanisms to ensure that its capital is used wisely and that its physical resources are protected for future use [21].

At the time of high profitability and abundant financial resources, the importance of financial performance decreases. So, at a time when most healthcare providers are billing based on the costs incurred, the role of finance becomes very low. In such cases, the most important function of finance will be the identification of costs, because considering costs is more important than controlling them. In response to existing requirements, healthcare providers are generating many reports both to comply with regulations and to maximize profits. The complexity of reimbursement means that a lot of time must be spent on accounting procedures, invoicing and document collection. Therefore, instead of focusing on value-adding activities, most financial work is focused on bureaucratic functions.

Currently, financial affairs functions are much more strategic and sophisticated in understanding the changes that have occurred in the healthcare sector. Although invoicing and collections are still important, for finance to be of greatest value to a company today, it must involve a much broader set of activities, including strategy development, cost containment efforts, insurance contract negotiations, joint venture decisions, risk management and clinical integrations which must be supported. In essence, financial affairs should help guide organizations into the future rather than merely record what happened in the past.

Financial performance is emphasized here, but there is no unimportant function in healthcare organizations. Senior managers must understand many other functions such as operations, marketing, facilities management, quality improvement and human resource management in addition to financial affairs. However, all business decisions have financial implications, so all managers (whether involved in financial affairs or not) must have sufficient knowledge of financial affairs to properly consider any financial implications in the decisions they make in their areas of expertise.

3 Non-profit Organizations and Their Financial Conditions

If an organization meets a set of strict requirements, it can be eligible to change to a tax-exempt or non-profit corporation. Tax-exempt corporations are sometimes called nonprofit corporations. Because nonprofit businesses, unlike charities such as the United Way, need profits to operate, and because it is difficult to explain why nonprofits need to make profits, the term nonprofit is better suited to healthcare companies.

Examples of non-profit healthcare companies include Kaiser Permanente (https://healthy.kaiserpermanente.org), Catholic Health Initiatives (www.catholichealthinitiatives.org), and Mayoclinic (www.mayoclinic.org).

Tax-exempt status is granted to corporations that meet the tax definition of a charitable organization under Internal Revenue Service (IRS) Tax Code section 501(c)(3) or 501(c)(4). Hence, such corporations are also known as 501(c)(3) or 501(c)(4) corporations [21].

The tax law defines a charitable organization as: "any corporation, social fund, fund, or foundation organized and operated exclusively for religious, charitable, scientific, public safety, literary, or educational purposes." Because health promotion is generally considered a charitable activity, a company providing healthcare services can qualify for a tax exemption, provided it meets other conditions.

In addition to its charitable purpose, a non-profit corporation must be organized and governed in such a way that it operates exclusively for the public and not for private benefit. Therefore, no profit can be used for private gain and no direct political activity can be done. Also, if the company is dissolved or sold to an investor-owned business, the proceeds from the liquidation or sale must be used for charitable purposes. Since individuals cannot benefit from the profits of non-profit corporations, such organizations cannot pay dividends. However, the prohibition of private benefit from the organization's profit does not prevent the organization's people, such as managers and doctors, from benefiting from the benefits of salaries, pensions, contracts and etc.

Non-profit companies are significantly different from investor-owned companies. Since non-profit corporations do not have shareholders, no group of individuals has the right to own the remaining profits of the corporation or exercise control over the corporation. Instead, control is exercised by a board of trustees that is not constrained by external oversight, as is the board of directors of a for-profit corporation that must answer to shareholders. Also, non-profit corporations are generally exempt from property and income taxes and have the right to issue tax-exempt debt (municipal bonds). Finally, individual contributions to nonprofits can be deducted from taxable income by the donor, so nonprofits have access to tax-subsidized partnership capital.

For-profit corporations must file an annual income tax return with the IRS. For nonprofit corporations, IRS Form 990, titled "Exempt Organization Return," is equivalent to an annual income tax return. The purpose of this form is to provide financial information about nonprofit organizations to the IRS and the general public and is often considered the only source of this type of information. In addition, this form is used by government organizations as a basis to prevent possible abuse of tax exemption by organizations. Form 990 requires disclosure of significant information regarding governance and board of trustees (https://www.irs.gov/forms-pubs/about-form-990). IRS regulations require nonprofits to make copies of their three most recent Forms 990 available to anyone who requests them, either in person or by mail, fax, or email. Form 990 is also available to the public through several online services.

The inherent differences between investor-owned and nonprofit organizations have profound implications for many elements of healthcare financial management including organizational goals, funding decisions and investment decisions [21].

4 The Necessity of Budgeting in General and Emphasizing its Need in Healthcare Environment

Financial planning and budgeting play a vital role in the financial performance of all healthcare organizations. In fact, it can be said that planning and budgeting are the most important tasks related to financial affairs.

Planning involves the overall process of preparing for the future. Because of its importance to organizational success, most healthcare managers, especially in large organizations, spend a lot of time on planning-related activities. Budgeting is a subset of the planning process. A set of budgets is a basic management accounting tool used to review planned operations and control them (with the possibility of comparing actual results with expected results). In general, organizational plans focus on the big long-term picture, while budgets deal with the details of planning for the near future and, through a control mechanism, ensure that current performance is consistent with organizational plans and goals.

5 The Importance of Management Accounting for Healthcare Managers

Healthcare managers have several duties. Some of the most important ones are planning, budgeting, and creating policies that control the organization's operations and oversee the daily activities of employees. All these activities require a large amount of information. This information should be presented in a format that facilitates analysis, interpretation and decision making. This is where management accounting helps managers. Without a timely and effective management accounting system, healthcare managers are unable to make appropriate decisions based on information. Of course, accurate information does not guarantee the right decision, but without it, it is almost impossible to make the right decision.

6 Necessary Financial Concepts in the Field of Healthcare

6.1 *Expense*

From the point of view of accounting, the word "Expense" has different meanings and definitions depending on the context of its application. In the accounting information system, the expense is generally crystallized in the form of cash outflow in the past or the obligation to pay it in the future or the expiration of the value and consumption of assets. But in cost accounting and management accounting in particular, the term expense is defined as follows:

A monetary measure of economic resources that have been consumed and sacrificed in the past, or are intended to be consumed in the future, to achieve a specific goal or a specific benefit.

6.2 *Cost, Expense and Loss*

The cost is the lost resources to acquire other resources, which is actually the change and conversion of assets from one type to another. For example, buying goods (converting cash to goods in the balance sheet); As long as the goods are not sold, a cost in the sense of application in financial accounting has not been realized. As soon as the goods are sold, the relevant consumed resources, as the cost of the goods sold, are converted into expense (in the common sense in financial accounting) and are reflected in the income statement, and those items that their economic benefits are not realized convert to loss. In fact, loss is the sacrifice of resources without gaining any benefit. Preoperational expenditures and the book value of machinery which are considered as the cost (asset), cost of goods sold and depreciation of machinery are expenses and waste and bad debts are examples of losses.

A cost has future benefits, while an expense does not have future benefits; But both have a purpose.

The expense has created a benefit in the past, it is targeted and controllable, but the loss has not resulted in a benefit in the past, it is involuntary and has little controllability.

Depending on the situation and management information needs, we can classify expenses in different ways. Expenses can be classified in different ways, some of these classifications are mentioned as follows.

6.3 *Classification of Costs to Direct and Indirect*

Direct costs refer to cost that can be related to a specific issue, such as raw materials used in a product unit.

Indirect costs refer to costs that cannot be related to a specific object, such as electricity used in the production of products.

Because indirect costs cannot be assigned to a specific object, they cannot be specifically related to an object, but these costs are generally shared between several cost objects. Indirect costs are allocated to different cost items such as products based on different allocation methods. In summary, it can be stated that direct costs are costs that can be easily tracked and allocated to a product, but indirect costs are costs that cannot be easily tracked and allocated to a product, but these costs must be allocated between products or in other words, different cost objects.

6.4 Classification of Costs Based on Product Components

6.4.1 Direct Material Costs

Direct material costs refer to items that can be easily tracked and allocated to a unit of manufactured product. These materials make up the appearance of the product and it is impossible to produce the product without using these materials, such as the cost of leather used in shoe production or fabric used in clothing production.

6.4.2 Direct Labor Cost

The salaries and wages of people who directly contributed to the production of the product and which can be easily traced and allocated to a product unit are called direct labor costs, such as the cost of wages and salaries of production workers. Any other type of direct cost can be easily allocated to a product unit if it has the characteristics and features of direct materials and direct labor, such as packaging materials used in product packages.

6.4.3 Manufacturing Overhead Costs/Indirect Costs

These costs usually include factory costs with the exception of direct material and direct labor, that is, costs that cannot be easily allocated to a product unit, and to allocate these costs to the product, the process of allocation and sharing should be used. Such as indirect material costs, indirect labor and other manufacturing costs. For the costs of indirect materials, for example, the cost of glue or thread used in the production of shoes can be mentioned, and for indirect labor, for example, salaries of the foreman, production manager, storekeeper, security guard and ... cited. Other manufacturing costs include all indirect costs except for indirect materials and indirect labor, such as the costs of repairing and maintaining machinery, the insurance cost of factory machinery, the cost of factory fuel, the cost of water and electricity, and the factory telephone and other indirect factory costs. The sum of direct material costs, direct labor costs and manufacturing overhead costs are addressed as production costs.

Prime cost is directly related to production and includes the costs of direct materials and direct labor.

Conversion cost relate to costs that convert direct materials into finished products, which include direct labor costs and factory overhead costs.

6.5 Classification of Costs into Product Costs and Period Costs

Product cost is the same as production cost, or in other words, the sum of all three costs of direct materials, direct labor and manufacturing overhead costs. Period cost refers to all costs that cannot be considered as product costs. These costs are reflected in the income statement in the period of occurrence and are classified under the title of operating costs, such as distribution and sales costs or general and administrative costs. Period costs are costs that are neither directly nor indirectly related to production.

6.6 Classification of Costs Based on Cost Behavior

Classification of costs in terms of cost behavior refers to how costs react to changes in the level or volume of activity. In other words, the purpose of cost behavior is a model based on which a specific cost reacts to a change in the activity level. In this type of classification, the issue is that the costs show their behavior in front of the changes in production or services provided, and they are divided into two categories: fixed costs and variable costs.

In this cost classification, the possible volume range should be determined first. The volume of activity (measured as number of patients per days, number of visits, number of registrants, number of laboratory tests, etc.) in the next time period is always uncertain. However, healthcare managers often have an idea of the potential range of volumes in the future time period. For example, the business manager of an urgent care clinic that is open seven days a week might estimate that the number of visits in the coming year will be between 10,000 and 12,000 (27–32 cases per day). A range of 10,000–12,000 visits defines the appropriate range for the clinic if there is a small chance that annual use will fall outside this range. Of course, this range is related to a specific time period and for other time periods, the relevant range may be different.

Fixed costs are costs that are unchanged regardless of changes in production volume in a certain range of production (relevant range), such as depreciation expense (straight line method), insurance expense, rent expense and toll expense. Fixed cost is fixed in a relevant domain, but changes in the production volume of fixed costs in different domains must be changed. Fixed costs at the level of production in a related domain, the higher the amount of production, the lower the fixed cost per unit. The fixed cost per unit is equal to the fixed cost divided by the amount of production.

Variable costs are costs that change according to the change in the production level. Variable costs are variable at the level of total production but fixed at the level of each unit.

6.7 Profit Analysis Based on Activity Volume

Profit analysis is an analytical technique that is mainly used to analyze the effects of changes in the volume of activity on profits. However, the same procedures can also be used to evaluate the effects of volume changes on costs, so this type of analysis is often called cost-volume-profit (CVP) analysis. CVP analysis allows managers to examine the effects of alternative assumptions on costs, volumes, and prices. Obviously, such information is useful when managers evaluate future trends in pricing and introducing new services.

6.8 Profit Margin

Profit margin is one of the profitability ratios obtained by dividing (net) profit by revenue or sales. Profit margin is expressed as a percentage and indicates how many cents of profit a company earns for every $1 of sales (revenue). For example, if a company's net profit margin is 20%, it means that the company earns $20 in net profit for every $100 in sales.

7 Other Terms Related to Cost

7.1 Cost Object

The cost object is anything that requires separate measurement of its costs. In other words, the cost object is the destination to which costs are attributed and allocated. A product unit of a manufacturing company is considered as the final cost object.

7.2 Cost Driver

A cost driver (cost generator) is a factor that affects the sum of costs. That is, a change in the amount and size of the cost driver causes a change in the total amount of costs related to the desired cost object. The first important step to understand the cost behavior in any organization is to identify the cost drivers.

7.3 Costing

The costing is to find the price of each product, service, activity, organizational unit and many other items that managers must know the price of the cost object for making decisions. In cost accounting, valuation is a process in which the price of an item is determined. In a costing system, the price of object is usually determined during the two stages of cost accumulation and cost allocation.

Cost accumulation means collecting information related to costs in an organized way and through the accounting system.

Cost Assignment means allocating the accumulated costs in the accumulation stage to the cost object and is done in two ways: (a) tracing the accumulated costs to a cost objects and (b) allocating the accumulated costs to various cost objects.

7.4 Cost Center

It is a place that is responsible for controlling its related expenses. Usually, the cost of each center is considered separately. Such as production departments, repair departments and etc.

7.5 Cost Pool

Accumulation of costs that are supposed to be allocated to a number of cost objects for specific purposes. Such as the initial allocation of construction overhead costs to departments. Each of the departments is considered as a cost object and the collected costs are considered as a cost pool. However, in the secondary allocation of overhead costs, service departments are considered as cost pools and service user departments are considered as cost objects.

7.6 Expired Cost and Unexpired Cost

The cost can be divided into "expired costs" whose benefit is only the income of the period that occurred, and does not extend to subsequent periods, and "unexpired costs" whose benefit is expected to extend to future periods as well. Unexpired expenses are considered as assets and are transferred to the next periods through reflection in the balance sheet. A clear example of these costs are inventories, pre payments of costs and property, plant and equipment. Expired costs are reflected in the income statement of the period of occurrence and are matched with the income of that period. Its examples include: the cost of water, electricity, advertising, and sales and administrative staff salaries. The purchase of machinery is considered as an asset and its annual depreciation expense at the end of each year is considered as the expired part of the cost of this asset. This classification is extremely important in terms of preparing financial statements at the end of each financial period.

7.7 Opportunity Cost

One of the tasks of management accounting as an information system is to provide information related to costs for various decisions of managers at different levels in economic enterprises. But different decisions require different information. "Lost opportunity cost" is one of the important and effective information in managers' decisions in various fields, including the pricing of internal transfers between different departments of an economic enterprises, accepting or rejecting a specific order and making a part in-house or buying It is from outside. In order to achieve their desired goals, economic enterprises have at their disposal resources that include cash, receivables, inventory of goods, property, plant and equipment, investment in shares of other companies and human resources. The use of any of these resources leads to the loss of the opportunity to use those resources in another way for economic enterprises. This means that if one of these resources is used for a specific purpose, that resource cannot be used for other purposes. It can be said simply, "lost opportunity cost" is the value of any opportunity that is given up in order to engage in another activity. In other words, the lost opportunity cost is defined as an advantage that is sacrificed by refraining from doing one way of doing something in order to do another.

7.8 Sunk Cost

A wasted or lost cost refers to a cost that occurred in the past and, as a result, has no effect on future decisions and costs, and it cannot be returned or changed through current or future actions. A clear example of such costs is the cost of acquiring equipment that has already been purchased and the cost of inventories that have already been acquired.

7.9 Differential Cost

Differential cost is the difference between the costs of two different solutions. When we are faced with the problem of choosing among various solutions, attention to differential costs is given priority instead of dealing with total and accumulated costs. In making various decisions, paying attention to the difference between the cost of different solutions and comparing them, keeping in mind the total cost of these solutions, is more expressive, convenient and effective. Differential cost is sometimes called incremental cost and marginal cost.

7.10 Avoidable Cost and Unavoidable Cost

Avoidable costs are costs that can be eliminated when choosing a solution from among different approaches.

Unavoidable costs are costs that remain constant between different solutions and do not change. In other words, the costs that will continue even with the removal of a part of the unit or an activity.

7.11 Relevant Cost

There are costs that become effective in specific decision-making conditions, and are related to a specific decision and are defined as future expected costs that cause the difference between different solutions. Therefore, it is effective in the specific decision-making of the management and is considered relevant and intended for the calculation of the cost. For each cost to be considered relevant, it must have the following two characteristics: (a) the occurrence of these items is expected in future financial periods and (b) the amount of these items should be different for each of the solutions.

7.12 Standard Cost

It refers to an estimated or budgeted cost of making a specific product unit or performing a service, which is used as a model and index to compare and evaluate performance. These target costs are often used in the budgeting process.

7.13 Joint Costs

The costs incurred in the joint manufacturing process and before the joint products appear separately and are identifiable. In other words, the sum of all the costs incurred in the joint manufacturing process up to the separation point is used to manufacture joint products.

7.14 Separable Costs

It refers to the costs that occur for the processing of joint products after the separation point. The feature of such costs is the ease of tracking them directly with each of the common products. These costs are not part of the costs of the joint manufacturing process and are related to the steps after the separation point of the joint products.

7.15 Mixed Costs

Mixed costs have characteristics of both variable and fixed costs. For example, on a range of production volume, the mixed cost remains constant in the sum of Dollars, and hence it will be a fixed cost. On the other range of production, the mixed cost may change in proportion to changes in the level of production, and hence it will be a variable cost. Mixed cost sometimes refers to semi-variable cost or semi-fixed cost. Such as water, electricity and telephone costs.

7.16 Semi-variable Costs

Some costs are increased with the increase in the level of activity (production), but its increase is not with a fixed ratio, such costs are called semi-variable costs, such as the bulk purchase of some necessities, or receiving services from service agencies reduce the rate by increasing the number of visits.

7.17 Semifixed (or Step Function) Cost

Semi-fixed costs remain constant in a range of activity, but increase in leaps and bounds with increasing activity. Many costs tend to be semi-fixed. Semi-fixed costs have the characteristics of both fixed and variable costs, like variable costs, they increase stepwise with the volume of activity, and like fixed costs, they are fixed within the limits of activity.

8 Budgeting

Budgeting consists of detailed plans, expressed in real terms that specify how resources will be acquired and used over a specified period of time in the future. It should be recognized that the budget is considered not only as an accounting tool but also as a management tool. In fact, budgets are more important to managers than to financial staff because budgets provide a means of planning and communicating operational expectations within an organization. In addition, the budgeting process and the resulting final budget provide a tool for top managers to allocate financial resources among multiple demands in an organization.

Although planning, communication, and allocation are important goals of the budgeting process, perhaps the greatest value of budgeting is that it establishes financial criteria for control. By comparing actual and budgeted results, managers are provided with feedback on the financial performance of the business unit for which they are responsible. Such comparisons help managers evaluate individual performance and identify areas that may need to be addressed.

When actual results differ from budgeted results, analysts use variance analysis to identify the factors that caused the different performance. In this way, management resources can be used in operational areas that need improvement. In addition, in the control process, information generated by comparing actual results with expected (planned) results is useful in improving the overall accuracy of the planning process. By examining the budget variance, managers may identify changes in the operating environment that they need to consider in the next planning cycle.

8.1 Prerequisites of Budgeting (Scheduling)

Almost all healthcare organizations set an annual budget for the following year. However, if budget feedback is provided only annually, it takes too long for managers to identify unfavorable trends, so most organizations also have quarterly budgets, while some have monthly, weekly, or even daily budgets. Not all existing budgets or sub-units of an organization use the same scheduling model. Some may use monthly budgets, while others use weekly budgets. In addition, many organizations prepare budgets for one or more years, which are more aligned with financial planning than with operational control.

8.2 Traditional Budgeting Versus Zero-based Budgeting

Most healthcare organizations use the traditional budgeting approach to develop their budgets. In this approach, the previous budget is used as a starting point for creating a new budget. Each line item in the previous budget is reviewed and then adjustments are made to reflect the changes in the new conditions. In this approach, usually many budget changes are applied more or less equally in departments and programs. For example, it may be assumed that labor costs increase at the same rate of inflation for all departments and programs of an organization. The main task under the traditional approach is to determine what (usually minor) changes must be made to the previous budget to account for changes in the operating environment. In other words, it is assumed that except for these changes, the current budget accurately reflects the organization's resource needs.

Conceptually, zero-based budgeting is superior to conventional budgeting. In fact, when zero-based budgeting was introduced in the 1970s, it was widely embraced. Zero-Based Budgeting is one of the budgeting methods in which all expenses are reviewed and calculated for each new period. This process starts from "base zero" and analyzes the needs and costs of each function in an organization or institution. After that, regardless of whether each budget is higher or lower than the previous budget; the budget required for the next period is determined. Unlike traditional budgeting, zero-based budgeting starts all calculations from zero and justifies all individual or public expenses in a period through a report. In this method of budgeting, instead of using incremental budgeting that exists in the traditional budgeting method, all small and large needs of the company are evaluated and analyzed. Basically, this type of budgeting will be very useful for a top-down strategic approach and performance analysis of a particular project.

Zero-based budgeting in an organization is such that in the budgeting process, high-level strategic goals are integrated with the specific tasks of that organization, and after that, costs are classified and then compared with previous results and current expectations. In this method, most of the programs and activities within the organization are evaluated or analyzed from the point of view of their effectiveness and efficiency. Then each of these activities and programs are prioritized based on their importance. Some activities may even be recognized as very low priority and of little value and finally eliminated. Eliminating items that are not necessary and do not have a high priority in a set can prevent additional costs and in the long run, significant savings for companies. With these savings, other departments that were mostly weak due to lack of attention from the managers and computing affairs units will be strengthened and will bring a lot of profits for the whole group. Because the excess costs spent on unimportant and necessary programs are now spent on these units.

Managers or leaders of a company can implement zero-based budgeting in their groups, but the process may take several years due to its detail-oriented nature. Zero-based budgeting can help reduce costs by avoiding the overall increase or decrease of the previous period's budget. However; This is a time-consuming process and will take much longer than traditional cost-based budgeting. Therefore, many organizations that initially adopt zero-based budgeting soon find that the benefits of this method do not outweigh the costs. However, many healthcare organizations are again using zero-based budgeting, largely because market forces require managers to implement cost control methods on a more or less continuous basis. As a solution, some healthcare organizations use conventional annual budgeting, but also use zero-based budgeting on a smaller scale, such as every five years. An alternative approach is to use the conventional approach for 80% of each year's budget and the zero-based approach for 20%. Then, in each five-year period, the entire budget is subjected to zero-based budgeting. This approach takes advantage of zero-based budgeting without creating a time-consuming budgeting process for managers each year.

Unlike zero-based budgeting, in traditional budgeting there should be a gradual increase in budget compared to previous budgets. For example; a 2% increase should be applied in the expenses and with this increase in expenses, appropriate budgeting should be considered for the new year.

Furthermore; in traditional budgeting, only new expenses are analyzed, while in zero-based budgeting, it is necessary to start from zero and in addition to new expenses, old and recurring expenses should also be justified. Note that the justification of costs in zero-based budgeting is the responsibility of the managers, and the optimization of costs and not just revenues bring great value to the organization or company.

Suppose a hospital is going to implement a zero-based budgeting process, which requires a more detailed examination of the costs of the laboratory department. This hospital realizes that some specific tests of its clients and patients are outsourced to another healthcare center, which increases the price by 5% every year.

By examining the details, the hospital observes that it is possible to perform these tests with the help of its own forces and by making some minor changes inside the hospital. Therefore, after evaluating the pros and cons of this issue, the hospital decides to conduct the tests itself to make it cheaper than the outside center.

Therefore; Instead of blindly increasing the budget by a certain percentage and hiding the increase in current costs, the hospital can identify important situations and decide whether it is able to perform tests at a lower cost or whether it is necessary to outsource certain tests for its patients.

In traditional budgeting, it is not possible to identify the positions and costs in each department. Zero-based budgeting is a more detailed process that aims to identify and justify all available costs. However; zero-based budgeting is more involved in a company's costs and can evaluate current costs against savings that may be identified in the process.

Zero-based budgeting, as a good accounting method, has many advantages, including centralized operations, lower costs, flexibility in the budgeting process, and strategic implementation of the process.

When the managers of a company think about how to spend every dollar in the operations of that company, operations that are less expensive and more profitable are more important to them. Furthermore; Zero-based budgeting will reduce costs and prevent misallocation of resources that may occur over time.

In addition to the advantages that we have listed, zero-based budgeting also has disadvantages. First, it depends on time and requires resources. Since a new budget must be prepared each period, the associated time cost may not be very worthwhile. Instead, it may be more beneficial to use a modified budgeting model in a particular situation. Second, areas such as research and development, or those for which an organization has a long-term vision, may be neglected, and short-term perspectives may be given more value by allocating more resources and receiving the highest revenue.

8.3 Top-Down Budgeting Versus Bottom-Up Budgeting

Budgets affect almost everyone in the organization, and how people react to the budgeting process can have a significant impact on the overall effectiveness of the organization. Therefore, one of the most important budgeting decisions is whether the budget should be created top-down or bottom-up.

With bottom-up or participatory budgeting, the budgeting process starts from the lower levels of the organization. In this approach, the budget is first formulated by department or program managers. Such individuals are likely to be knowledgeable about the financial needs of their departments or programs. The budget of the department is presented to the finance department for review and compilation in the organizational budget, which must be approved by senior management. Unfortunately, combining departmental or program budgets often results in an organizational budget that is not financially feasible. In such cases, the budgets of the various parts of the organization must be returned to the main providers for revision, which begins a negotiation process with the goal of creating a budget acceptable to all parties, or at least to many parties.

A more authoritative approach to budgeting is a top-down approach in which little negotiation takes place between middle and upper management. With top-down budgeting, budget goals are generally set at the top management level of the organization and for each major department or activity within the organization. Then, the budget of each unit of the organization is given to the managers of that department, and they must prepare a budget according to the goals imposed on them from above. Similarly, when budgets are set at the departmental level, targets are given to managers lower in the organizational hierarchy. These managers are then required to prepare budgets that will achieve the desired goals for their operational area.

This approach has the advantages that it is relatively quick, requires less planning, reflects the view of senior management from the beginning, and senior management can use top-down budgets to impose their views. However, by limiting participation and communication, a top-down approach often results in less commitment among middle managers and employees than a bottom-up approach. Bottom-up budgeting takes much more time and may be revised several times until the budget draft is properly coordinated, but the idea of participatory budgeting is to involve as many managers and even employees as possible in the process. Budgeting is involved because people are likely to perform better and put more effort into achieving budget goals if they have a prominent role in setting these goals. Also, this approach reflects the views and expectations of managers who are closer to operations and therefore may have a better understanding of what is not achievable.

9 Types of Budgets

Although an organization's future financial expectations are expressed in a document called a budget, in most organizations, the "master budget" is actually made up of several different budgets. Unlike an organization's financial statements, a specific form and format for the budget is not determined by generally accepted accounting principles, so the content and format of the budget is dictated by the organization's mission and structure and management preferences. It should be noted that several types of budgets are used in almost all healthcare organizations, either formally or informally.

9.1 Statistical Budget

The statistical budget is the cornerstone of the budgeting process, as it defines the patient volume and resource assumptions used in other budgets. Since the statistical budget is included in other budgets, accuracy in its preparation is of particular importance. A statistical budget does not provide detailed information about required resources, such as staffing needs or short-term operating assets, but provides general guidance.

Some organizations, particularly smaller ones, may not have a separate statistical budget, but instead may incorporate data directly into revenue and expense budgets, or perhaps into an operating budget. The advantage of having a separate statistical budget is that, in large organizations, it forces all other budgets to use the same set of patient volume assumptions and resources. Unfortunately, estimating patient volume, which is the heart of statistical budgeting and drives all other projections, is extremely difficult. To illustrate the complexities of forecasting patient volume, consider the procedures a hospital follows when preparing its statistical budget. To begin with, demand for services is divided into four major groups: inpatient, outpatient, ancillary, and other services. The trend of the volume of patients in each of these regions during the last five years is drawn and the first approximate forecast is made assuming the continuation of the past trend. In the next step, the level of population growth and disease trends are predicted. For example, how much will the population over 60 grow in the hospital's service area? These predictions are used to develop patient volumes for core diagnoses and to differentiate between routine services and intensive care services. Hospital managers then analyze the competitive environment. Consideration is given to factors such as the hospital's inpatient and outpatient capacities, the capacities of competitors, and new or improved services that the hospital or its competitors may develop. Next, managers consider the impact of the hospital's budgeted pricing actions on patient volume. For example, does the hospital have plans to increase outpatient costs to increase profit margins, or reduce costs to gain market share and use excess capacity? If such measures are expected to affect patient volume forecasts, these forecasts should be revised to reflect the expected impact.

If the forecast of the volume of hospital patients is less than the allowed limit, it can have serious consequences. If the market for any particular service expands beyond what the hospital expected and planned for, the hospital will not be able to meet the needs of its patients, and potential patients will eventually go to competitors, and the hospital will lose market share. He may miss a great opportunity. However, if its projections are too optimistic, the hospital could end the budget period with excess capacity, which means higher-than-necessary costs due to additional facilities and staff.

9.2 Budget Based on Revenues

Detailed information from the statistical budget is transferred to the revenue budget, which combines patient volume and reimbursement information to develop revenue projections. Hospital planners consider their pricing strategy for managed care programs, traditional fee-for-service contracts, and private care patients, as well as inflation trends and insurance reimbursements, all of which affect operating income.

The result of this process is a set of operating income forecasts based on services, which are both aggregated (such as inpatient income) and based on individual diagnosis. Individual diagnosis forecasts are summarized and compared to service group forecasts. The differences are reconciled and the result is a forecast of operating income for the hospital as a total income, disaggregated by service categories and individual diagnoses. In addition to operating income, other incomes such as profits from investments and rent payments for medical office buildings should also be anticipated. Note that in all income projections, both amount and time are important. Therefore, the revenue budget should not only predict the amount of revenue, but also when the revenue is expected to occur, which is usually monthly.

9.3 Budget Based on Expenses

Like the revenue budget, the expense budget is also obtained from the data in the statistical budget. Here the focus is on the expenses of providing the service rather than the revenues generated from it. Expense-based budgeting is usually divided into labor and non-labor. Labor expenses include salaries and other benefits such as travel and education, and non-labor components include expenses related to things like depreciation, rent, utilities, medical and office supplies. Expenses are usually divided into fixed and variable components.

9.4 Operating Budget

For large organizations, operating budgets come from revenue and expense budgets. For smaller businesses, data typically found in statistical, revenue, and expense budgets are used to create an operating budget in one step. Since the operating budget (including revenue and expense budgets) is prepared using accrual accounting methods, it can be thought of almost as a projected income statement. However, unlike the income statement, which is usually prepared at the organizational level, operating budgets are prepared at the sub-unit level, such as a division or product line.

10 Budget Deviation Analysis

Budget deviation analysis, which focuses on the differences (variances) between realized values and forecasts, is an important technique for controlling operations. In accounting, a variance is the difference between actual (realized) amounts and budgeted amounts, often called standard amounts. Of course, the definition of deviation in accounting is different from the statistical definition, although both meanings indicate a difference from a base value. In fact, deviation analysis examines and interprets the differences between what actually happened and what was planned. If the budget is based on realistic expectations, variance analysis can provide managers with useful information. Deviation analysis doesn't provide all the answers, but it helps managers ask the right questions. Deviation analysis is essential for the management control process. Actions taken in response to deviation analysis often have the potential to significantly improve an organization's operations and financial performance. For example, many deviations are controllable and correctable with management actions, so managers can take steps to prevent undesirable deviations in the future. Deviation analysis should not seek to find the culprit for unfavorable results. Rather, the purpose of deviation analysis is to discover the cause of operational problems so that these problems can be corrected as quickly as possible and avoided or at least minimized in the future. Unfortunately, not all deviations can be controlled by management. Nevertheless, awareness of such deviations is essential for the overall management and welfare of the organization.

10.1 Fixed Budgets Versus Flexible Budgets

For managers to get the most out of it, deviation analysis should be systematically reviewed. The starting point for such analyzes is the fixed budget. This budget is the same as the original approved budget, in which the difference between the volume of planned and actual (realized) patients is not taken into account. However, at the end of a budget period, realized volume is unlikely to equal forecasted volume, and it is useful to know which deviations are due to volume forecast error and which deviations are due to other factors.

To illustrate this concept, consider the operating budget of a clinic in 2022. Assume that $100,000 in profit is projected based on certain patient volume assumptions: 45,000 visits for agency contracts and 62,000 visits for the expected per capita rate of the clinic's geographic area population. At the end of the year, the managers compare the actual profit with the budgeted profit, and it is very unlikely that the actual profit will come exactly from the 45,000 referrals from the organizations and 54,000 referrals from the population of the region. The number of hits achieved in each category may be higher or lower than expected, and they may use the service at a different rate than what is considered in the fixed budget. Therefore, if clinic managers simply compare realized profit with a profit of $100,000 in a fixed budget, they do not know whether the difference in profit is due to differences in forecasted and realized patient volumes or to underlying operational differences.

Clinic managers should prepare a flexible budget to account for factors that cause profit deviations. A flexible budget is a budget in which the fixed budget is adjusted to reflect the actual volume achieved during the budget period. Basically, flexible budgeting is a tool that tells managers what results will be below actual volume levels, assuming other budgeting assumptions are held constant. Flexible budgeting provides a more accurate analysis than when variance analysis is achieved using only comparisons of actual results with a fixed budget. However, a flexible budget only manipulates variable costs, so it requires the identification of variable and fixed costs and places a greater burden on the management accounting system of the organization.

In the clinic's flexible budget, data used for variance analysis is tracked in its management accounting information system throughout the year, and variance analysis is performed monthly. This allows managers to take the necessary actions throughout the year to positively impact annual results.

11 Making Decisions About Capital Investments

With the tremendous technological advances in the field of improving the methods of producing goods and services, various business units invest huge sums of money in facilities, machinery, equipment, environmental protection and other new assets every year. Unlike current assets, long-term assets, which are called capital assets, are used by the business unit in the physical process of producing goods and services during several different periods. Considering that the amounts spent on acquiring capital assets are generally significant, business units usually carefully plan and evaluate such expenses before making them. The planning of said expenses is called capital budgeting. Determining the amount of expenses for the collection of capital assets and the type of assets to be collected is also referred to as capital budgeting.

The capital budget represents the estimate of total costs that are expected to be invested in fixed assets during the budget period. It should be noted that the budget period of capital expenses may be different from the period of other expenses because the capital budget is usually predicted for the next few years, for example in three-year, five-year or even ten-year periods, in which case for Control divides it into short-term annual periods.

Capital budgeting decisions are one of the most critical decisions that healthcare managers must make. Because the results of these decisions generally affect the business for a long time. If a business invests too much in facilities and equipment (fixed assets), it will have too much capacity and too many costs. On the other hand, a business that invests very little in fixed assets may face the two problems of technology obsolescence and insufficient capacity. A healthcare provider without the latest technology is losing patients to more up-to-date competitors and depriving their patients of the best available health diagnoses and treatments.

Effective capital budgeting provides many benefits to businesses. A business that anticipates its needs for capital assets can plan its purchases carefully, thereby negotiating the highest quality assets at the best price. In addition, asset development usually involves significant expenses and, since large amounts of cash are not usually available, must be sourced from outside the organization. Good capital budgeting practices allow a business to identify its financing needs and resources in advance, which ensures the lowest possible financing expenses as well as the availability of required funds.

11.1 Capital Budgeting Basics

Capital budgeting is the planning, evaluation and selection of investment plans that have returns in the long term. Capital budgeting, in fact, is the decision-making process for providing capital expenditures in the budget period or the process of identifying, evaluating, planning and financial support of major investment projects of business units.

In all companies, a list of plans and projects is prepared to estimate capital costs by middle and operational managers, and after conducting reviews and holding meetings, some of these plans are selected, then a capital budget is prepared and presented to the board of directors for approval.

The purpose of budgeting is to identify and determine opportunities and plans whose value is more than their cost, but in addition, the purpose of capital budgeting is to maximize shareholder wealth.

Capital budgeting is one of the most important parts of decision making and management. The importance of the funds (resources) used as well as the time required to recover the investments make it necessary to carry out detailed analyzes and valid judgments. Capital expenditures create long-term obligations in order to acquire future benefits. These expenses affect the basic goals of the business unit and have long-term and major effects on the economic position of the company.

Since the benefits from capital costs are obtained over a relatively long period of time, management mistakes in this field can cause the business unit to incur huge costs over many years.

Capital budgeting is the process of diagnosis, evaluation, planning and financial support of investment projects in organizational units. Decisions made in connection with capital budgeting largely affect the organization's success in achieving the set goals, therefore capital budgeting plays a major role in the long-term success of these units.

11.2 The Importance of Cash Flows from Investment

Cash is one of the important and vital resources of any profit-making unit, and creating a balance between available cash and cash needs is the most important factor in the economic health of any profit-making unit. Cash is brought into the for-profit unit through normal operations and other financing sources and is used to implement operations, pay interest, repay debts, and develop the for-profit unit and invest. The flow of entry and exit in each profit-making unit reflects management's decision-making regarding short-term, long-term, operational planning and investment and financing plans. The importance of cash has increased to such an extent that the management is not able to make efficient and effective decisions without knowing its status. Because every decision depends on the amount and availability of cash or cash that is expected to be available in the future.

The data used to judge and evaluate investment proposals are cash flows, not profit figures. Because the company needs cash to pay investors' profits and expenses, and if it cannot get cash returns from investments, sooner or later it will go bankrupt. Cash inflows and outflows are calculated annually, that is, cash flows into or out of the company only once a year. Usually, any type of investment starts with cash outflow, and the budget resulting from the implementation of the project represents the cash flow coming into the company.

12 Project Risk Assessment and its Application in the Capital Investment Decision Making Process

Risk in the project means unknown events or possible situations that, if they happen, will have negative or positive consequences on the project's goals. Each of these events or situations has specific causes and identifiable consequences. The consequences of these events directly affect the time, cost and quality of the project. Therefore, it is very important to identify the risk and determine the amount of its positive and negative consequences on the project goals. Therefore, project risk is an inseparable phenomenon from the project, so it must be managed. The purpose of project risk management is to plan, organize, direct and control the activities and processes of a project, so that the positive effects (opportunities) are maximized and the negative effects (threats) are minimized. In fact, risk management is a systematic process of planning to identify, analyze, respond and monitor project risk. This management includes processes, tools and techniques that help the project manager to maximize the probability of positive event outcomes and minimize the probability of negative event outcomes.

In capital investments, identifying potential and unpleasant events that can affect the main projects or business plans requires preparing oneself and the organization to deal with them. Risk analysis provides companies with knowledge and information about some long-term investments that they can use in their important decisions. Capital budgeting can be an investment in uncertainty, but organizations can cover all their essential areas by conducting a professional risk analysis. Identifying and understanding the expected outcomes puts companies in a better position to move forward with a full understanding of all potential risks.

To determine the validity of long-term investments, risk analysis is not enough in terms of objective risk factor assessments and measurements. Therefore, protecting the company with expert insight into investment results can be a smart way to do business in today's world of market uncertainty and uncertainty about future.

For example, if the organization is part of the healthcare industry, risk analysis can be useful for establishing positions related to the organization's advanced medical technologies. In capital budgeting, allocating resources for necessary capital expenditures can increase value for stakeholders, but this is only acceptable if the company has taken prudent investment actions.

Therefore, risk analysis is essential for making long-term investment decisions. By establishing a process for evaluating new opportunities, organizations can estimate long-term goals and future cash flows and control capital expenditures.

12.1 Classification of Capital Projects

Although careful analysis of investment proposals has many advantages, such an approach also entails many costs. For certain projects, detailed analysis may be required, but for other projects, simpler methods can be used. Accordingly, healthcare businesses generally classify projects into categories and then analyze them differently within each category. For example, a hospital uses the following classifications:

- Mandatory replacement: This category includes the costs required to replace worn or damaged equipment necessary for hospital operations. Because these costs are mandatory, they are usually done with only limited analysis and decision-making processes.
- Optional replacement: This category includes the costs that are made to replace repairable but old equipment. These projects generally aim to reduce costs or provide more effective clinical services. Because this category projects are not mandatory, a more rigorous decision-making process is usually required to justify costs than mandatory replacement projects.
- Expansion of services or existing markets: The costs of increasing the capacity or expansion in the markets that are currently provided by the hospital are included in this category. These decisions are more complex, so more detailed analysis is required and the final decision is made at a higher level in the organization.
- Expansion of services or new markets: These are projects that are necessary to provide new services or expand into geographic areas that are not currently served. Such projects involve strategic decisions that can fundamentally change the nature of the hospital and usually require large sums of money to be spent over long periods of time. Invariably, a detailed and specific analysis is required, and the board of trustees generally makes the final decision as part of the hospital's strategic plan.
- Safety or environmental projects: This category includes expenses necessary to comply with government orders, labor contracts, accreditation requirements and etc. If these expenses are large, the expenses of this category are considered as expenses of mandatory replacement.
- Other projects: This category is for projects that are not regularly placed in another category. The main determinant of how to evaluate this category projects is the amount of funding required.

In general, relatively simple analyzes and only a few supporting documents are needed for alternative decisions and safety or environmental projects, especially those that are mandatory. More detailed analysis is required for development and other projects.

Within each category, projects are classified by size: larger projects require more detailed analysis and approval at a higher level within the hospital. For example, department heads can spend up to a certain amount on discretionary replacement projects, while expansion projects costing more than 20 times that cap must be approved by the entire board [21].

12.2 *The Role of Financial Analysis in Healthcare Capital Budgeting*

For investor-owned businesses, where maximizing owner wealth is the primary goal, the role of financial analysis in investment decisions is clear. Projects that help increase the owner's wealth should be undertaken, while projects that do not should be ignored. But in the case of non-profit businesses whose goal is not to maximize wealth, an appropriate goal is to provide high-quality, cost-effective services to the communities served. In this situation, capital budgeting decisions should consider many factors in addition to the financial consequences of the project. For example, the needs of the healthcare staff and the welfare of the community should also be considered. In many cases, non-economic factors outweigh financial considerations.

However, good decision-making and sustainability of healthcare businesses require that the financial impact of capital investments be fully recognized. If a healthcare provider undertakes a series of highly unprofitable projects that meet non-financial goals and such projects are not offset by profitable projects, the company's financial position will get worse and worse. If this situation continues over time, the provider will eventually lose its financial viability and may even be forced into bankruptcy and closure. Of course, non-profit businesses can offset some of the project's losses with contributions and donations. However, long-term financial sustainability is best ensured by striving for operational profitability rather than depending on less reliable sources of finance.

Because bankrupt companies cannot meet the needs of a community, even nonprofit business managers must consider the potential impact of a project on the company's finances. Managers may make a conscious decision to accept a project with poor financial projections because of their non-financial preferences, but it is important for managers to know the financial impact in advance, rather than being surprised when the project drains the company's financial resources.

Financial analysis provides managers with relevant information about the financial impact of the project and helps managers make better decisions, including those based primarily on non-financial considerations.

12.3 *Cash Flow Forecast*

The most critical and also the most difficult stage in the evaluation of long-term (capital) investment proposals is the estimation of the project's cash flows. This step includes estimating investment costs, expected annual net operating cash flows when the project begins, and cash flows associated with its completion.

Many variables are involved in cash flow estimation and many people and departments are involved in this process. It is very difficult to accurately predict the costs and revenues associated with a large and complex project, and the error caused by the prediction can also be large. Therefore, it is necessary to carry out risk analysis in prospective projects. The difficulty and importance of cash flow estimation cannot be exaggerated, but if the concepts discussed in the following sections are followed, the errors that often occur can be minimized.

12.3.1 Incremental Cash Flows

The relevant cash flows to consider when evaluating a new investment are the project's incremental cash flows, defined as the business's cash flows in each period if the project is implemented, minus the cash flows if the project is not implemented:

$$\textbf{Incremental}\, CFt = CFt\,\textbf{(Business with project)} - CFt\,\textbf{(Business without project)}$$

In this equation, t specifies a period of time, which is often annual.

CF_0 is the incremental cash flow during year zero, which is usually assumed to be the start of the project. CF_1 is the incremental cash flow during the first year and CF_2 is the incremental cash flow during the second year.

In practice, initial incremental cash flows, especially in year zero, are usually cash outflows that include costs associated with setting up and running the project. As the project begins to generate revenue, incremental cash flows typically become positive. In practice, it is usually not possible to predict the cash flows of a business with and without a new project. Therefore, the real estimation process focuses on the specific cash flows of the project being evaluated.

12.3.2 Income Statement and Cash Flows (Annual and Non-annual Schedule Based on GAAP)

An accounting income statement prepared in accordance with generally accepted accounting principles (GAAP) is in some ways like a combination of several disparate factors. Accountants deduct labor costs, which are cash outflows, from revenues that may not be entirely cash. For example, for healthcare providers, most receipts are from insurance companies, which may not be received for several months after services are provided. Also, the income statement does not recognize capital expenditures that are cash flows but deducts depreciation expense that is not a cash flow.

In investment decisions, it is very important that the decisions are based on the inflows and outflows of cash from the business, because in addition to the issue of profitability of a business, the ability to provide medical services also depends on the cash flows. Of course, according to generally accepted accounting principles, accounting items can affect cash flows, because non-cash items such as depreciation can affect cash flows such as taxes.

Financial analysts should also pay attention to the timing of cash flows. Accounting income statements are prepared for annual periods and do not accurately reflect when revenues and expenses occur during the period. In theory, capital budgeting cash flows should be analyzed exactly as they occur. Of course, a kind of balance should be created between being precise and practical. A timeline provides the most accuracy for daily cash flows, but daily cash flow estimates are difficult to use and will likely be less accurate than annual cash flows. Of course, in most cases, analysts use annual cash flow information at the end of each year. However, for projects that have regular and predictable cash flows throughout the year, it may be more appropriate to assume that cash flows occur every six months, quarterly, or even monthly.

12.3.3 Sunk Costs

A sunk or lost cost (mentioned earlier) is the cost of acquiring equipment that has already been purchased or the cost of inventory that has already been acquired. For example, suppose in 2022, a public hospital is considering purchasing an MRI system. To make better decisions, the hospital will contract with a consultant in 2021 and pay him $5000 to conduct a marketing study. This cash flow is irrelevant for investment decisions. Because the hospital cannot recover such cost regardless of whether it purchased the MRI or not. Cash flows that are not relevant to the analysis are called non-incremental cash flows.

12.3.4 Opportunity Cost

One of the tasks of management accounting as an information system is to provide information related to costs for various decisions of managers at different levels in economic units. But different decisions require different information. "Lost opportunity cost" is one of the important and effective information in managers' decisions in various fields, including the pricing of internal transfers between different departments of an economic enterprise, accepting or rejecting a specific order and making a part in-house or buying It is from outside. In order to achieve their desired goals, economic units have at their disposal resources that include cash, receivables, inventory of goods, property, plant and equipment, investment in shares of other companies and human resources. The use of any of these resources leads to the loss of the opportunity to use those resources in another way for economic units. This means that if one of these resources is used for a specific purpose, that resource cannot be used for other purposes. For example, suppose that a hospital's MRI is being installed at a separate location, and the hospital already owns the land where the required MRI facility will be built. The hospital purchased the land ten years ago for $20,000, but the current market value of the land after deducting legal and real estate costs is $150,000. When considering the purchase of an MRI, the value of the land cannot be overlooked because using it for an MRI facility would preclude the hospital from using it for other purposes. The land may be used for a walk-in clinic, an ambulatory surgery center, or a parking lot instead of being sold. But the best measure of its value to the hospital, and thus the inherent opportunity cost of its use, is the cash flow that can be obtained by selling it. Therefore, the MRI project has a lost opportunity cost of $150,000. The opportunity cost of $150,000 is the net market value of the land, regardless of whether the land was purchased for $20,000 or $200,000.

12.3.5 Terminal Value

The value of an asset, a project or a business can be predicted after a certain period, with the help of which future cash flows can be estimated. This value is called the terminal value (TV). The terminal value assumes that the business in question will continue to grow at a specified growth rate after a forecast period. The forecasting process will be more difficult in businesses with longer time horizons. An example of this can be clearly seen in finance, when it comes to estimating the company's future cash flows. But anyway, every business need valuation; thus, in order to solve such problems, analysts use financial models such as discounted cash flow (DFC) in addition to specific assumptions to obtain the final value of a project or business. Cash flow discount is one of the common methods that is widely used in the valuation of stocks in the financial markets. The theory of this method is based on the fact that the value of an asset is equal to the future cash flows obtained from that asset. This cash flow should be discounted at a discount rate that reflects the cost of capital, such as the interest rate. Cash flow discounting has two important parts: the forecast period and the terminal value.

One of the first decisions to be made in project cash flow forecasting is project life. How many years of cash flow forecast is enough? Many projects, such as a new hospital or ambulatory care clinic, have a long useful life. In theory, the cash flow forecast should last for the life of the project, yet most managers do not have much confidence in any long-term cash flow forecast. Therefore, most organizations consider an arbitrary limit for the life of the project that they consider in capital budgeting analyses, and usually forecast periods are 5 years. If the time period exceeds this range, the accuracy of the predictions will decrease. This is exactly were calculating the terminal value (TV) becomes important.

To calculate the terminal value, there are two common methods, which are: constant growth and exit coefficient.

In the perpetual growth method, it is assumed that the cash flow in a company will continue at a constant rate forever. But in the exit coefficient method; it is assumed that in the end the business in question will be handed over in exchange for some market criteria and its life will end.

12.3.6 Salvage Value

Salvage value is the amount of the net value of the asset after the end of the useful life of the asset, which is earned by the organization after deducting the percentage of depreciation and the costs of selling the asset. Failure to use the asset or the end of its useful life causes the asset to be discarded, which is called a depreciated fixed asset.

In fact, salvage value is the remaining value of an asset after scrapping and when it is destroyed. Some projects have a short life and some assets may have residual value until the end of the project, which should be considered in the reviews and evaluations of the cash flows resulting from the sale or transfer of these assets.

12.3.7 Effects of Inflation

The effects of inflation can have a significant impact on the profitability of a project, so inflation must be properly considered in any capital budgeting analysis. A company's cost of capital is the weighted average of its debt and equity costs. These costs are estimated based on the expected rates of return of investors and financiers, which include an inflation premium in their rates. For example, a financier might accept a 5% yield on a ten-year bond if inflation is taken into account. However, if inflation is expected to average 4% over the next ten years, the financier will have an expected return of 9%. Equity and debt investors therefore add an inflation premium to their expected rate of return to protect against the loss of purchasing power caused by inflation. Since the effects of inflation are already included in the company's cost of capital, and since this cost is used as the starting point for discounting cash flows in profitability metrics, the effects of inflation must also be included in the project's estimated cash flows. If the cash flow estimates do not include the effects of inflation, but a discount rate is used that includes the effects of inflation, the profitability of the project will be lower. The most effective way to deal with inflation is to apply inflation effects to each cash flow component using the best available information on how each component is affected. Since it is impossible to estimate future inflation rates with great accuracy, deviations are likely to occur. Inflation is often assumed to be neutral, that is, inflation is assumed to affect all components of income and expenditure equally, except depreciation. However, at certain times, expenses may increase faster than income or vice versa. Therefore, in general, it is better to apply a different inflation rate to each cash flow component. For example, net income is expected to increase at a rate of 3%, while labor costs may increase at a rate of 5%. Inflation adds to the uncertainty and risk of the project under consideration, as well as to the complexity of the capital budget analysis. Fortunately, computers and spreadsheet programs can easily handle the mechanics of inflation analysis.

12.3.8 Strategic Value

Sometimes a project has value in its cash flows in addition to its intrinsic value. Strategic value is the value that arises from future investment opportunities and is only possible if the project under consideration is accepted. To illustrate this concept, consider a hospital management company that is analyzing a management contract for a hospital in Malaysia, the first step towards Asia. On its own, this project may not be profitable, but it may provide entry into the Asian market, which could open the door to a wide range of highly profitable new projects. Or suppose a hospital is looking to start a kidney transplant program with state-of-the-art equipment and a financial analysis of the project shows that the program is not profitable, but hospital managers believe that kidney transplantation will enhance the hospital's reputation for technological and clinical excellence. As a result, it helps the overall profitability of the hospital. Theoretically, the best way to assess strategic value is to forecast the cash flows from subsequent projects, estimate the probability of their occurrence, and then add the expected cash flows from the subsequent projects to the cash flows of the project under consideration. In practice, however, this is usually impossible to do because either future cash flows are too uncertain or the number of potential future projects is too large. At the very least, decision makers should recognize that some projects have strategic value and that value should be considered qualitatively when making capital budgeting decisions.

12.4 Break-Even Point Analysis

In healthcare financial management, break-even analysis is considered in many different situations, so it is essential to fully understand the meaning of the term break-even. Break-even analysis is one of the analytical tools used by management for short-term operational decisions, which helps management in profit planning and can be based on historical information (i.e., past operations) or sales forecasts and made future expenses. Calculating the break-even point in business units is of great importance, because by having information about the break-even point, management decisions for things such as increasing or decreasing the volume of production and sales and increasing or decreasing costs are easy and the effects of decisions on profit can also be calculated.

Break-even analysis can check the success of business ideas, help approve or reject a new product introduction, or show what happens if you change your pricing strategy. The break-even point is the point where the total cost and total revenue of the business are equal and there is no loss. In other words, it shows when you reach a level of production where the cost of producing a product equals its revenue. Businesses use this analysis to find out how many units of a product or service they need to sell to break even. Break-even analysis determines whether it makes sense to produce new products by showing the number of units needed to be sold to cover costs.

The break-even analysis discussed here is actually a part of cost-volume-profit analysis (CVP). In the break-even point analysis, the relationship between sales, expenses and profitability, as well as their mutual effects on each other, is examined. By knowing the specific relationships between expenses and revenues, this study informs the managers that by determining the amount of production, sales and profits can be brought to the highest possible level. Therefore, it can be applied not only to entire businesses, but also to sub-units within businesses such as individual departments and services.

The break-even point analysis can be examined from two accounting and economic points of view, and in accounting, break-even analysis can be done in three ways.

First in the form of production level or percentage of operating capacity, in this case, the production level is determined in which the total cost of the plan is equal to the total income of the plan. In this case, the break-even point is determined by the relationship between the fixed costs and the difference in the unit sales price and the unit variable costs, and three practical results are obtained from the analysis of the break-even point in this case. The higher the fixed costs, the higher the break-even point. The greater the difference between the unit sales price and the variable operational costs, the lower the break-even point will be, and in this case, the fixed costs are absorbed faster through the difference between the unit sales price and the unit variable costs. A high break-even point is disproportionate because it makes the company vulnerable to changes in production (sales) levels.

The second in the form of income or sales level, in this case, the income level is determined in which the profit of the plan is zero. Calculating the break-even point based on the monetary value of sales (rather than sales volume) is often useful. The main advantage of this method is that it calculates a total break-even point for institutions that have several products with different selling prices. In addition, this method requires very limited information. Only three values of sales, fixed costs and variable costs are necessary.

The third one in the form of the product price level, in this case, the price level is determined where the total income of the plan is equal to the total cost.

In the analysis of the economic break-even point, the volume required to produce a certain level of profit is considered, that is, the volume that creates an income equal to the accounting costs plus some desired profit.

According to the stated content, the break-even point is the risk assessment point for the business unit, and if the income or sales level of the business unit is predicted to be less than the break-even point, the managers should be worried and think of a solution. However, under normal conditions, managers plan to achieve profit and use break-even analysis to determine at which point in the sales volume they will achieve a certain profit.

12.5 Analysis of Return on Investments (ROI)

Investigating the rate of return of an investment is one of the first steps to be taken before investing. The rate of return on investment is an important criterion for evaluating the performance of a project or an investment situation, which measures the amount of profit obtained from the investment compared to the total investment amount. When you enter a particular investment, you have a certain prediction in mind about the future of the asset in question and expect a good return from it. If the desired investment cannot achieve the return you want, you will probably go for better investment opportunities. In other words, the return on investment is used as a measure of the effectiveness of an investment.

The rate of return on investment or ROI is a measure of performance that is used to evaluate the efficiency of an investment or to compare the returns of several different investments. The rate of return on investment measures the rate of return on an investment in proportion to the costs incurred for that investment. To calculate the rate of return on an investment, the profit or return of an investment is divided by the cost of the investment, and the result is expressed as a percentage or ratio. The rate of return on investment is calculated by the following formula:

$$\mathbf{ROI} = \mathbf{Net\ income/Cost\ of\ investment} \times 100$$

In the above formula, net income or "investment income" refers to the income from the sale of the investment. Because ROI is measured as a percentage, it can be easily compared to the rate of return on other investments, and as a result, a person can compare different types of investments. The rate of return on investment is a popular measure because of its flexibility and simplicity. This rate can necessarily be used as an initial measure of the profitability of an investment. Calculating investment return rate is very easy and can be applied in various ways. This means that if an investment does not have a positive ROI, or if the investor has other opportunities with a higher ROI, this metric can show him which investments are preferable to others.

Considering the many advantages of the investment return rate, such as versatility, simplicity and ease of use, the possibility of simple interpretation of the results, and the most important advantage of the investment return rate being percentage and comparative, there are also limitations in this return rate and this means that investments should not be compared using only ROI and a limited view of it. The problem of time in the investment return rate is one of the most important problems. When we are going to compare the investment returns of two projects, we will not understand how long each of the return rates will be effective. One solution is to equalize the time of the calculated rates, for example, if one project takes one month and the other project takes three months, the rate calculated in the second project can be divided by 3 to get the time be the same as the first project. Another solution is to use ROI along with other evaluation metrics that include time in their calculations.

12.6 Net Present Value (NPV)

NPV or Net Present Value is a method of evaluating capital expenditures. Net present value is used to determine whether investments or projects are profitable or not, as well as when they will be profitable. The net present value method is one of the best criteria for evaluating investment projects and is used when the company's expected rate of return for investment projects is known. In this method, it is assumed that all receipts and payments take place reliably and all the resulting funds are reinvested at a rate equal to the expected rate of return (financing expense rate). It is necessary to explain that some business units may use a discount rate higher than the expected rate of return to calculate the present value. Determining the discount rate depends on the probability of risk, uncertainty and other characteristics of the investment under consideration, but in order to maintain uniformity and the possibility of comparability of investment projects, it is better that all projects use the same rate, such as the financing expense rate which is discounted.

NPV is the difference between the present value of incoming cash flows and the present value of outgoing cash flows in a certain period of time, which is obtained from the following relationship where PV is the present value of cash inflows and I is the initial investment amount.

$$\mathbf{NPV = PV - I}$$

It is worth noting that in the calculation of NPV, all sources that create cash flow, such as operations, purchase or sale of equipment, and recycling of working capital, are taken into account, and the concept of accrual accounting is not used in it regarding revenues and expenses, and for this reason depreciation expense is not included in NPV calculation. Also, the calculation of NPV is done in a certain period of time so that the company knows when it can expect the return of its investment. To express net present value results, currency symbols are used instead of percentages. Typically, this method is thought to be easier to understand for people without a major in finance.

The NPV of a project may be positive, negative or zero. If the NPV is positive, it means that the actual rate of return of the project is higher than the rate of its financing expense, and therefore the investment is affordable. But if the NPV is negative, it means that the real rate of return of the project is lower than the expense of financing it, and it means that the investment project is uneconomic, in other words, the amount spent to provide the required capital is more than the amount that will be spent on the implementation of the project. It is worth noting that in cases where the NPV is zero, it indicates that the real rate of return of the project is equal to the rate of its financing expense, in which case this rate is called the internal rate of return.

In calculating NPV, the time value of money is considered and future cash flows are expressed based on today's value of money. The time value of money means that the money you have now is better and more valuable than the money you will have in the future. For example, \$100 this year is not equivalent to \$100 next year; because it is possible to earn income and increase its value by investing money, and also the value of money decreases due to inflation. For this reason, the discount rate is used in calculating the net present value. In financial analysis, to eliminate the time factor in calculations, the value of future cash flows is converted to present value using a discount rate. Also, by calculating the net present value, managers can easily compare the initial cash invested amount with the present value of the return on investment. In order to calculate the net present value, the following steps must be taken:

- Determining the amount of initial capital: The first step to calculate NPV is to determine the amount of money that needs to be invested in the project. Suppose the hospital wants to invest in the purchase of equipment for the operating room. The managers decide to use the net present value formula to calculate the NPV of the equipment with an initial capital of 200,000 units.
- Determining the expected net cash inflow: It must be determined how much money is expected to be obtained from the project or investment. Suppose the hospital predicts that with this investment, their cash income will increase by 40,000 currency units per month for 1 year.
- Decide on the time period: Decide in what time frame the return on the investment is going to be achieved, for a few months or even a few years. For example, the hospital wants to see the return on its investment after 12 months.
- Determining the discount rate: The discount rate is the rate of return that is needed to earn money from the project or investment. Common methods of calculating the discount rate include using the expected return of other investment options with similar risk (the rate of return that investors would expect), or the expense associated with borrowing the money needed to finance the project. Suppose the hospital needs a rate of return of 12% to make the project worth doing.

The advantage of the net present value method is that it takes into account the time value of money and the timing of cash flows, as well as the profitability of the project throughout its lifetime. The main drawbacks of this method are that if the investment projects compared have different initial investment amounts, the project that is more profitable based on this method is not necessarily the best project, because the difference in the initial investment amount is not taken into account, and also when dealing with different projects that have different economic lives, the results can be misleading. For example, a project with a higher NPV may be less popular than a project with a shorter economic life due to its longer economic life. Also, measuring the profitability of an investment with NPV relies heavily on assumptions and estimates, so there may be considerable room for error. Estimated factors include investment costs, discount rates and expected returns. A project may also often require unforeseen expenses.

12.7 Internal Rate of Return (IRR)

The internal rate of return (IRR) is the rate by which the present value of the project's incoming cash flows equals the initial investment amount. In other words, the internal rate of return is the rate at which NPV becomes zero. In the internal rate of return method, which is also called the discounted cash flow method, the present value theory is used and it is assumed that the cash flows from the project will be reinvested with the internal rate of return. In this method, the internal rate of return of the projects is compared with each other and a project is selected for investment whose IRR is higher than other projects, provided that the IRR is not lower than the financing expense rate, because in this case the implementation of the project will not be cost-effective. IRR calculation will be as follows:

$$\mathbf{NPV = 0;\ \ PV = I}$$

When you calculate IRR, you define it as a separate criterion for investment decisions. For example, your organization may specify that it only implements projects that have a return of more than 15%. Some people also know IRR as break-even interest rate. This method is popular among investors who want to achieve a certain rate of return on their investments. A quick calculation shows what rate of return a particular investment will bring over a specified period of time.

Of course, calculating the internal rate of return is not a simple calculation. For example, your hospital offers a $3000 investment that will earn $1300 a year over the next three years. You can't get the total cash flow by adding up three years' worth of income (i.e., $3900) and calculating the rate of return, because that income is spread over three years. Instead, you should use an iterative process and try different expected rates of return or annual interest rates until the net present value is zero. Fortunately, you can easily calculate the internal rate of return with Microsoft Excel software or a financial calculator. You don't even need to get involved in mathematical calculations; all these steps are done electronically [21].

The advantage of the internal rate of return method is that it takes into account the time value of money and the timing of cash flows, as well as the profitability of the project throughout its life. Also, the calculated internal rate of return may mean more to management than the net present value amount. This method also enables logical and uniform classification of investment projects. The main drawback of the internal rate of return method is that it is difficult to use compared to other methods, especially in cases where the cash flows of the project are not the same, and also the assumption of reinvesting the cash flows from the project with the internal rate of return, to especially in cases where the internal rate of return is relatively high, it is combined with optimism and in reality, such a thing is less possible.

In reviewing investment projects and comparing them, the biggest mistake is to exclusively use the internal rate of return. It is better to use at least one other method such as net present value to analyze the project. Using the internal rate of return alone and without considering other methods, makes you unable to make a correct investment decision, especially when you compare projects that have different durations.

For example, suppose you have two projects; one is a one-year project with an internal rate of return of 20% and the other is a ten-year project with an internal rate of return of 13%. If you base your decision on the internal rate of return, you might consider a project that has a 20% internal rate of return. But this is not the right choice. Considering that the expected rate of return in your company during this period of time is 10%, it is better for your internal rate of return for ten years to be 13% rather than 20% for a one-year project [21].

You should also consider how the internal rate of return takes into account the time value of money. In the internal rate of return, it is assumed that the future cash flow obtained from a project will be reinvested at the internal rate of return, not at the company's cost of capital. Therefore, to the extent that the net present value is related to the cost of capital and the time value of money, the internal rate of return is not dependent on these two factors. The adjusted internal rate of return, which considers positive cash flow as reinvested in the firm's cost of capital, better reflects the cost and profitability of a project.

All in all, consider the general principle of using internal rate of return along with net present value to get an overall and accurate picture of a company's investment and return on investment.

12.8 NPV Versus IRR

The internal rate of return is the rate that determines the profit and loss of a project. Economic analysts usually use this factor along with net present value. This is because both methods are similar but have different variables. With the help of the net present value, a specific discount rate can be arrived at for the company and then the present value of the investment can be calculated. But in the internal rate of return, one must calculate the actual return of the project's cash flows and then compare this rate of return with the company's expected rate of return. If the internal rate of return is higher, the company's investment will be a worthwhile investment. Companies usually use both factors, i.e.; internal rate of return and net present value, to evaluate investments. Net present value provides more information about the expected return on an investment, but economic analysts often use the internal rate of return to report to people who are not financial experts because the internal rate of return is more understandable and easier to understand.

If we have a project with an internal rate of return of 14% and an expected rate of return of 10%, the audience will think that we have achieved success and we have a 4% more return on investment in this project. Whereas if you say that the net present value of this project is $2 million, the audience will ask you about the net present value, and you explain that this amount is the present value of the future cash flow in this project, which, taking into account the expected rate of return of 10%, is the initial investment brings it to two million dollars. The only downside is that IRR is more conceptual than net present value. The internal rate of return does not specify the exact amount of income generated. For example, suppose that the internal rate of return is 20%. This 20% does not give you any information about how much money you have earned.

Regarding the relationship between the net present value and the internal rate of return, it can be said that if the NPV of an investment project is greater than zero, the IRR of that project will be greater than the expected rate of return, and if the NPV of the project is less than zero, the IRR of the project will be smaller than the expected rate of return. If the NPV of the project is equal to zero, then the IRR will be equal to the expected rate of return.

12.9 *Modified Internal Rate of Return (MIRR)*

In calculating the internal rate of return (IRR), all expenses and revenues of cash flows are discounted to the present value at a constant rate, which must be obtained in the equation, which is the IRR. The internal rate of return is determined in such a way that the algebraic sum of the present value of all cash flows equals zero. But based on the market conditions, the discount rate of expenses and revenues may have a significant difference, in which case the rate of each of these two flows should be determined separately and according to that, the internal rate of return index should be calculated (MIRR).

The modified internal rate of return, abbreviated as MIRR, is the real internal rate of return, taking into account reinvestment. In the calculation of IRR, one of the problems that exists is that in these calculations, the reinvestment rate for the received funds is assumed to be equal to the internal rate of return. But in MIRR calculations, it is assumed that the received funds are reinvested with another investment rate, which shows a more realistic and correct rate for investment returns and project profit estimation.

In order to calculate the MIRR rate related to the cash flows of an investment project, the Borrowing Rate and also the Reinvestment Rate should be determined based on the capital market conditions. Borrowing rate means the rate that can be used to finance the project from available sources such as the bank. It should be seen at what cost the project will be financed. Normally, the rate of receiving loans from banks and credit institutions is higher than the rate of investment in them, and therefore the cost of financing will be more than the profit from its investment. Of course, it is clear that these conditions must prevail, otherwise, by receiving a loan and reinvesting it in the bank, you can earn money from the difference in investment and borrowing rates without any economic activity.

In calculating the MIRR, all negative cash flows related to each of the years of construction or operation, which are actually expenses and must be financed, using the borrowing rate, at the present value. Of course, it should be noted that the goal is the final cash flow of each year. Because there are both expenses and revenues for the company every year. The algebraic sum of these expenses and revenues represents the net cash flow for that year, and the criterion in these calculations is the net cash flow. If this cash flow is negative, it is converted to present value using the borrowing rate. After that, all the cash flows converted to present value are added together.

After performing the above calculations, at this stage, each of the cash flows related to each of the years, which has reached a positive cash flow from the algebraic sum of expenses and revenues in that year, based on the reinvestment rate, are converted to the future value. Considering that the reinvestment rate is smaller than the borrowing rate, therefore the calculation of the future value of positive cash flows in comparison will reach a smaller number, and in fact, by determining the exact rate of borrowing and investment, the time value of money for each of the cash flows in a way It is more accurate. By performing the above calculations, we will finally reach two figures.

The first figure Present Value (PV) is equivalent to the total daily value of negative cash flows with the borrowing rate and the second figure Future Value (FV) is equivalent to the sum of the future value of positive cash flows with the reinvestment rate. Therefore, we have a present value that is converted into a future value based on a discount rate and after a certain period of time. The discount rate that made this conversion is called the modified internal rate of return (MIRR).

12.10 Net Present Social Value Model

The financial analysis techniques discussed so far have focused exclusively on the cash flow implications of a proposed project. Some health care businesses, especially nonprofit providers, aim to produce community services alongside commercial services. For such companies, a proper analysis of proposed projects should systematically consider the social value of a project along with its purely financial or cash flow value.

When social value is considered, the total net present value (TNPV) of a project can be expressed as follows:

$$\mathbf{TNPV} = \mathbf{NPV} + \mathbf{NPSV}$$

where NPV represents the typical NPV of the project's cash flows and NPSV is the project's net present social value. The term NPSV, which indicates managers' assessment of the social value of a project, clearly distinguishes capital budgeting in nonprofit firms from budgeting in investor-owned firms. In the evaluation of each project, a project whose TNPV is greater than or equal to zero is acceptable. This means that the sum of the financial and social values of the project is at least zero, so when both aspects of value are considered, the project has positive or at least non-negative value. Probably not all projects have social value, but if a project has social value, it is formally considered in this decision-making model. However, no project should be accepted if its NPSV is negative, even if its TNPV is positive [21].

13 Conclusion

The budget of non-profit organizations is a financial document that shows the organization's spending plan and includes expenses, investments and revenues, or in general, the organization's inputs and outputs. The budget should be adjusted according to the main goals of the organization. Having a budget plan shows transparency and responsibility. Benefactors and sponsors look for these two features before trusting the company. They want to know what happens to their money. A good budget assures donors that the nonprofit organization has carefully considered the budgeting process. Having a good budget also helps the board of directors to be more confident about the organization's plans and their implementation.

Maintaining the budget allows the board of directors to have the necessary control. The budget accurately shows the amount of income and expenditure and is the basis of the work of the board of directors in making decisions and preventing mistakes. Budgeting allows the board of directors to limit some expenses if needed and to try to increase revenue sources when faced with a lack of resources. Monitoring the budget gives the board the opportunity to allocate money to different and appropriate areas by changing the financial flow. Most importantly, the budget should be adjusted around the plans and activities of the company so that the company remains focused on its goals.

In order to thrive, non-profit organizations must have revenues from several different sources. The budget lists all these sources and shows the amount of revenue expected for each of the financial sources. Fundraising is a key activity for non-profit organizations. These donations come from ticket sales, membership fees, auctions, charity events, sales of products or services, or other charitable activities.

Under the heading of expenses, the board of directors should allocate expenses to their programs and activities. Expenditures include direct costs, such as the cost of hiring new staff, ordering products, preparing brochures or other press, and travel. The cost required for buying or maintaining fixed assets, such as repairing or maintaining buildings, land, and cars, is one of the capital costs. Indirect cost (overhead) includes items such as bills, internet and postage.

As mentioned, the operating budget is different from the capital budget and plays an important role in the budgeting of non-profit centers. Capital budgeting includes projects that have a permanent impact on your performance. The capital budget is also used to plan the main costs, such as construction costs and other large costs that take more than one fiscal year to implement. The difference between the operating budget and the capital budget is that this budget shows the distribution of expected annual expenses and revenues according to different financial sources, the operating expenses of each program and overhead expenses.

The operational budget shows you the financial picture of the company's activities for the next year. The board of directors also uses this budget to show different amounts of income and financial resources. As it can be seen, the operational budget shows the amount of expected cost for the company's activities in the next year. Budgeting should always be consistent with the strategic plan and be effective in advancing the company's goals. Due to the factors such as rapid changes in the field of health care, the expansion of markets based on health tourism, developments based on reducing the role of human labor and upgrading the position of new equipment and technologies, the necessity of transformation in the system is inevitable. It is obvious that the existing patterns in financial system of health is not able to guide the decision makers of this field and it makes the need to create interdisciplinary knowledge to meet these information needs more clear [1, 9–20, 22–27].

References

1. Abbasi, F., Allahviranloo, T.: Conception and implementation of a new data-driven fuzzy method for reliability and safety analysis. New Math. Nat. Comput. **16**(02), 339–361 (2020). https://doi.org/10.1142/s1793005720500210
2. Abbasi, F., Allahviranloo, T.: The fuzzy arithmetic operations of transmission average on pseudo-hexagonal fuzzy numbers and its application in fuzzy system reliability analysis. Fuzzy Inf. Eng. **13**(1), 58–78 (2021). https://doi.org/10.1080/16168658.2021.1915449
3. Abbasi, F., Allahviranloo, T.: Realistic solution of fuzzy critical path problems, case study: the airport's cargo ground operation systems. Granular Comput. **8**(3), 617–632 (2022). https://doi.org/10.1007/s41066-022-00347-w
4. Akram, M., Shahzadi, S., Shah, S.M.U., Allahviranloo, T.: A fully Fermatean fuzzy multi-objective transportation model using an extended DEA technique. Granular Comput. (2023). https://doi.org/10.1007/s41066-023-00399-6
5. Allahviranloo, T., Abbasi, F.: A new estimation of failure analysis in fuzzy environment, case study: the electrical model failure for the football stadium. New Math. Nat. Comput. **18**(03), 791–817 (2022). https://doi.org/10.1142/s1793005722500387
6. Amirteimoori, A., Allahviranloo, T., Kordrostami, S., Bagheri, S.F.: Improving decision-making units in performance analysis methods: a data envelopment analysis approach. Math. Sci. (2023). https://doi.org/10.1007/s40096-023-00512-5
7. Amirteimoori, A., Allahviranloo, T., Zadmirzaei, M.: Scale elasticity and technical efficiency analysis in the European forest sector: a stochastic value-based approach. Eur. J. Forest Res. (2023). https://doi.org/10.1007/s10342-023-01589-2
8. Amirteimoori, A., Allahviranloo, T., Zadmirzaei, M., Hasanzadeh, F.: On the environmental performance analysis: a combined fuzzy data envelopment analysis and artificial intelligence algorithms. Expert Syst. Appl. **224**, 119953 (2023). https://doi.org/10.1016/j.eswa.2023.119953
9. Banker, R.D., Amirteimoori, A., Allahviranloo, T., Sinha, R.P.: Performance analysis and managerial ability in the general insurance market: a study of India and Iran. Inf. Technol. Manage. (2023). https://doi.org/10.1007/s10799-023-00405-y
10. Bjørnenak, T., Mitchell, F.: The development of activity-based costing journal literature, 1987–2000. Eur. Account. Rev. **11**(3), 481–508 (2002)
11. Chehlabi, M., Allahviranloo, T.: Concreted solutions to fuzzy linear fractional differential equations. Appl. Soft Comput. **44**, 108–116 (2016)
12. da Silva Etges, A.P.B., Cruz, L.N., Notti, R.K., Neyeloff, J.L., Schlatter, R.P., Astigarraga, C.C., Polanczyk, C.A., et al.: An 8-step framework for implementing time-driven activity-based costing in healthcare studies. Eur. J. Health Econ. **20**(8), 1133–1145 (2019)
13. Hammad, S.A., Jusoh, R., Yen Nee Oon, E.: Management accounting system for hospitals: a research framework. Ind. Manage. Data Syst. **110**(5), 762–784 (2010)
14. Kieso, D.E., Weygandt, J.J., Warfield, T.D., Wiecek, I.M., McConomy, B.J.: Intermediate Accounting, vol. 1. Wiley & Sons (2019)
15. Lueg, R., Storgaard, N.: The adoption and implementation of activity-based costing: a systematic literature review. Int. J. Strateg. Manage. **17**(2), 7–24 (2017)
16. Mahmoodirad, A., Allahviranloo, T., Niroomand, S.: A new effective solution method for fully intuitionistic fuzzy transportation problem. Soft. Comput. **23**(12), 4521–4530 (2019)
17. Moloudzadeh, S., Allahviranloo, T., Darabi, P.: A new method for solving an arbitrary fully fuzzy linear system. Soft. Comput. **17**(9), 1725–1731 (2013)
18. Öker, F., Özyapici, H.: A new costing model in hospital management: time-driven activity-based costing system. Health Prog. **32**(1), 23–36 (2013)
19. Quesado, P., Silva, R.: Activity-based costing (ABC) and its implication for open innovation. J. Open Innov. Technol. Market Complex. **7**(1), 41 (2021)
20. Rahmani, A., Lotfi, F.H., Rostamy-Malkhalifeh, M., Allahviranloo, T.: A new method for defuzzification and ranking of fuzzy numbers based on the statistical beta distribution. Adv. Fuzzy Syst. **2016**, 1–8 (2016)

21. Reiter, K.L., Song, P.H.: Gapenski's Healthcare Finance: An Introduction to Accounting and Financial Management. Health Administration Press (2021)
22. Seyyedabbasi, A.: WOASCALF: a new hybrid whale optimization algorithm based on sine cosine algorithm and levy flight to solve global optimization problems. Adv. Eng. Softw. **173**, 103272 (2022). https://doi.org/10.1016/j.advengsoft.2022.103272
23. Seyyedabbasi, A.: A reinforcement learning-based metaheuristic algorithm for solving global optimization problems. Adv. Eng. Softw. **178**, 103411 (2023). https://doi.org/10.1016/j.advengsoft.2023.10341
24. Seyyedabbasi, A.: Binary sand cat swarm optimization algorithm for wrapper feature selection on biological data. Biomimetics **8**(3), 310 (2023)
25. Seyyedabbasi, A., Kiani, F., Allahviranloo, T., Fernandez-Gamiz, U., Noeiaghdam, S.: Optimal data transmission and pathfinding for WSN and decentralized IoT systems using I-GWO and Ex-GWO algorithms. Alex. Eng. J. **63**, 339–357 (2023)
26. Siguenza-Guzman, L., Van den Abbeele, A., Vandewalle, J., Verhaaren, H., Cattrysse, D.: Recent evolutions in costing systems: a literature review of time-driven activity-based costing. Rev. Bus. Econ. Lit. **58**(1), 34–64 (2013)
27. Smith, P.: Introduction. In: Smith, P., Mossialos, E.M., Papanicolas, I., Leatherman, S. (eds.) Performance Measurement for Health System Improvement Experiences, Challenges and Prospects (2009)

Sleep Disorders Detection and Classification Using Random Forests Algorithm

Wadhah Zeyad Tareq Tareq

Abstract Insomnia and Sleep Apnea are popular sleep disorders. Sleep detection is an important step, especially in the earliest diagnosis of mental disease analysis. Moreover, sleep disorders affect body health such as blood pressure and stroke. Traditional detection methods are expensive and time-consuming due to devices required to read signals and experts for understanding and analyzing these signals. Therefore, different automatic systems based on machine learning algorithms have been developed to detect sleep disorders based on pre-assembled data from different clinics. In this chapter, a sleep disorders forecasting model is implemented using a Random Forests Classifier algorithm. The model is trained and tested using Sleep Health and Lifestyle dataset. The Sleep Health and Lifestyle dataset includes three classes Insomnia, Sleep Apnea, and None. Each class is featured with 12 different values such as gender, Sleep Duration, and Quality of Sleep. The detection accuracy of the Random Forests Classifier algorithm is recorded to be 88% on the sleep Health and Lifestyle dataset. Moreover, different algorithms were trained and tested on the same dataset to measure the performance of the selected algorithm. The result showed that the Random Forests Classifier algorithm is better than the other algorithms.

Keywords Machine learning · Classification · Random forest · Health dataset

1 Introduction and Motivation

Sleep is a natural phenomenon that plays a vital role in the lifespan of living beings. Different body functions and organics parts face different situations due to changes in awareness and sensual drive. These changes produce many diseases, some of which are very dangerous and may lead to death. The International Classification of Sleep Disorders divided these diseases into seven categories with more than 60 different sleep disorders [1]. Sleep Apnea and Insomnia are common sleep disorders

W. Z. T. Tareq (✉)
Faculty of Engineering and Natural Sciences, Istinye University, Istanbul, Turkey
e-mail: wadhah.tareq@istinye.edu.tr

T. Allahviranloo et al. (eds.), *Decision Making in Healthcare Systems*,
Studies in Systems, Decision and Control 513,
https://doi.org/10.1007/978-3-031-46735-6_10

that affect men and women at different age levels. Sleep apnea is characterized by abnormal breath pauses or reductions during sleep [2]. Insomnia patients cannot sleep properly due to stress, heart failure, heartburn, and drugs such as alcohol [3]. Traditionally, sleep disorders diagnosis occurs by observation of the patient's polysomnography (PSG) signals. Observing PSG signals requires an expert physician and many different resources. Such diagnosis is expensive due to the used resource. Moreover, the results depend on the experiences of the physician. So, the foregoing limits are evidence of the need for more practical diagnosis systems to reduce costs and provide reliable results [4].

In past years, different artificial intelligence (AI) approaches based on machine learning algorithms proposed to detect and diagnose sleep disorders. These approaches identify different disorders including Apnea and Insomnia based on different inputs. Some approaches used Age, weight, lifestyle, depression, and physical data to accurately predict or detect whether a person has a risk of a sleep disorder. Other approaches used machine learning algorithms to detect sleep disorders based on data received from different devices such as electrocardiographs (ECG) [5] and pulse oximetry [6]. Some approaches used data from questionnaires [7] and snoring [8] as input for algorithms to diagnose sleep disorders.

The AI model developed in this chapter is based on raw data to detect both Apnea and Insomnia disorders. The used dataset involves many features about the patient including age, gender, occupation, quality of sleep, sleep duration, physical activity level, body mass index, stress level, blood pressure, daily steps, and heart rate. All these features enable the model to predict accurately if a person suffers from sleep disorders or not. In order to understand the data and the effect of each feature on the final decision, different analysis methods were applied to the dataset. After that and depending on the analysis results, a classification supervised learning algorithm is applied. Supervised learning is used when there is a training dataset that has a well-defined relationship between each input and expected output. The rest of this chapter is organized as follows. In Sect. 2, the related works are described briefly. Section 3 describes the dataset and different analysis methods applied to it. Section 4 shows the experiments and the obtained results from these experiments. Finally, Sect. 5 concludes this chapter.

2 Literature Review

In previous studies, Tsinalis [9] used convolutional neural networks (CNNs) for sleep-stage scoring using electroencephalography (EEG) signals. The dataset was public and contained 20 records for 20 adults. Their work achieved 74% overall accuracy with a range between 71 and 76% overall records. Supratak et al. [10] proposed the DeepSleepNet model to learn sleep stages automatically using convolutional neural networks. They extracted extract time-invariant features to learn transition rules among sleep stages automatically from EEG epochs. Their results showed that the proposed model achieved similar overall accuracy compared with the different methods on the same dataset. Chambon et al. [11] introduced an end-to-end sleep stage classifier based on deep learning approaches. They used multi-modal polysomnography (PSG) signals including EEG, electromyography (EMG), and electrooculography (EOG). Olesen et al. [12] implemented a deep neural network with fifteen thousand polysomnography studies from several groups. They applied different scenarios such as measuring the performance of a single group on other groups, comparing the performance of using single data and mixed data, and finally the impact of timescales on the results. Their overall accuracy increased by 25% compared with related approaches.

Xu et al. [13] applied four CNNs on a sleep heart health study dataset to classify sleep stages. The results showed that the long short-term memory (LSTM) network had a better classification performance than the CNNs. Sridhar et al. [14] utilized a deep learning approach to build a model that uses instantaneous heart rate (IHR) extracted ECG to sleep stage scoring. They used data set with 10,000 records. The overall performance of the algorithm was 0.77 and they classified sleep into four main classes: wake, light sleep, deep sleep, and rapid eye movement (REM). Peter-Derex et al. [15] aimed to evaluate the performance of the single-channel automatic sleep staging (AS software ASEEGA in patients diagnosed with different sleep disorders. They used 95 patients' records including 23 patients with Insomnia, 24 patients with Hypersomnia, 24 patients with Narcolepsy, and 24 patients with Obstructive sleep apnea. Visual staging (VS was performed by two experts (VS1 and VS2 and AS was based on the analysis of a single electroencephalogram channel (Cz-Pz, without any information from electrooculography or electromyography. They compared pairwise (VS1-VS2, AS-VS1, AS-VS2 and between AS and consensual VS. The comparing results were: AS and VS1 78.6%, AS and VS2 75.0%; and VS1 and VS2 79.5%. The comparison between AS and 1 VS was 85.6% with the following distribution: insomnia 85.5%, narcolepsy 83.8%, idiopathic hypersomnia 86.1%, and obstructive sleep disorder 87.2%.

Sharma et al. [16] focused on the detection of several sleep disorders such as bruxism, insomnia, nocturnal frontal lobe epilepsy (NFLE), narcolepsy, rapid eye movement (REM), periodic leg movement (PLM), sleep-disordered breathing, and behavioral disorder. They used the cyclic alternating pattern (CAP) open-source dataset to train and test supervised machine learning classifiers. Their model accuracy was 85.3% for unbalanced datasets and 92.8% for balanced datasets. Perslev et al. [17] presented a deep learning system known as U-Sleep for sleep stages classification. U-Sleep used fully convolutional neural network architecture and trained using 15,660 data records from 16 different clinical. U-sleep works by using EEG and EOG signals and provides an accurate classification for different sleep stages. Goshtasbi et al. [18] introduced the SleepFCN approach based on convolutional neural network architecture to classify sleep stages into five classes. The input of the SleepFCN is single-channel electroencephalograms (EEGs) and the output is the predicted class. They used multi-scale feature extraction (MSFE) for feature extraction and residual dilated causal convolutions (ResDC) for temporal sequence encoding. They tested their approach using two different datasets: Sleep-EDF and Sleep Heart Health Study

(SHHS). Their results showed that their model outperformed the other models in both accuracy and speed.

3 Sleep Health Dataset

For this chapter, Sleep Health and Lifestyle (SHL) dataset [19] is used. The SHL contains 374 records with 12 features with three sleep conditions: Insomnia, Sleep Apnea, or None. Each sleep disorder is diagnosed based on Gender, Age, Occupation, Sleep Duration (hours), Quality of Sleep (scale from 1 to 10), Physical Activity Level (minutes/day), Stress Level (scale from 1 to 10), Body Mass Index (BMI), Blood Pressure (systolic/diastolic), Heart Rate (beats per minute), and Daily Steps. The sleep conditions represent three different situations: None means the individual does not exhibit any specific sleep disorder. Insomnia means the individual experiences difficulty falling asleep or staying asleep, leading to inadequate or poor-quality sleep. Sleep Apnea means the individual suffers from pauses in breathing during sleep, resulting in disrupted sleep patterns and potential health risks. Table 1 shows the first 5 records and the last 5 records for the SHL dataset. The dataset has no missed value. All features are assigned with correct real values. However, the dataset suffers from class imbalance where there are 219 patients without sleep disorder or with normal cases, 78 patients with apnea disorder, and 77 patients with insomnia disorder.

Table 2 shows a general statistical description of the data. The statistical description includes the number of non-empty features, the average value for a particular feature for all patients, the standard deviation for that feature, the minimum and maximum values, and the interpreted data distributions. Figure 1 shows relationship between the age and sleep disorders. Finally, Fig. 2 shows the mutual information matrix between variables and how each variable affects other variables.

4 Experiments and Results

The literature mentioned many different works to optimize different problems such as [20–23]. In this chapter, the Random forests classifier (RFC) algorithm is used for building a prediction model. The RFC algorithm was implemented by Leo Breiman in 2001 [24]. RFC is a popular machine learning algorithm used in different applications such as pattern recognition, classification, and skewed problems. RFC was built based on a decision tree algorithm where RFC contains one or many decision trees with various parameters. Consider a dataset $D = ((M_1, N_1), \ldots, (M_n, N_n))$ made of n records. $X \in M$ and $Y \in N$ where X and Y are sets of observations and class labels respectively. RFC mapping each observation for a label $X \rightarrow Y$ using an individual tree of the forest. Each tree produces a certain classification result. After each iteration, RFC selects the class decision with the highest ratio across all trees in the forest [25].

Table 1 First and last 5 samples from sleep health and lifestyle dataset

Gender	*Age*	*Occupation*	*Sleep duration*	*Quality of sleep*	*Physical activity level*
Male	27	Software engineer	6.10	6	42
Male	28	Doctor	6.20	6	60
Male	28	Doctor	6.20	6	60
Male	28	Sales representative	5.90	4	30
Male	28	Sales representative	5.90	4	30
…	…	…	…	…	…
…	…	…	…	…	…
…	…	…	…	…	…
Female	59	Nurse	8.10	9	75
Female	59	Nurse	8.00	9	75
Female	59	Nurse	8.10	9	75
Female	59	Nurse	8.10	9	75
Female	59	Nurse	8.10	9	75
Stress level	*BMI category*	*Blood pressure*	*Heart rate*	*Daily steps*	*Sleep disorder*
6	Overweight	126/83	77	4200	None
8	Normal	125/80	75	10,000	None
8	Normal	125/80	75	10,000	None
8	Obese	140/90	85	3000	Sleep apnea
8	Obese	140/90	85	3000	Sleep apnea
…	…	…	…	…	…
3	Overweight	140/95	68	7000	Sleep apnea
3	Overweight	140/95	68	7000	Sleep apnea
3	Overweight	140/95	68	7000	Sleep apnea
3	Overweight	140/95	68	7000	Sleep apnea
3	Overweight	140/95	68	7000	Sleep apnea

Before training the algorithm, we split the Sleep Health and Lifestyle dataset into training and testing datasets. The training data set contains 80% of the total dataset records, and the testing dataset contains the remaining 20%. We used the Scikit-Learn library to implement the RFC algorithm. Scikit-Learn is a free library for different machine learning algorithms written using Python programming language. Scikit-Learn provides different algorithms for different tasks such as regression, classification, and clustering. After training the model, the test dataset is used to measure the prediction accuracy for unseen data. The summary of precision, recall,

Table 2 General statistical description of the data

	Age	Sleep duration	Quality of sleep	Physical activity level	Stress level	Heart rate	Daily steps
Count	374	374	374	374	374	374	374
Mean	42.1	7.1	7.3	59.1	5.3	70.1	6816.8
std	8.6	0.7	1.1	20.8	1.7	4.1	1617.9
min	27	5.8	4	30	3	65	3000
25%	35.2	6.4	6	45	4	68	5600
50%	43	7.2	7	60	5	70	7000
75%	50	7.8	8	75	7	72	8000
max	59	8.5	9	90	8	86	10,000

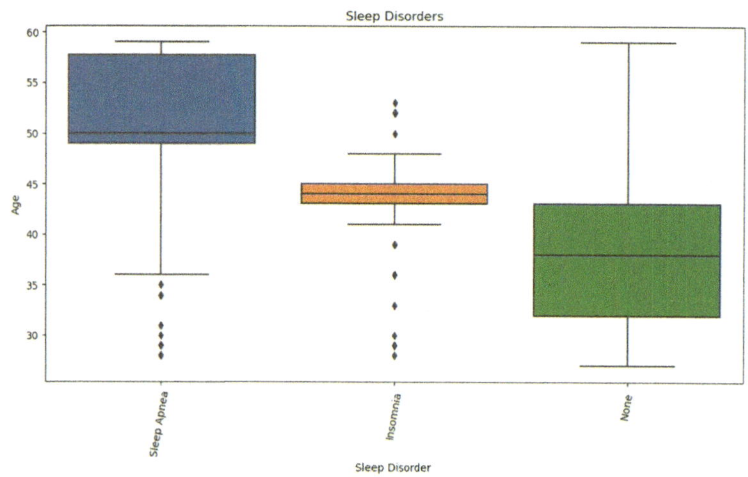

Fig. 1 Relationship between the age and the sleep disorders

and F1 scores for each class is presented in Table 3. Moreover, the unweighted and weighted averages per label are shown in the same table.

In Table 4, we compared the performance of the RFC algorithm with different machine learning algorithms such as LightGBM Classifier, Extra Tree Classifier, Bernoulli Naive Bayes, K-Nearest Neighbors (KNN) Classification, Support Vector Classification, Nearest Centroid Classifier, Nu-Support Vector Classification, AdaBoost Classifier, Gaussian Naive Bayes, Quadratic Discriminant Analysis, and Dummy Classifier. All these algorithms trained and tested using the same training set and test set. Random Forest Classifier has the highest accuracy compared with other algorithms. However, there are many other algorithms may perform better.

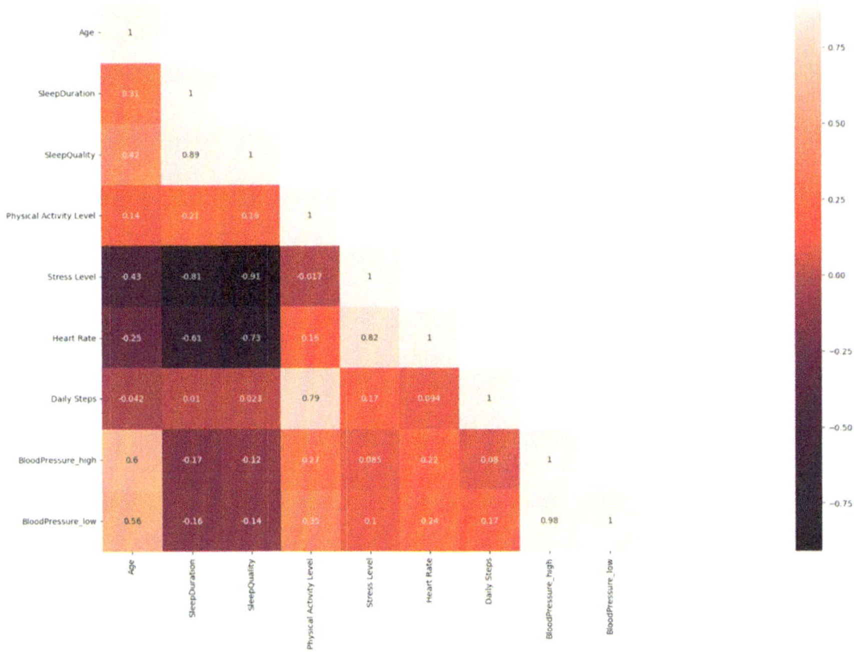

Fig. 2 Mutual information matrix between variables

Table 3 Summary of the main classification metrics

	Precision	Recall	F1-score	Support
Insomnia	0.72	0.81	0.76	16
None	0.95	0.98	0.97	43
Sleep apnea	0.85	0.69	0.76	16
Accuracy			0.88	75
Unweighted	0.84	0.83	0.83	75
Weighted	0.88	0.88	0.88	75

Table 4 Comparing RFC with different machine learning algorithms

Algorithm name	Accuracy
RandomForestClassifier	0.88
LGBMClassifier	0.88
ExtraTreeClassifier	0.88
BernoulliNB	0.88
KNeighborsClassifier	0.87
SVC	0.87
NearestCentroid	0.85
NuSVC	0.85
AdaBoostClassifier	0.75
GaussianNB	0.39
QuadraticDiscriminantAnalysis	0.56
DummyClassifier	0.57

5 Conclusion

This chapter concludes that it is possible to diagnose sleep disorders based on general features such as Gender, Age, Occupation, Sleep Duration, Quality of Sleep, Physical Activity Level, Stress Level, Body Mass Index, Blood Pressure, Heart Rate, and Daily Steps. The implemented approach proved that is reliable to detect sleep disorders without the need for an expert or plugged-in devices. It is easy to measure all mentioned features using simple devices. The diagnosis approach was developed using the Random forests classifier (RFC) algorithm. RFC algorithm is a machine learning classification algorithm based on decision tree concepts. The RFC algorithm was trained and tested using the Sleep Health and Lifestyle (SHL) dataset. The RFC classifier accuracy is found to be 88%. Therefore, it will be easy to detect different sleep disorders with simple information as discussed above.

References

1. Mendonça, F., Mostafa, S.S., Ravelo-García, A.G., Morgado-Dias, F., Penzel, T.: A review of obstructive sleep apnea detection approaches. IEEE J. Biomed. Health Inform. **23**(2), 825–837 (2019). https://doi.org/10.1109/jbhi.2018.2823265
2. Xie, B., Minn, H.: Real-time sleep apnea detection by classifier combination. IEEE Trans. Inf. Technol. Biomed. **16**(3), 469–477 (2012). https://doi.org/10.1109/titb.2012.2188299
3. Tripathi, P., Ansari, M.A., Gandhi, T.K., Mehrotra, R., Heyat, B.B., Akhtar, F., Ukwuoma, C.C., Muaad, A., Kadah, Y.M., Kim, T., Li, J.: Ensemble computational intelligent for insomnia sleep stage detection via the sleep ECG signal. IEEE Access **10**, 108710–108721 (2022). https://doi.org/10.1109/access.2022.3212120
4. Hassan, A.R.: Computer-aided obstructive sleep apnea detection using normal inverse Gaussian parameters and adaptive boosting. Biomed. Signal Process. Control **29**, 22–30 (2016). https://doi.org/10.1016/j.bspc.2016.05.009

5. McNames, J., Fraser, A.G.: Obstructive sleep apnea classification based on spectrogram patterns in the electrocardiogram (2000). https://doi.org/10.1109/cic.2000.898633
6. Magalang, U.J., Dmochowski, J.P., Veeramachaneni, S.B., Draw, A., Mador, M.J., El-Solh, A.A., Grant, B.J.B.: Prediction of the apnea-hypopnea index from overnight pulse oximetry*. Chest **124**(5), 1694–1701 (2003). https://doi.org/10.1378/chest.124.5.1694
7. Netzer, N.C., Stoohs, R., Netzer, C., Clark, K., Strohl, K.P.: Using the Berlin questionnaire to identify patients at risk for the sleep apnea syndrome. Ann. Intern. Med. **131**(7), 485 (1999). https://doi.org/10.7326/0003-4819-131-7-199910050-00002
8. Ng, A.K., Koh, T.S., Baey, E., Puvanendran, K.: Speech-like analysis of snore signals for the detection of obstructive sleep apnea. In: IEEE Conference Publication | IEEE Xplore (2006). https://ieeexplore.ieee.org/abstract/document/4155871
9. Tsinalis, O.. Automatic Sleep Stage Scoring with Single-Channel EEG Using Convolutional Neural Networks. arXiv.org. https://doi.org/10.1016/j.swevo.2018.09.008
10. Supratak, A., Dong, H., Li, V.C., Guo, Y.: DeepSleepNet: a model for automatic sleep stage scoring based on raw single-channel EEG. IEEE Trans. Neural Syst. Rehab. Eng. **25**(11), 1998–2008 (2017). https://doi.org/10.1109/tnsre.2017.2721116
11. Chambon, S., Galtier, M., Arnal, P.J., Wainrib, G., Gramfort, A.: A deep learning architecture for temporal sleep stage classification using multivariate and multimodal time series. IEEE Trans. Neural Syst. Rehab. Eng. **26**(4), 758–769 (2018). https://doi.org/10.1109/tnsre.2018.2813138
12. Olesen, A.N., Jennum, P., Mignot, E., Sørensen, H.B.D.: Automatic sleep stage classification with deep residual networks in a mixed-cohort setting. Sleep **44**(1) (2020). https://doi.org/10.1093/sleep/zsaa161
13. Xu, Z., Yang, X., Sun, J., Liu, P., Qin, W.: Sleep stage classification using time-frequency spectra from consecutive multi-time points. Front. Neurosci. **14**(2020).https://doi.org/10.3389/fnins.2020.00014
14. Sridhar, N., Shoeb, A., Stephens, P.J., Kharbouch, A., Shimol, D.B., Burkart, J., Ghoreyshi, A., Myers, L.J.: Deep learning for automated sleep staging using instantaneous heart rate. NPJ Digit. Med. **3**(1) (2020). https://doi.org/10.1038/s41746-020-0291-x
15. Peter-Derex, L., Berthomier, C., Taillard, J., Berthomier, P., Bouet, R., Mattout, J., Brandewinder, M., Bastuji, H.: Automatic analysis of single-channel sleep EEG in a large spectrum of sleep disorders. J. Clin. Sleep Med. **17**(3), 393–402 (2021). https://doi.org/10.5664/jcsm.8864
16. Sharma, M., Tiwari, J., Acharya, U.R.: Automatic sleep-stage scoring in healthy and sleep disorder patients using optimal wavelet filter bank technique with EEG signals. Int. J. Environ. Res. Public Health **18**(6), 3087 (2021). https://doi.org/10.3390/ijerph18063087
17. Perslev, M., Darkner, S., Kempfner, L., Nikolic, M., Jennum, P., Igel, C.: U-Sleep: resilient high-frequency sleep staging. NPJ Digit. Med. **4**(1) (2021). https://doi.org/10.1038/s41746-021-00440-5
18. Goshtasbi, N., Boostani, R., Sanei, S.: SleepFCN: a fully convolutional deep learning framework for sleep stage classification using single-channel electroencephalograms. IEEE Trans. Neural Syst. Rehabil. Eng. **30**, 2088–2096 (2022). https://doi.org/10.1109/tnsre.2022.3192988
19. Sleep Health and Lifestyle Dataset.: Kaggle (2023). https://www.kaggle.com/datasets/uom190346a/sleep-health-and-lifestyle-dataset
20. Seyyedabbasi, A.: WOASCALF: a new hybrid whale optimization algorithm based on sine cosine algorithm and levy flight to solve global optimization problems. Adv. Eng. Softw. **173**, 103272 (2022). https://doi.org/10.1016/j.advengsoft.2022.103272
21. Seyyedabbasi, A.: A reinforcement learning-based metaheuristic algorithm for solving global optimization problems. Adv. Eng. Softw. **178**, 103411 (2023). https://doi.org/10.1016/j.advengsoft.2023.10341
22. Seyyedabbasi, A.: Binary sand cat swarm optimization algorithm for wrapper feature selection on biological data. Biomimetics **8**(3), 310 (2023)
23. Seyyedabbasi, A., Kiani, F., Allahviranloo, T., Fernandez-Gamiz, U., Noeiaghdam, S.: Optimal data transmission and pathfinding for WSN and decentralized IoT systems using I-GWO and Ex-GWO algorithms. Alex. Eng. J. **63**, 339–357 (2023)

24. Breiman, L.: Random forests. Mach. Learn. **45**(1), 5–32 (2001). https://doi.org/10.1023/a:1010933404324
25. Azar, A.T., Elshazly, H.I., Hassanien, A.E., Elkorany, A.S.: A random forest classifier for lymph diseases. Comput. Methods Programs Biomed. **113**(2), 465–473 (2014). https://doi.org/10.1016/j.cmpb.2013.11.004

Green Supply Chain in Medicine

Mehdi Fadaei Eshkiki and Mahdi Homayounfar

Abstract A green supply chain in medicine refers to the integration of environmentally practices into the pharmaceutical industry's supply chain processes. This involves reducing the environmental impact of the sourcing, manufacturing, distribution, and disposal of medicines by incorporating eco-friendly methods, materials, and processes. Since, the pharmaceutical industry ranks 8th in terms of carbon dioxide production and 6th in terms of hazardous waste generation among various industries, paying attention to environmental issues is of great importance in this industry. The implementation of a green supply chain in medicine can result in reduced waste and pollution, improved patient safety, increased efficiency and cost savings, and enhanced stakeholder reputation. However, there are also challenges involved in implementing such practices, including regulatory compliance, cost considerations, and the need for collaboration across the supply chain. Overall, a green supply chain in medicine has the potential to benefit both the environment and the healthcare industry. Du to its importance, in this study the benefits, challenges and opportunities of medicine supply chain are discussed in different sections. Then, a conceptual model is developed for further analysis of medicine green supply chain (GSC) in terms of causes, contextual factors, interventions, strategies and outcomes. Finally, some medicine organizations that successfully have implemented green supply chain practices, are introduced as case studies.

Keywords Supply chain management · Healthcare · Medicine · Green · Environmental issues

M. F. Eshkiki (✉) · M. Homayounfar
Department of Industrial Management, Rasht Branch, Islamic Azad University, Rasht, Iran
e-mail: fadaei@iaurasht.ac.ir

T. Allahviranloo et al. (eds.), *Decision Making in Healthcare Systems*,
Studies in Systems, Decision and Control 513,
https://doi.org/10.1007/978-3-031-46735-6_11

1 Introduction

With the growing concern for the environment, there is an increasing need for the healthcare industry to adopt green practices. The supply chain in medicine plays a vital role in achieving green goals. However, the sector's growth and expansion have led to environmental degradation, posing significant risks to human health and the planet's ecosystem. As such, there is an increasing need for the healthcare industry to adopt green practices that reduce its environmental footprint. The concept of a green supply chain in medicine involves the integration of environmentally friendly practices in the sourcing, manufacturing, distribution, and disposal of medical products. It involves using sustainable materials, reducing waste, and minimizing carbon emissions through the adoption of eco-friendly practices. The implementation of a green supply chain in medicine can significantly reduce the environmental impact of the healthcare industry and contribute to the achievement of global sustainability goals. This chapter provides an overview of the green supply chain in medicine and its significance in the healthcare industry. One of the techniques for decision making is Data Envelopment Analysis (DEA), and many researchers have conducted research on this topic. Several recent papers have been cited to mention their research area, [1–4]. Some authors have explored the topic in a different way: safety analysis and reliability, [5–9].

2 Medicine Supply Chain

The medicine supply chain refers to the complex network of processes, activities, and stakeholders involved in the production, distribution, and delivery of pharmaceuticals and medical products from component producer, manufacturers to end users, such as patients and healthcare providers [10]. This includes the flow of raw materials, intermediate products, finished goods, and information throughout the supply chain to ensure that safe and effective medicines are available when and where they are needed. Several key elements are involved in the medicine supply chain, including component suppliers, medicine manufacturers, wholesalers, distributors, retailers, pharmacies, hospitals, clinics, and patients. Efficient supply chain management is crucial to ensure that medicines are produced, stored, transported, and dispensed in a timely and efficient manner while maintaining quality and safety standards. A simple scheme of a medicine supply chain is presented in Fig. 1.

- Manufacturers contract with wholesalers to distribute their products. These contracts may include provisions for bulk-purchasing discounts or discounts for immediate payment, but the specific terms are typically negotiated on a case-by-case basis. In addition to these discounts, manufacturers pay wholesalers a service fee to manage inventory, financial transactions, distribution, and data processing.

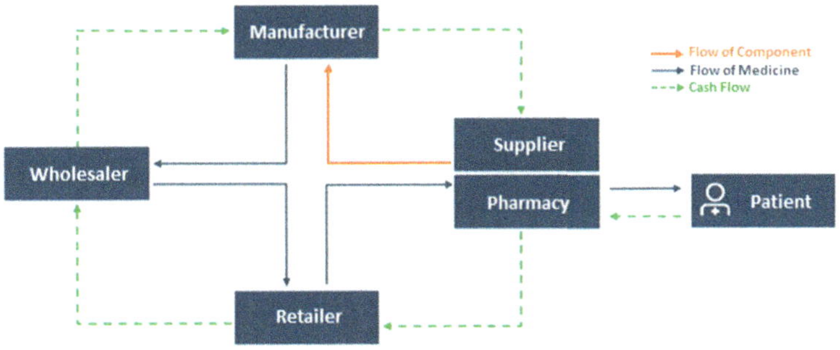

Fig. 1 Medicine supply chain

- Wholesalers are responsible for purchasing drugs from manufacturers and distributing them to various customers, including independent, chain, or mail-order pharmacies, hospitals, long-term care facilities, and other medical facilities. Wholesalers may specialize in selling certain products, such as biologic products, or to specific customers in addition to providing more specialized services. Wholesalers typically purchase drugs at the wholesale acquisition cost (WAC), adjusted for any negotiated purchase discounts.
- Pharmacies purchase drugs from wholesalers, and occasionally directly from manufacturers. After purchasing these drugs, pharmacies must safely store and dispense them to patients. Pharmacies typically purchase drugs at WAC, adjusted for any purchase discounts. The negotiated percentage is often influenced by a pharmacy's volume of purchases.

Medicine supply chain is critical for ensuring the availability and accessibility of essential medicines to patients in need. A well-functioning medicine supply chain involves the efficient and effective management of the flow of medicines from manufacturers to patients, including procurement, storage, transportation, distribution, and inventory management. A reliable medicine supply chain is essential for the timely delivery of high-quality medicines, especially in emergencies or during disease outbreaks. It also plays a crucial role in reducing medicine stock-outs, ensuring the availability of essential medicines, and preventing the circulation of counterfeit or substandard medicines. In addition, an optimized medicine supply chain can help reduce waste, lower costs, and improve patient safety by ensuring the proper handling and storage of medicines. It can also facilitate the implementation of public health programs and support the achievement of global health goals, such as the sustainable development goals.

However, the medicine supply chain faces various challenges, including inadequate infrastructure, lack of resources and capacity, inefficient logistics, and weak regulatory systems. These challenges can result in medicine shortages, stock-outs, delays, and quality issues, which can have severe consequences for patients' health and well-being. Therefore, there is a need for ongoing efforts to strengthen the medicine supply chain, including investments in infrastructure and technology, capacity building, and regulatory reforms. Such efforts can help ensure the availability, accessibility, affordability, and quality of essential medicines to patients in need, and ultimately contribute to improving global health outcomes. In Table 1, the main industries of the world are compared based upon the various indicators [11].

Note that because of the high difference between energy industry with the other industries in green indicators, it was not considered in the Figs. 2 and 3.

3 Green Supply Chain in Medicine

The increasing concern about environmental warnings and efforts to reduce as much as possible the bio-environmental pollutants has led to the emergence of new concepts such as GSCM. It was first introduced by the Industrial Research Society of the University of Michigan in 1996 as a novel management model for the environment protection [12].

Green supply chain management (GSCM) as an emerging approach aims to reduce the environmental impact of supply chains while improving their efficiency and effectiveness. In the medicine industry. In the medicine industry, a green supply chain management involves designing and managing the entire supply chain process with a focus on minimizing its environmental impact. This can include reducing energy

Table 1 Evaluation of the world main industries in 2021

Criteria	Annual revenue (billions USD)	Number of employees (millions)	Carbon emissions (metric tons CO2 equivalent)	Water consumption (billions of gallons per year)	Hazardous waste generated (millions of tons)
Pharmaceutical	1,430.30	4.4	45.7	1.6	0.1
Automotive	2,564.90	1.3	118.5	5.5	0.05
Aerospace and defense	439.6	3.1	98.9	5.6	0.3
Electronics	5,196.50	10.7	163.8	6.5	0.02
Information technology (IT)	5,188.70	14.5	264.7	3.6	0.05
Energy	5,762.70	5.8	1,954.20	40.7	1.3
Telecommunications	1,064.70	2.2	132.2	1.4	0.2
Construction	1,275.70	7.2	127.5	4.4	0.2
Agriculture	2,712.70	1.4	473.5	2,677.50	0.2
Banking and finance	4,687.70	0.4	160.5	1.6	0.02
Tourism and hospitality	837.4	4.4	177.6	0.7	0.01

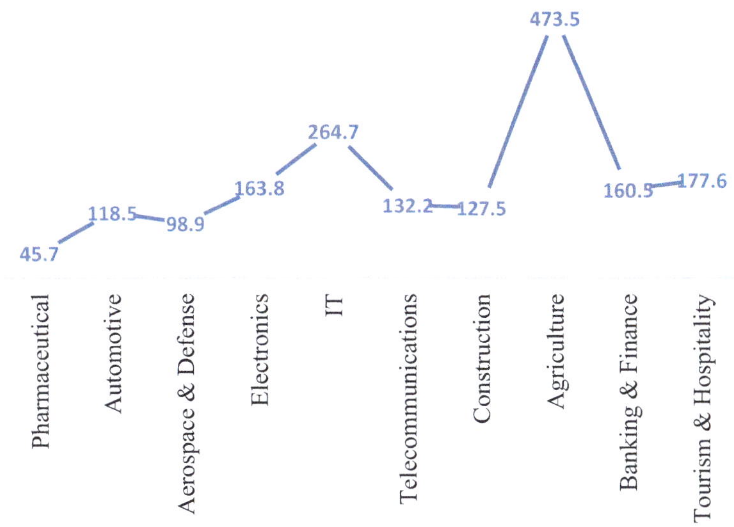

Fig. 2 Carbon emissions (in metric tons CO2 equivalent)

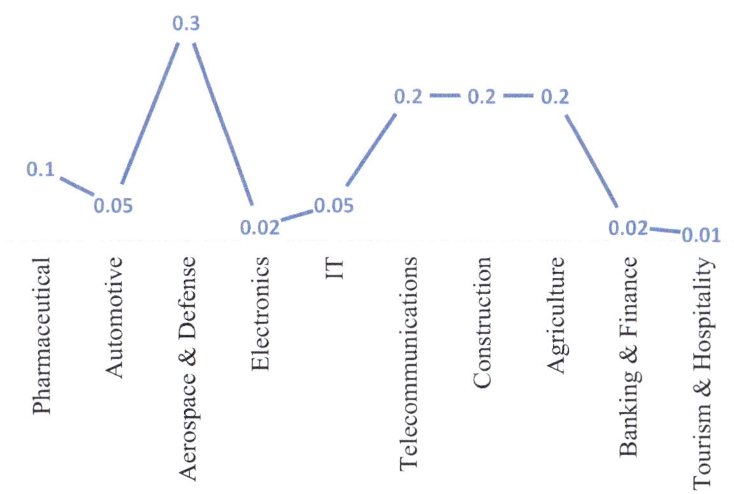

Fig. 3 Hazardous waste generated (in millions of tons)

consumption, decreasing carbon emissions, and minimizing waste throughout the production, transportation, and disposal of medical products [13].

The implementation of GSCM practices has various benefits for the healthcare industry, including reducing the environmental impact, enhancing the reputation of healthcare organizations, and improving operational efficiency [14].

- Reducing the Environmental Impact

The healthcare industry has a significant impact on the environment due to the generation of medical waste, high energy consumption, and the use of hazardous materials. The implementation of GSCM practices can significantly reduce the environmental impact of the healthcare industry. For instance, healthcare organizations can reduce energy consumption by adopting energy-efficient technologies, reduce waste generation by using recyclable and biodegradable materials, and minimize the use of hazardous materials by adopting safer alternatives. These practices can reduce the environmental impact of the healthcare industry and promote sustainability [15, 16].

- Enhancing the Reputation of Healthcare Organizations

The implementation of GSCM practices can enhance the reputation of medicine organizations. Consumers are becoming increasingly aware of the environmental impact of their purchasing decisions, and environmentally conscious consumers prefer to purchase products from sustainable organizations. Healthcare organizations that adopt GSCM practices can attract environmentally conscious consumers and enhance their reputation. This can result in increased customer loyalty, improved brand image, and increased revenue.

- Improving Operational Efficiency

The implementation of GSCM practices can also improve the operational efficiency of medicine organizations. For instance, adopting energy-efficient technologies can reduce energy consumption and lower operational costs. Adopting sustainable waste management practices can reduce waste generation and lower disposal costs. Moreover, adopting GSCM practices can improve supply chain visibility, enhance communication and collaboration between stakeholders, and improve supply chain performance.

- Compliance with Environmental Regulations

The implementation of GSCM practices can help healthcare organizations comply with environmental regulations. Governments are increasingly implementing regulations to reduce the environmental impact of various industries, including the healthcare industry. By adopting GSCM practices, healthcare organizations can comply with environmental regulations and avoid penalties and legal issues. Studies on personnel employment and planning in hospitals and other health institutions are still among the important studies today. Provide timely and good quality care to sick individuals. When making these choices, it is important to note that most hospitals are obliged to have 24-h staff in their nursing and emergency units. There are also many pressures to reduce the costs of health care. Health care providers should control the cost. An element that has a significant impact on cost is the staff.

3.1 Sourcing in Medicine GSC

The use of eco-friendly materials and green sourcing practices can significantly reduce the environmental impact of the healthcare industry. Medical equipment and devices can be made from recycled materials or sourced from suppliers who prioritize green practices. Additionally, the use of renewable energy sources such as solar or wind power in manufacturing can reduce carbon emissions.

Sourcing in GSC involves selecting suppliers that have implemented environmental management practices and have demonstrated their commitment to greenness. Medicine manufacturers need to identify suppliers that are willing to work towards reducing their environmental footprint such as waste and greenhouse gas emissions, and collaborate with them to develop strategies to reduce their impact. Sourcing green materials, healthcare manufacturers can reduce costs associated with waste disposal, increase efficiency, and enhance their reputation. Collaborating with suppliers to develop green strategies can lead to long-term partnerships that benefit both parties.

Suppliers can also benefit from green sourcing in supply chain. Implementing green practices, suppliers can enhance their reputation and attract more customers. Moreover, by collaborating with medicine manufacturers to develop sustainable strategies, suppliers can gain access to new markets and increase their competitiveness. In addition, through the sourcing environmentally compatible materials such as recyclable plastics, biodegradable packaging, and reusable products can significantly reduce the environmental impact of the medicine industry. Finally, sourcing from local suppliers can reduce transportation emissions, which contribute significantly to the carbon footprint of the healthcare industry.

3.2 Manufacturing in Medicine GSC

Green production in the medicine industry involves the implementation of environmentally-friendly practices throughout the entire production process. This includes the use of sustainable materials, reducing waste and pollution, and minimizing the carbon footprint of the production process. Green production also involves ensuring that the end product is safe and healthy for both patients and the environment [17].

One of the ways that the medicine industry can implement green production practices is by using sustainable and biodegradable materials in packaging and production. For example, using plant-based materials for capsules and packaging materials made from recycled or biodegradable materials can significantly reduce the environmental impact of medicine production. Another important aspect of green production in the medicine industry is reducing waste and pollution. This can be achieved by using energy-efficient technologies, renewable energy sources recycling or repurposing waste materials, and reducing the use of harmful chemicals in the production process. Green manufacturing, and includes the use of, reducing water consumption, minimizing waste, and adopting green technologies [18, 19].

Green production practices in the medicine industry can also contribute to improving the health and safety of patients. By reducing the use of harmful chemicals and implementing more sustainable practices, medicine manufacturers can minimize the negative impact of their products on the environment and the health of the individuals who use them.

Adapting green manufacturing, in addition to reduce costs associated with waste disposal, manufacturers could increase their operational efficiency, enhance their reputation and attract environmentally conscious consumers. However, implementing green manufacturing practices in the medicine industry can be challenging. Healthcare organizations need to invest in research and development to identify green technologies and practices. Moreover, green manufacturing practices may require significant capital investments, which may deter suppliers from adopting them. The implementation of lean manufacturing practices in medicine industry as a manufacturing philosophy can also reduce waste and improve efficiency.

3.3 Distribution in Medicine GSC

The green distribution of medicine industry involves adopting green transportation, storage, and delivery of medical supplies, equipment, and pharmaceutical products that reduce the environmental impact of the traditional transportation methods. The use of green transportation options such as electric or hybrid vehicles can significantly reduce carbon emissions. Using the green fuels such as low-sulfur and alternative fuels such as liquefied natural gases, and the promotion of environmentally friendly driving to reduce fuel consumption. Efficient supply chain management can optimize delivery routes and reduce transportation costs, further contributing to sustainability goals [20].

Another important component of green distribution is the adoption of sustainable packaging materials. This can include the use of biodegradable or recyclable materials, as well as the reduction of excess packaging. The proper disposal of packaging waste is also a critical element of green distribution, as it ensures that the waste does not end up in landfills or pollute the environment.

Adopting green transportation practices requires collaboration between healthcare manufacturers and suppliers to develop strategies that promote sustainability and reduce the environmental impact of distribution processes. However, Green transportation has been given the least attention from medicine organizations and has been considered as a general concept, while the transportation system has significant environmental impacts. Deaths and dangers from toxic gases in transportation, which are never covered by companies [21].

3.4 Disposal in Medicine GSC

Disposal is a critical aspect of the medicine industry that requires strict adherence to regulations and guidelines. Medicine waste can contain hazardous substances that pose a threat to the ecosystem and the population. Therefore, the medicine industry must employ proper disposal methods to ensure the safety of the environment and public health.

The disposal of medicine waste involves several stages, including segregation, collection, transportation, treatment, and final disposal. At the segregation stage, waste is sorted based on its properties and potential hazards. This step ensures that hazardous and non-hazardous waste is separated, and the proper disposal method is employed. The collection stage involves the proper storage and labeling of the waste. This ensures that the waste is easily identifiable and that the proper disposal method is employed. Transportation is the stage where the waste is moved from the point of generation to the treatment site. The transportation process must follow strict regulations to prevent accidents and ensure the safe handling of the waste. At the treatment stage, the waste undergoes various processes, including incineration, chemical treatment, or biological treatment. The final disposal stage involves the safe and environmentally sound disposal of the treated waste. The medicine industry must ensure that the final disposal method is consistent with the regulations and guidelines set by the government. While an effective disposal system has significant benefits for medicine organizations, improper disposal of medical waste can have severe environmental consequences such as loss of reputation and fall in loyal consumers.

4 Challenges/Opportunities of Medicine GSC

Medicine supply chains face several challenges in implementing their green practices [17]. Implementation of a green supply chain requires significant investments in eco-friendly technology and infrastructure. Additionally, the adoption of sustainable practices can require changes in organizational culture and supply chain management practices. Medicine organizations must also ensure compliance with regulations related to environmental sustainability. Following, the main challenges of GSCM in medicine are presented and the impact of these challenges on the medicine industry is described [22].

- Cost Considerations.

GSCM practices often require significant investments in technologies, training, and infrastructure. Moreover, adopting green practices may result in higher operational costs in the short term. Medicine organizations often have limited resources, and the adoption of GSCM practices may not be a top priority. Therefore, medicine organizations may be reluctant to adopt GSCM practices due to cost considerations.

- Lack of Standards and Regulations

The medicine industry lacks specific guidelines and regulations for environmentally friendly practices. This lack of standards and regulations makes it challenging for medicine organizations to measure and evaluate their environmental performance. Moreover, healthcare organizations may face difficulties in identifying and selecting green suppliers due to the lack of industry standards [23].

- Limited Stakeholder Engagement

The successful implementation of GSCM practices in medicine industry requires engagement and collaboration between stakeholders, including healthcare organizations, suppliers, regulators, and customers. However, limited stakeholder engagement is a significant challenge of GSCM in the medicine industry. Suppliers may not have the resources or knowledge to adopt environmentally friendly practices. Regulators may not provide adequate support or incentives for medicine organizations to adopt GSCM practices. Customers may not be aware of the environmental impact of their purchasing decisions.

- Complex and Fragmented Supply Chain

The medicine supply chain is complex and fragmented, involving multiple stakeholders, including manufacturers, distributors, wholesalers, and retailers. This complexity and fragmentation make it challenging to implement GSCM practices effectively. For instance, medicine organizations may face difficulties in monitoring and controlling environmental practices across the supply chain. Moreover, medicine organizations may face challenges in identifying and selecting environmentally friendly suppliers across the supply chain.

Despite of the challenges that green supply chains are faced in medicine industry, adopting green supply chain practices can help medicine organizations reduce their environmental impacts and promote sustainability. Some potential opportunities and benefits for implementing the green supply chain in medicine are listed below.

- Sustainable Procurement

One of the significant opportunities for implementing a green supply chain in medicine is sustainable procurement. Sustainable procurement involves selecting suppliers who demonstrate environmentally friendly practices, such as using renewable energy, reducing waste, and minimizing their carbon footprint. By selecting green suppliers, medicine organizations can promote sustainability throughout the supply chain.

- Energy Efficiency

Another opportunity for implementing a green supply chain in medicine is energy efficiency. Healthcare facilities are significant energy users, and energy efficiency measures can help reduce energy consumption and associated carbon emissions. Energy-efficient practices can include implementing renewable energy sources, upgrading lighting and HVAC systems, and using energy-efficient equipment.

- Waste Reduction and Recycling

Reducing waste and increasing recycling are critical opportunities for implementing a green supply chain in medicine. Medicine organizations generate significant amounts of waste, including hazardous materials, medical equipment, and pharmaceuticals. Implementing waste reduction and recycling practices can help medicine organizations minimize their environmental impacts and reduce their carbon footprint.

- Green Transportation

Transportation is a significant contributor to the carbon emissions associated with the healthcare industry. Implementing green transportation practices can help healthcare organizations reduce their environmental impacts. Examples of green transportation practices include using low-emission vehicles, optimizing transportation routes, and promoting alternative transportation methods such as cycling or public transit.

- Stakeholder Engagement

Effective stakeholder engagement is critical for implementing a green supply chain in medicine. Engaging stakeholders such as suppliers, employees, and customers can help promote sustainability and environmental awareness.

5 Conceptual Model of the Medicine GSC

In this section, to better understand the dimensions of the medicine green supply chain, a qualitative approach, namely grounded theory (GT) is employed. GT first developed by Glaser and Strauss in the 1960 to systematically generating theories or explanations from data collected through empirical research. Since 1960s, it has been widely used in various fields, including social sciences, healthcare, business, and education.

The basic process of grounded theory involves collecting and analyzing data inductively, allowing theories or concepts to emerge from the data rather than being imposed a priori. The researcher starts with an open mind, without preconceived theories or hypotheses, and engages in a cyclic process of data collection, coding, and analysis to identify patterns, concepts, and relationships. This process typically involves several stages, including data coding, constant comparison, theoretical sampling, and theoretical saturation.

GT is characterized by its emphasis on theoretical development from the data itself, rather than relying solely on existing theories or prior knowledge. It aims to generate theories that are grounded in the lived experiences and perspectives of the participants, allowing for a deep understanding of the phenomenon under study. Grounded theory is often used to explore complex social processes, uncover new insights, and generate theories that can be further tested or refined in future research. The main components of a GT model are:

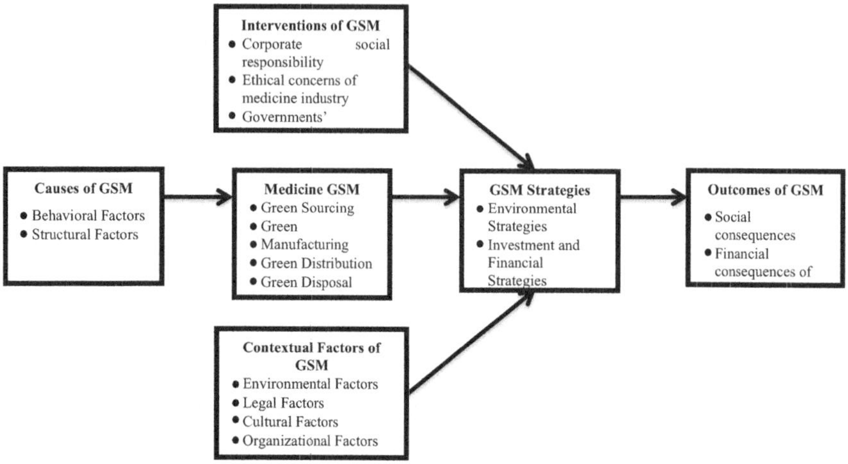

Fig. 4 The Conceptual model of green supply chain in medicine

- Causes: This category includes factors that contribute to the phenomenon under study. These may be individual, environmental, or social factors that have an impact on the phenomenon.
- Contextual factors: This category includes factors that are unique to the context in which the phenomenon is observed. This may include cultural, social, or historical factors that influence the phenomenon.
- Interventions: This category includes strategies or actions that are implemented to address the phenomenon. This may include policies, programs, or other interventions that are designed to mitigate the effects of the phenomenon.
- Strategies: This category includes specific actions or approaches that are used to address the phenomenon. This may include specific methods or techniques that are used to address the causes or effects of the phenomenon.
- Outcomes: This category includes the results or consequences of the phenomenon. This may include short-term or long-term outcomes that are related to the phenomenon.

Implementing the GT approach, the following table and conceptual model are proposed for the green supply chain of medicine (Fig. 4 and Table 2).

6 Case Studies

Green supply chain management practices are increasingly being adopted by some of the biggest pharmaceutical organizations worldwide to promote sustainability and reduce environmental impacts [24]. In this section, we will examine some case studies of medicine organizations that have implemented green supply chain practices.

Table 2 The components of green supply chain model in medicine

Component	Sub category	Category
Causes	Structural factors	Alignment of organizational and environmental goals
		Program for reducing energy consumption in the pharmaceutical industry
		Environmental impact assessment system for medicines
		Green supplier evaluation system
		Establishment of a green monitoring team
		Implementation of pharmaceutical waste management
		Monitoring of greenhouse gases in the pharmaceutical industry
		Planning to avoid the production of pharmaceutical waste
	Behavioral factors	Leadership style supportive of green sourcing in the pharmaceutical industry
		Culture of support for green supply chain in the industry
Green SCM	Green sourcing	Purchasing recycled materials for production
		Purchasing biodegradable material for packaging
		Coordinating with green suppliers
		Purchasing renewable energy sources
		Sourcing from local suppliers to reduce transportation emissions
	Green manufacturing	Using green materials for production
		Implementing lean manufacturing practices to reduce waste
		Minimizing the pollution of production process
		Producing safe and healthy medicine for both patients and the environment
		Using energy-efficient technologies
		Using biodegradable materials in packaging
		Using renewable energy sources for production
		Recycling or repurposing waste materials
		Reducing the use of harmful chemicals in the production process
		Reducing water consumption
	Green distribution	Adopting green transportation, storage, and delivery of medical supplies and products
		Use of electric or hybrid vehicles for transportation
		Promotion of environmentally friendly driving to reduce fuel consumption
		Optimizing the delivery routes
		Deaths and dangers from toxic material in transportation

(continued)

Table 2 (continued)

Component	Sub category	Category
	Green disposal	Sorting waste based on its properties and potential hazards at the segregation stage
		Separating hazardous and non-hazardous waste
		Proper storage and labelling of the waste in collection stage
		Following strict regulations to prevent accidents and ensure the safe handling of the waste
		Chemical or biological treatment of the waste under various processes
		Safe and environmentally sound disposal of the treated waste
		Disposal consistent with the governmental regulations and guidelines
Intervention		Low commitment to social responsibility
		Decrease in ethical concerns of the medicine industry
		Government weakness in environmental support
		Weak infrastructures for green supply
Contextual	Environmental factor	Utilization of renewable energy sources
		Presence of environmental management systems
		Ecological design
	Legal factors	Environmental laws and regulations
	Cultural factors	Training and development of human resources
		Supportive management atmosphere for green systems
	Organizational factors	Waste management/ disposal
		Management systems utilization of sustainable resource
	Technological factors	Utilization of green technologies
Strategies	Environmental strategy	Environmental impact assessments
		Implementation of waste reduction and recycling programs
		Establishment of environmental management systems
		Commitment to the environmental regulations and standards
		Development of green logistics and transportation strategies
	Financial strategy	Collaboration with suppliers for sustainable investment in renewable energy and technologies
		Development of shareholder participation strategies for sustainability
	HRM strategy	Training and participation of employees in sustainable practices
	Marketing strategy	Development and design of green products and packaging
		Design of a green supply chain network
Outcomes	Social	Improvement of environmental outcomes for the community

(continued)

Table 2 (continued)

Component	Sub category	Category
		Enhancement of public health
	Financial	Increase in resource efficiency in the pharmaceutical industry
		Cost savings
	Non-financial	Improvement of risk management
		Transparency of the supply chain
		Optimal communication with stakeholders
		Increase in company credibility
		Shareholder satisfaction
		Resilience of the pharmaceutical industry

- Novo Nordisk

Novo Nordisk is a global healthcare company headquartered in Bagsværd, Denmark. It is a leading global provider of diabetes care and other serious chronic conditions, with a focus on research, development, and commercialization of innovative pharmaceuticals and devices. Novo Nordisk was founded in 1923 and has a long history of expertise in diabetes care. The company's mission is to drive change to defeat diabetes and other serious chronic conditions such as obesity, hemophilia, and growth disorders. It has implemented a comprehensive green supply chain program. They have set targets to improve energy efficiency, reduce waste generation, and promote responsible sourcing. As part of their initiatives, Novartis has invested in renewable energy sources, optimized packaging, and implemented waste reduction programs. The company's goal is to reduce carbon emissions from its supply chain by 60% by 2030. To achieve this goal, Novo Nordisk has implemented a range of initiatives, including the use of renewable energy sources, optimization of transport routes, and the implementation of sustainable packaging materials. As of 2021, the company had already achieved a 24% reduction in carbon emissions from its supply chain compared to its 2015 baseline. In 2020, Novartis sourced 99% of their electricity from renewable sources. In 2020, they also reduced their waste generation by 4% compared to the previous year.

- Novartis

Novartis International AG is a Swiss multinational pharmaceutical company headquartered in Basel, Switzerland. It is one of the largest pharmaceutical companies in the world, with a global presence and a diverse portfolio of pharmaceuticals, generics, eye care, and other healthcare products. Novartis has implemented a wide range of green supply chain initiatives. Novartis conducts research, development, manufacturing, and marketing of a wide range of innovative prescription drugs, over-the-counter (OTC) medicines, and generic drugs. Novartis has set a target to reduce its absolute GHG emissions by 35% by 2020 compared to a 2010 baseline. As of

2020, Novartis has already achieved a reduction of 46% in absolute GHG emissions, surpassing its target. In 2020, It also sourced 83% of its electricity from renewable sources, such as wind, solar, and hydropower. As of 2020, Novartis achieved a waste recycling rate of 78%, with a goal to reach 90% by 2020. between 2015 and 2020, Novartis reduced its water consumption by 16%.

- Johnson & Johnson

Johnson & Johnson (J&J) is a multinational healthcare company headquartered in New Brunswick, New Jersey, United States. J&J was founded in 1886 and after 140 years activity accounts one of the leading-edge companies in health industry. Its businesses are organized into three segments: Pharmaceutical, Medical Devices, and Consumer Health. J&J's pharmaceutical segment focuses on the research, development, and commercialization of prescription medicines in therapeutic areas such as oncology, immunology, neuroscience, and infectious diseases. I&J pharmaceutical company that has implemented a range of green supply chain initiatives. As part of their green supply chain initiatives, they have implemented various measures, such as optimizing transportation routes, reducing packaging materials, and promoting recycling. For instance, in 2019, Johnson & Johnson reduced their absolute carbon emissions by 5.6% compared to the previous year, saving 64,000 metric tons of CO2. The company's aims to source 100% renewable energy for its global operations by 2050. As of 2021, Johnson & Johnson achieved a 30% reduction in carbon emissions from its global operations compared to its 2010 baseline.

- Pfizer

Pfizer Inc. is a global pharmaceutical company headquartered in New York City, United States. It was founded in 1849 and already is one of the largest pharmaceutical companies in the world, with a wide range of prescription medicines, vaccines, and consumer healthcare products. The company focuses on research and development to bring innovative treatments and therapies to patients in areas such as oncology, immunology, cardiovascular health, rare diseases, and more. Pfizer has a strong portfolio of both small molecule and biologic medicines, as well as a leading position in vaccines. It has implemented a range of green supply chain initiatives. For example, the company has set a goal to reduce its carbon emissions from its operations by 20% by 2025. To achieve this goal, Pfizer has implemented initiatives such as the use of renewable energy sources, optimization of transport routes, and the implementation of sustainable packaging materials. As part of its initiatives, Pfizer has implemented energy-saving initiatives, such as LED lighting and advanced building management systems, and optimized their transportation routes to reduce emissions. In 2019, Pfizer reduced their greenhouse gas emissions by 18% compared to the baseline year of 2012.

- AstraZeneca

AstraZeneca is a global pharmaceutical company headquartered in Cambridge, United Kingdom, with operations in over 100 countries. It was founded in 1999 through the merger of Astra AB (a Swedish pharmaceutical company) and Zeneca

Group plc (a UK-based pharmaceutical company). It is a leading biopharmaceutical company that specializes in the research, development, and commercialization of prescription medicines in various therapeutic areas, including oncology, cardiovascular, respiratory, neuroscience, and more. In recent decades, AstraZeneca is recognized for its commitment to sustainability and green supply chain. As a global pharmaceutical company, has implemented green supply chain practices to reduce their environmental impact and improve sustainability. AstraZeneca has implemented energy-saving measures, such as upgrading equipment and optimizing processes, and implemented waste reduction programs. The company has set a goal to reduce its CO2 emissions by 30% by 2025, compared to its 2015 baseline. In 2019 and 2020, AstraZeneca achieved a 22.6 and 29% respectively reduced in its CO2 emissions compared to its 2015 baseline. The company has implemented a range of initiatives, including the use of renewable energy, the optimization of logistics, and the reduction of waste. In 2020, AstraZeneca reduced their greenhouse gas emissions by 29% compared to the baseline year of 2015.

- GlaxoSmithKline (GSK)

GlaxoSmithKline (GSK) is a global pharmaceutical company headquartered in Brentford, London, United Kingdom. It was formed in 2000 through the merger of Glaxo Wellcome and SmithKline Beecham, two leading pharmaceutical companies. The company operates in over 150 countries and has a diverse portfolio of products that span various therapeutic areas, including respiratory, HIV/AIDS, vaccines, oncology, and more. GlaxoSmithKline has implemented a number of green supply chain initiatives. They set targets to reduce carbon emissions, waste generation, and water consumption. For example, the company has set a goal to reduce its carbon emissions from its supply chain by 25% by 2025. To achieve this goal, GlaxoSmithKline has implemented a range of initiatives, including the use of electric vehicles for transportation and the optimization of supply chain processes to reduce waste. As of 2021, the company had already achieved a 16% reduction in carbon emissions from its supply chain compared to its 2016 baseline.

- Merck & Co., Inc.

Merck & Co., Inc., commonly known as Merck, is a global pharmaceutical company headquartered in Kenilworth, New Jersey, United States. It is one of the largest pharmaceutical companies in the world, with operations in over 140 countries and a diverse portfolio of prescription medicines, vaccines, biologic therapies, and animal health products. As a global pharmaceutical company, Merck has implemented green supply chain practices to reduce their environmental footprint and enhance sustainability and set targets to improve energy efficiency, reduce waste generation, and promote responsible sourcing. Merck has implemented energy-saving measures, such as upgrading equipment and optimizing processes, and implemented waste reduction programs. In 2020, Merck reduced their waste generation by 13% compared to the previous year.

- Roche

Roche Holding AG is a global pharmaceutical company headquartered in Basel, Switzerland, with operations in over 150 countries. It was founded in 1896 and has grown to become one of the world's leading pharmaceutical companies. Roche is also known for its commitment to sustainability and green supply chain practices. The company has made significant efforts in implementing green practices to reduce its environmental impact. For example, Roche has set ambitious targets to reduce its greenhouse gas emissions, water usage, and waste generation. As of 2020, Roche has reduced its greenhouse gas emissions by 65% compared to its 2006 baseline, and aims to be carbon–neutral by 2025. The company has also reduced its water usage by 52% and achieved a recycling rate of 94% for its waste. These efforts highlight Roche's commitment to sustainability and environmental responsibility in its operations.

- Sanofi

Sanofi is a global pharmaceutical company headquartered in Paris, France, with operations in over 170 countries. It was founded in 1973 and is known for its research, development, and commercialization of pharmaceuticals in areas such as diabetes, vaccines, rare diseases, and more. Sanofi is also dedicated to sustainability and has implemented green supply chain practices to minimize its environmental footprint. The company has set targets to reduce its greenhouse gas emissions, water usage, and waste generation. For example, Sanofi aims to achieve a 55% reduction in its greenhouse gas emissions by 2025 compared to its 2015 baseline. The company has also set a target to reduce its water consumption by 30% by 2025. In addition, Sanofi has implemented waste reduction programs and recycling initiatives in its operations, with the aim of achieving zero waste to landfill at its major sites. Sanofi's commitment to sustainability is also reflected in its inclusion in the Dow Jones Sustainability Index, a recognized benchmark for corporate sustainability performance.

- Gilead Sciences

Gilead Sciences, Inc. is a biopharmaceutical company headquartered in Foster City, California, United States, with global operations. It was founded in 1987 and specializes in the research, development, and commercialization of therapeutics in areas such as HIV/AIDS, liver diseases, oncology, and more stewardship, and advance sustainability initiatives in the biopharmaceutical industry. The company has implemented green practices to reduce its environmental impact, particularly in the areas of energy usage and waste reduction. Gilead has set targets to reduce its greenhouse gas emissions, energy consumption, and waste generation. For example, the company has committed to a 25% reduction in its Scope 1 and Scope 2 greenhouse gas emissions by 2025 compared to its 2016 baseline. Gilead also promotes waste reduction and recycling initiatives in its operations, with the aim of reducing its overall waste generation. These efforts demonstrate Gilead's commitment to environmental sustainability and responsible business practices.

- Moderna

Moderna, Inc. is a biotechnology company headquartered in Cambridge, Massachusetts, United States, with a global presence. It was founded in 2010 and is known for its pioneering work in mRNA technology and the development of the COVID-19 mRNA vaccine. The company has shown a commitment to sustainability and green practices through its environmental initiatives. Moderna has set targets to reduce its greenhouse gas emissions, energy usage, and waste generation. For example, the company has committed to achieving a 100% renewable electricity supply for its operations by 2023. Moderna also promotes waste reduction and recycling initiatives in its operations, with the aim of minimizing its environmental impact. These efforts highlight Moderna's dedication to sustainability and its recognition of the importance of environmental responsibility in its operations.

7 Conclusion

Green supply chain management (GSCM) has become increasingly popular as an approach to reduce the environmental impacts of supply chain activities while simultaneously creating value for companies. The medicine industry is one of the most significant contributors to environmental pollution, and as such, the adoption of GSCM practices is critical to minimizing environmental impacts. To be more successful in medicine supply chain, some issues must be considered in supply chains. The commitment of top management to environment and social responsibility is one of the critical success factors in green supply chains. This includes companies' commitment to reduce greenhouse gas emissions, minimizing waste generation, conservation of the natural resources, and promotion of the using environmentally friendly materials and technologies. When leaders set clear goals and provide the necessary resources, it helps to create a culture of social responsibility throughout the organization. Integrating environmental commitments and CSR principles into the supply chain strategy and operations is an important factor for a green supply chain in medicine. This includes setting and achieving sustainability goals, measuring and reporting environmental performance, and engaging in community initiatives related to environmental conservation.

To be more successful, organizations should also set sustainability targets, measure their performance, and continuously improve their environmental performance through regular monitoring and reporting. Successful green supply chain also requires collaboration and partnerships with suppliers, customers, employees and other stakeholders. Especially, employees' engagement in green supply chain through training, education, and incentives can help to create a sense of ownership and commitment to greenness goals.

Another critical factor for achieving success in medicine green supply chain is establishing clear metrics and measurement systems for tracking environmental performance. This allows companies to monitor progress, identify areas for improvement, and demonstrate the value of sustainability efforts to stakeholders. Compliance with environmental regulations and standards is a factor which frequently mentioned as the success of medicine green supply chain. Organizations need to be aware of the regulatory requirements related to environmental sustainability, such as waste disposal, emissions control, and hazardous materials handling. They should ensure that their supply chain operations comply with applicable laws, regulations, and industry standards at all stages of the medicine supply chain. Non-compliance can result in legal penalties, reputational damage, and loss of business opportunities. Therefore, organizations need to establish robust systems for monitoring and managing regulatory compliance and ensure that their suppliers and partners also adhere to the same standards. Innovation is another key success factor for GSCM in medicine [25]. Organizations need to continuously explore and adopt innovative technologies, processes. Adoption of innovative technologies and practices can enhance the sustainability of the supply chain in medicine. This includes using advanced analytics and data-driven decision-making, leveraging Internet of Things (IoT) for real-time monitoring and optimization, and adopting green transportation technologies such as electric vehicles. The integration of the mentioned practices in sourcing, manufacturing, distribution, and disposal of medical products can significantly reduce the environmental impact of the healthcare industry.

References

1. Akram, M., Shahzadi, S., Shah, S.M.U., Allahviranloo, T.: A fully fermatean fuzzy multi-objective transportation model using an extended DEA technique. Granul. Comp. (2023). https://doi.org/10.1007/s41066-023-00399-6
2. Amirteimoori, A., Allahviranloo, T., Kordrostami, S., Bagheri, S.F.: Improving decision-making units in performance analysis methods: a data envelopment analysis approach. Math. Sci. (2023a). https://doi.org/10.1007/s40096-023-00512-5
3. Amirteimoori, A., Allahviranloo, T., Zadmirzaei, M.: Scale elasticity and technical efficiency analysis in the European forest sector: a stochastic value-based approach. Eur. J. Forest Res. (2023b). https://doi.org/10.1007/s10342-023-01589-2
4. Amirteimoori, A., Allahviranloo, T., Zadmirzaei, M., Hasanzadeh, F.: On the environmental performance analysis: a combined fuzzy data envelopment analysis and artificial intelligence algorithms. Expert Syst. Appl. **224**, 119953 (2023c). https://doi.org/10.1016/j.eswa.2023.119953
5. Abbasi, F., Allahviranloo, T.: The fuzzy arithmetic operations of transmission average on Pseudo-Hexagonal fuzzy numbers and its application in fuzzy system reliability analysis. Fuzzy Inform. Eng. **13**(1), 58–78 (2021). https://doi.org/10.1080/16168658.2021.1915449
6. Abbasi, F., Allahviranloo, T.: Realistic solution of fuzzy critical path problems, case study: the airport's cargo ground operation systems. Granul. Comp. **8**(3), 617–632 (2022). https://doi.org/10.1007/s41066-022-00347-w
7. Allahviranloo, T., Abbasi, F.: A new estimation of failure analysis in fuzzy environment, case study: the electrical model failure for the football stadium. New Math. Nat. Comp. **18**(03), 791–817 (2022). https://doi.org/10.1142/s1793005722500387

8. Abbasi, F., Allahviranloo, T.: Conception and implementation of a new data-driven fuzzy method for reliability and safety analysis. New Math. Nat. Comp. **16**(02), 339–361 (2020). https://doi.org/10.1142/s1793005720500210
9. Banker, R.D., Amirteimoori, A., Allahviranloo, T., Sinha, R.P.: Performance analysis and managerial ability in the general insurance market: a study of India and Iran. Inf. Technol. Manage. (2023). https://doi.org/10.1007/s10799-023-00405-y
10. Gao, Y., Bai, C., Guo, J., Li, J., Yan, C.: Green supply chain management in healthcare sector: a systematic literature review. J. Clean. Prod. **239**, 118064 (2019)
11. Statistics & Facts.: Statista. https://www.statista.com. (2021)
12. Holm, E.: Greening the healthcare supply chain: case studies and resources. J. Healthcare Contract. **21**(3), 26–33 (2019)
13. Longoni, A., Cagliano, R., Caron, F.: Understanding the benefits and drivers of sustainable supply chain management in the healthcare industry. Supply Chain Manag. Int. J. **20**(3), 324–339 (2015)
14. Lam, S.S.K., Lai, K.H.: An empirical study on implementing green supply chain management practices in the Hong Kong logistics industry. Int. J. Prod. Econ. **137**(1), 49–61 (2012)
15. Choy, K.L., Lee, W.B.: Sustainable supply chain management in the healthcare sector: an innovative approach. Expert Syst. Appl. **40**(18), 7301–7310 (2013)
16. Gunasekaran, A., Spalanzani, A.: Sustainability of manufacturing and services: investigations for research and applications. Int. J. Prod. Econ. **140**(1), 35–47 (2012)
17. Bhat, M.I., Khan, A.M.: A review of green supply chain management practices in healthcare industry. J. Clean. Prod. **183**, 595–606 (2018)
18. Banomyong, R., Supatn, N.: Green supply chain management in the healthcare industry: an empirical study. Int. J. Prod. Econ. **181**, 34–45 (2016)
19. Bhatia, S., Jain, V., Sharma, S., Sharma, P.: Green supply chain management in healthcare: a review. Int. J. Healthcare Manag. **10**(2), 78–89 (2017)
20. Mahmoodirad, A., Allahviranloo, T., Niroomand, S.: A new effective solution method for fully intuitionistic fuzzy transportation problem. Soft. Comput. **23**(12), 4521–4530 (2019). https://doi.org/10.1007/s00500-018-3115-z
21. Bhagat, R.B., Hassan, M.K.: Green distribution management in supply chain: a review. J. Clean. Prod. **256**, 1–21 (2020)
22. Subramanian, N., Abdulrahman, M.D.: Determinants of green supply chain management practices in healthcare sector: an ISM-TISM approach. J. Clean. Prod. **230**, 1261–1279 (2019)
23. Hsu, C.W., Kuo, T.C., Hu, A.H.: The linkages between green supply chain management and performance outcomes: a meta-analysis. J. Clean. Prod. **108**, 483–498 (2015)
24. Prakash, A., Singh, R.K.: Green supply chain management practices in healthcare sector: a systematic literature review. J. Clean. Prod. **139**, 362–377 (2016)
25. Cheng, Y., Choi, T.Y.: The impact of green supply chain management practices on firm performance: the role of collaboration intensity, decision comprehensiveness, and supplier environmental innovation. Int. J. Prod. Econ. **210**, 1–15 (2019)

Statistical Analysis and Structural Equations on Influential Parameters in Health

Mahdi Homayounfar, Mehdi Fadaei Eshkiki, and Sara Namdar

Abstract Statistics, as an applied science for data analysis, plays a fundamental role in all sciences, especially in the field of health. By using statistical methods, researchers can quantify the extent to which each variable impacts health and identify the most significant factors. Structural equation modeling takes this a step further by allowing researchers to examine how different variables interact with each other and the pathways through which they operate. These approaches can help healthcare professionals develop more effective interventions for preventing and treating diseases, as well as informing public health policies. In this chapter, statistical analysis and structural equation modeling play a crucial role in understanding the complex interplay between various factors that influence health outcomes. In this section, after a brief description of statistics and statistical tests, a general classification of statistical tests and their assumptions are presented. Then, after examining various approaches to structural equation modeling (SEM), an empirical example is provided to demonstrate the application of SEM in health. The presented model investigates the effect of contextual factors on individuals' preventive behavior during the COVID-19 pandemic. In the proposed model, preventive behavior includes 3 variables of personal protection behavior, social distancing behavior and social responsibility awareness, contextual factors include three variables of health literacy, social norms and information sources. In addition, COVID-19 knowledge and risk perception are considered as mediator variables between contextual factors and preventive behaviors. Material status and education are also moderator variables. The model implemented based on the Smart PLS software and the results are described in details.

Keywords Statistical analysis · Structural equation modeling · Healthcare · COVID 19

M. Homayounfar (✉) · M. F. Eshkiki
Department of Industrial Management, Rasht Branch, Islamic Azad University, Rasht, Iran
e-mail: homayounfar@iaurasht.ac.ir

S. Namdar
Department of Accounting, Rasht Branch, Islamic Azad University, Rasht, Iran

T. Allahviranloo et al. (eds.), *Decision Making in Healthcare Systems*,
Studies in Systems, Decision and Control 513,
https://doi.org/10.1007/978-3-031-46735-6_12

1 Introduction

In healthcare, the use of statistics is essential for understanding and improving health outcomes for individuals and populations. It includes the collection, analysis, interpretation, and presentation of data in a way that enables healthcare professionals to make informed decisions and improve patient outcomes. Munro [1] describes statistics as a "powerful tool for investigating and understanding complex issues in healthcare".

One important aspect of statistics in healthcare is the ability to identify patterns and trends in disease incidence and prevalence. This information can be used to develop targeted prevention strategies and interventions to reduce the burden of disease. For example, statistical analysis can be used to identify risk factors for certain diseases, such as smoking for lung cancer, and develop targeted prevention programs to reduce the incidence of the disease.

Statistics is also important for evaluating the effectiveness of healthcare interventions. Through the use of clinical trials and other research studies, statistical analysis can be used to determine whether a particular treatment or intervention is effective in improving patient outcomes. According to a study published in the Journal of the American Medical Association, 30-day readmission rates for heart failure patients decreased from 21.3 to 18.4% after the implementation of a quality improvement initiative. This shows how statistical analysis can help identify effective interventions to improve patient outcomes.

Statistics is also important for healthcare policy decisions. By analyzing healthcare costs and outcomes, statistical data can inform decisions about resource allocation and spending. For example, in the United States, healthcare spending is estimated to be $3.8 trillion in 2022, accounting for 18.4% of the country's GDP. Statistical analysis of healthcare costs and outcomes can help policymakers make informed decisions about resource allocation and spending. Statistics can be used to identify risk factors and patterns of these diseases, enabling healthcare professionals to develop targeted prevention strategies. According to the world Health Organization, non-communicable diseases (NCDs) such as heart disease, cancer, diabetes, and respiratory disease are responsible for 71% of global deaths.

Additionally, statistical analysis can help identify factors contributing to the high prevalence of obesity, such as sedentary lifestyles and unhealthy diets. For example, the centers for Disease control and prevention (CDC) reported that in the United States, the prevalence of obesity among adults was 42.4% between 2017 and 2018. Moreover, statistics is used to monitor public health trends and identify emerging health threats. For instance, during the COVID-19 pandemic, statistical analysis was used to track the spread of the virus and monitor vaccination coverage rates. According to the World Health Organization, as of March 20, 2023, there have been over 466 million confirmed cases of COVID-19 and over 6.1 million deaths globally. Statistical analysis has been crucial in understanding the spread of the virus and informing public health policies. In this chapter, after a brief review of statistical tests, the application of the structural equation modeling in a real case study in healthcare, is studied.

Recent research points out that most mathematical models like dynamic systems and also linear systems get involved with real-world problems. Since their related information has different forms like certainty and uncertainty, the uncertain version of these models does have more importance in the applications. In health problems, two types of mathematical models; fuzzy dynamic systems and fuzzy linear programming problems even transportation problems, play an important role, on the other hand, the main and basic model of fuzzy linear programming problems is fuzzy linear systems.

In conclusion, fuzzy differential equations (as a special version of dynamic systems) [2–5], and fuzzy linear systems (as a basic model of fuzzy linear programming problems) [6], have an important role in this research. Recently several research has been done on investigating the advanced version of the uncertain information [4, 7–9], and moreover the above-mentioned basic models.

2 Statistics

Statistics is often known as one of the most versatile and useful areas of Mathematics. Statistics is a branch of science which deals with collection and analysis of data and interprets the resulted information. It helps us to make educated guesses about the unknown and find very useful information in this very ocean of data. Statistics play very important role in some critical decision-making situations. Generally, statistics can be broken down into the two main areas: (1) descriptive statistics makes use of the data to provide brief descriptions of the population, either through numerical calculations or graphs or tables. The main purpose of this type of statistics is present data in a way that will help in describing the data with help of graphs to facilitate easy understanding.

Descriptive statistics make the data we get easier to digest, even though some information about individual data points may be lost. Descriptive statistics is all about summarizing or highlighting most important aspects of the collected data such as central, variation, skewedness and kurtosis parameters. When people think of statistics, they often think about the descriptive statistics. (2) Inferential statistics makes good inferences and near perfect predictions about a population based on a sample of data selected from the population. Inferential statistics help to make decisions about data's uncertainty. Inferential Statistics helps in making predictions from data. So, in inferential statistics the goal is to take just a small bit of information, analyze it thoroughly, and then see what conclusions we can draw based on available information or infer about the bigger picture for future. This part of statistics is most enigmatic, but in actual certainty, it is one of the most powerful tools and it allows us to find even more information from the data that we have already collected.

3 Description of Variables

In statistical analysis, a variable is any characteristic or attribute that can vary or take on different values. Describing a variable involves identifying and summarizing its key characteristics, such as its type, scale of measurement, and distribution. Here are some steps you can follow to describe a variable:

- Identify the type of variable: There are two main types of variables in statistics: categorical and numerical. Categorical variables are qualitative in nature and represent groups or categories, while numerical variables are quantitative and represent numeric values.
- Determine the scale of measurement: If the variable is numerical, you need to determine its scale of measurement. The four main scales of measurement are nominal, ordinal, interval, and ratio. Nominal variables have no inherent order or numerical value, while ordinal variables have a natural order but no meaningful distance between values. Interval variables have a meaningful distance between values but no true zero point, while ratio variables have a true zero point.
- Summarize the distribution: If the variable is numerical, you can summarize its distribution using measures such as the mean, median, mode, and standard deviation. These measures provide information about the central tendency, variability, and shape of the distribution.
- Identify any outliers: Outliers are values that are significantly different from the other values in the dataset. Identifying and handling outliers is important in statistical analysis as they can affect the validity of your results.
- Describe any missing values: Missing values are data points that are not present in the dataset. It is important to describe the proportion of missing values and how they were handled in the analysis.

4 Statistical Test

A statistical test provides a mechanism for making quantitative decisions about a process or processes. The objective is to determine whether there is enough evidence to "reject" a conjecture or hypothesis about the process. The conjecture is called the null hypothesis. Not rejecting may be a good result if we want to continue to act as if we "believe" the null hypothesis is true. Or it may be a disappointing result, possibly indicating we may not yet have enough data to "prove" something by rejecting the null hypothesis. A statistical test requires a pair of hypotheses; namely, null and alternative hypotheses.

H_0: null hypothesis.
H_1: alternative hypothesis.

The null hypothesis is a statement about a belief. We may doubt that the null hypothesis is true, which might be why we are "testing" it. The alternative hypothesis might, in fact, be what we believe to be true. The test procedure is constructed so that the risk of rejecting the null hypothesis, when it is in fact true, is small. This risk, α, is often referred to as the significance level of the test. By having a test with a small value of α, we feel that we have actually "proved" something when we reject the null hypothesis.

The risk of failing to reject the null hypothesis when it is in fact false is not chosen by the user but is determined, as one might expect, by the magnitude of the real discrepancy. This risk, β, is usually referred to as the type II error. Large discrepancies between reality and the null hypothesis are easier to detect and lead to small type I error; while small discrepancies are more difficult to detect and lead to large type II error. Also, the risk β increases as the risk α decreases.

5 Statistical Methods and Assumptions

Choosing the appropriate statistical test is crucial in ensuring the accuracy and validity of the analysis requires careful consideration of the research question, type of data, number of variables, assumptions, and available statistical tests. Here are some general steps that can help you choose the appropriate statistical test:

- Identify your research question: Your research question should guide the selection of the appropriate statistical test. Ask yourself what you are trying to investigate or test, and what type of data you have collected.
- Identify the type of data: Determine whether your data is categorical or continuous. Categorical data includes variables that have distinct categories, such as gender or political affiliation, while continuous data includes variables that can take any value within a range, such as age or weight.
- Determine the number of variables: Consider whether you have one or more variables. For example, if you are examining the relationship between two variables, you will need to choose a different test than if you are only examining one variable.
- Consider the assumptions of the test: Different statistical tests have different assumptions, such as normality or homogeneity of variance. It is important to ensure that your data meets these assumptions before conducting the test.
- Choose the appropriate test: Once you have identified your research question, type of data, number of variables, and assumptions, you can select the appropriate statistical test. There are many statistical tests available, such as t-tests, ANOVA, chi-square tests, correlation analysis, and regression analysis, among others.
- Verify the results: After conducting the statistical test, it is important to verify the results to ensure that they are reliable and valid. This may involve checking for outliers, examining effect sizes, or conducting post-hoc analyses.

Table 12.1 describes some of the commonly used statistical tests in healthcare research, their assumptions, and appropriate usage. Please note that this is not an exhaustive list and there may be other statistical tests that are appropriate depending on the specific research question and data type.

Table 12.1 Classification of statistical tests

Test	Types	Conditions of use	Assumptions
t-test	One-sample t-test	Used to determine if the mean of a sample is significantly different from a known or hypothesized population mean	Random sampling, independent observations, normality
	Independent samples t-test	Used to determine if the means of two independent samples are significantly different from each other	Random sampling, independent observations, normality, variances of the two samples must be assumed to be equal[1] (can be tested using Levene's test), approximately equal sample sizes
	Paired samples t-test	Used to determine if the means of two dependent samples (e.g., pre-test and post-test measurements) are significantly different from each other	The two samples must be matched (or paired), random sampling, independent observations, normal distribution
ANOVA	One-way ANOVA	Used to test for mean differences between more than two independent groups	Normality, homogeneity of variances, independence of observations, continuity of variable
	Two-way ANOVA	Used to test for differences between two or more independent groups (or levels) on two continuous dependent variables, and to determine if there is an interaction between the two independent variables	
	Repeated measures ANOVA	Used to test for differences between more than two conditions (or treatments), where the same participants are measured at multiple time points (or under multiple conditions)	Sphericity (i.e., the variances of the differences between all possible pairs of conditions are equal), normality, independence of observations, continuity of variable
	Mixed design ANOVA	Used to test for differences between two or more conditions (or treatments), where there are both between-subjects and within-subjects factors	Sphericity, normality, homogeneity of variances, independence of observations, continuity of variable

(continued)

[1] Welch's t-test for unequal variances must be used.

Table 12.1 (continued)

Test	Types	Conditions of use	Assumptions
Regression analysis	Simple linear regression	Used to model the relationship between one continuous dependent variable and one continuous or categorical independent variable	Linearity, independence of observations, homoscedasticity (constant variance), normality and no auto-regression of residuals
	Multiple linear regression	Used to model the relationship between one continuous dependent variable and two or more continuous or categorical independent variables	Linearity, independence of observations, homoscedasticity, normality of residuals, no multicollinearity
	Logistic regression	Used to model the relationship between a binary dependent variable and one or more continuous or categorical independent variables	Linearity, independence of observations no outliers, no multicollinearity, absence of perfect separation
	Poisson regression	Used to model the relationship between a count-dependent variable and one or more continuous or categorical independent variables	Linearity, independence of observations, no multicollinearity, equality of means and variances, absence of overdispersion
	Nonlinear regression	Used to model the relationship between one continuous dependent variable and two or more continuous or categorical independent variables	Nonlinearity, independence of observations, no multicollinearity, equality of means and variances, absence of overdispersion
Correlation analysis	Pearson correlation	Used to measure the linear relationship between two continuous variables	Linearity, normality, homoscedasticity, absence of outliers
	Spearman correlation	Used to measure the monotonic relationship between two continuous or ordinal variables	Monotonicity, independence of observations
	Kendall correlation	Used to measure the rank-based association between two continuous or ordinal variables	Independence of observations, no tied ranks
	Point biserial correlation	Used to measure the association between one continuous variable and one dichotomous variable	Linearity, normality, homoscedasticity, absence of outliers

(continued)

Table 12.1 (continued)

Test	Types	Conditions of use	Assumptions
	Phi coefficient	Used to measure the association between two dichotomous variables	Independence of observations, no cell counts less than 5
	Cramer's V	Used to measure the association between two categorical variables	
Multivariate analysis	Cluster analysis	Used to group observations into clusters based on their similarity on multiple variables	Similarity or dissimilarity measures, no predetermined number of clusters
	Canonical correlation	Used to examine the relationship between multiple independent variables and multiple dependent variables	Linearity, normality, absence of multicollinearity, independence of observations
	Discriminant analysis	Used to classify observations into groups based on multiple predictor variables	Linearity, normality, homoscedasticity, absence of multicollinearity, independence of observations
	Factor analysis	Used to identify patterns in the correlations between multiple variables and reduce the dimensionality of the data	Linearity, normality, sampling adequacy, absence of multicollinearity, independence of observations
	Principal component analysis		
Time series	Naive	Used as a baseline model for time series forecasting	None
	Moving Average (MA)	Used to model and forecast time series data with no trend or seasonality	Stationarity, independence of observations, no autocorrelation in residuals
	Autoregressive (AR)	Used to model and forecast time series data with a strong trend	
	Autoregressive Moving Average (ARMA)	Used to model and forecast time series data with both trend and seasonality	
	Exponential Smoothing (ES)	Used to model and forecast time series data with trend and/or seasonality	
	Autoregressive Integrated Moving Average (ARIMA)	Used to model and forecast stationary time series data	
	Seasonal ARIMA (SARIMA)	Used to model and forecast seasonal time series data	

(continued)

Table 12.1 (continued)

Test	Types	Conditions of use	Assumptions
	Vector Autoregression (VAR)	Used to model and forecast multiple time series data that influence each other	
Chi-square tests	Goodness-of-fit test	Used to test whether the observed data fits a specific theoretical distribution	Independence of observations, expected frequencies are not too small (i.e., no more than 20% of the expected frequencies are less than 5)
		Used to test whether the observed frequencies match the expected frequencies	
	Test for independence	Used to test for association between two categorical variables	The data are in the form of a contingency table, independence of observations, The expected frequencies are not too small (i.e., no more than 20% of the expected frequencies are less than 5)
	Test for homogeneity	Used to test whether the distributions of two or more groups are homogeneous	
Sign test	One-sample mean test	Used to determine if the mean of a sample is significantly different from a known or hypothesized population mean	Random sampling, independent observations, ordinal or continuous data, non-normality
Mann–Whitney U test	Independent samples mean test	To determine if there is a significant difference between two independent groups on a continuous dependent variable when the assumptions for the t-test are not met	Independent or unrelated samples, ordinal data, continuous or discrete data, non-normality, unequal variances
Wilcoxon rank-sum test	Paired samples mean test	To test for significant differences between two related samples when assumptions of the paired t-test are not met	Dependent or related samples, ordinal data, continuous or discrete data non-normality
McNamar's test	Paired samples mean test	To test for significant differences between two dichotomous (categorical with 2 categories) variables on the same sample	Categorical data, dependent samples
Kruskal-Walli's test	K samples mean test (K > 2)	To test for differences between three or more independent groups on a continuous dependent variable when the assumptions for one way ANOVA are not met	Independent samples, ordinal data, continuous or discrete data (assuming the underlying distributions are similar), non-normality, unequal variances

(continued)

Table 12.1 (continued)

Test	Types	Conditions of use	Assumptions
Friedman test	K related samples mean test (K > 2)	To test for significant differences between three or more related samples when assumptions of ANOVA are not met	Continuity of variable, non-normally
	Homogeneity of k distribution	Used to determine if three or more dependent samples are drawn from populations with the same distribution or not	Dependent observations, three or more groups, equal variance in each group, ordinal or continuous data. Non-normality
Kendall's ι coefficient	Correlation coefficient	Used to determine the strength and direction of the relationship between two variables	Monotonic relationship between variables

6 Structural Equation Modelling (SEM)

Structural equations are mathematical models that are used to represent the relationships between variables in a system. These equations can be written in a variety of ways, including using matrices, path diagrams, or regression equations.

The goal of the SEM is to estimate the parameters of the model, which include the strength of the relationships between the variables and the variances and covariances of the latent variables. Latent variables and observable variables are two fundamental concepts in statistical analysis, especially in the context of factor analysis and structural equation modeling. Latent variables, are variables that cannot be directly observed, such as stress variable. One cannot directly observe and measure an individual's stress. Therefore, to measure latent variables, researchers use observable variables that could be measured through the questionnaire questions. For example, anxiety, impatience at aggression, and similar variables are observable variables used to measure the latent variable of burnout. Following, the design of a structural equation model is explained with an example. In a study, the relationship between three latent variables A, B, and C is investigated (Fig. 12.1).

The relationship among these variables is considered as follows:

- Latent variable A is an independent variable and has an effect on both latent variables B and C.
- Two observed variables A1 and A2 are used to measure latent variable A.
- Two observed variables B1 and B2 are used to measure latent variable B.
- Three observed variables C1, C2, and C3 are used to measure latent variable C.

The general model of structural equations follows the pattern shown above. The rules of this pattern are:

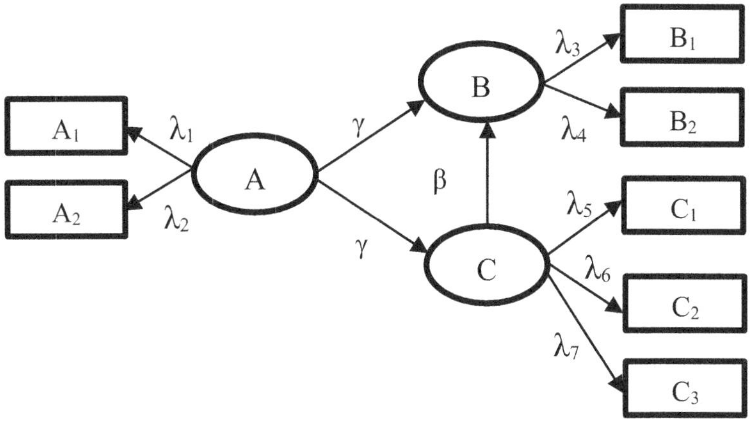

Fig. 12.1 A schematic SEM model

- Each ellipse in the structural equation model represents a latent variable.
- Each rectangle in the structural equation model represents an observable variable.
- An arrow which goes out from each ellipse to each rectangle, represented by λ, is called the factor loading.
- The path coefficient of the relationship between two independent latent variables is represented by γ.
- The coefficient of the relationship between two dependent latent variables is represented by β.

6.1 SEM Applications

Structural Equation Modeling (SEM) has several applications in various fields. It is a powerful tool for analyzing complex data structures and can be applied in a wide range of research areas, including psychology, sociology, economics, education, and public health. Some of the common applications of SEM are:

- Testing theories and models: SEM is often used to test theories and models in social and behavioral sciences. Researchers can use SEM to evaluate the fit of a model to the data, determine whether the relationships among variables are significant, and refine or revise theories.
- Measurement modeling: SEM can be used to model the relationships between observed and unobserved variables. This enables researchers to develop more accurate and reliable measures of the concepts they are studying.
- Causal modeling: SEM can be used to model causal relationships between variables. This allows researchers to investigate how one variable affects another while controlling for the effects of other variables.

- Multilevel modeling: SEM can be used to analyze data with a hierarchical structure, such as data collected from individuals nested within groups or clusters. This allows researchers to examine both within-group and between-group effects.
- Longitudinal modeling: SEM can be used to analyze data collected over time, such as repeated measures data or panel data. This allows researchers to examine how variables change over time and to investigate causal relationships that may change over time.

6.2 SEM Approaches

There are several approaches to SEM, each with its own strengths and limitations. Some of the common approaches to SEM are:

6.2.1 Covariance- Based SEM

Covariance-based SEM (CB-SEM) is an approach that is based on the covariance matrix of the observed variables. It is a popular approach because it can handle complex models that include multiple latent variables, as well as observed variables with multiple indicators. CB-SEM is often used in social and behavioral sciences to study complex relationships between variables.

The CB-SEM approach involves two key components: measurement models and structural models. The measurement model specifies the relationships between the latent variables and their observed indicators, while the structural model specifies the relationships between the latent variables themselves.

In the measurement model, the latent variables are assumed to underlie the observed variables, and are typically represented as circles in SEM diagrams. The observed variables, which are represented as rectangles in SEM diagrams, are considered to be indicators of the latent variables. The measurement model specifies how the observed variables are related to the latent variables, typically through a set of regression equations. These equations describe how the latent variables are estimated from the observed variables, and are known as factor loadings.

The structural model specifies the relationships between the latent variables, which are typically represented as arrows in SEM diagrams. The structural model describes how the latent variables influence one another, either directly or indirectly through other latent variables. The relationships between the latent variables are typically represented as a set of regression equations.

Once the measurement and structural models have been specified, the next step is to estimate the model parameters. The most common method for estimating CB-SEM models is maximum likelihood estimation, which involves finding the parameter estimates that maximize the likelihood of obtaining the observed data given the model.

After the model has been estimated, it is evaluated for goodness of fit using various fit indices, such as the chi-square test, the root mean square error of approximation (RMSEA), the comparative fit index (CFI), and the Tucker-Lewis index (TLI). These fit indices provide information about how well the model fits the data, with higher values indicating better fit.

6.2.2 Partial Least Squares (PLS)

Partial least squares structural equation modeling (PLS-SEM) is an approach to SEM that is based on latent variable models. It is a popular approach in fields such as management, marketing, and information systems, where the focus is often on predicting outcomes rather than testing complex models.

PLS-SEM is different from CB-SEM in several ways. Unlike CB-SEM, PLS-SEM does not rely on the assumption of multivariate normality and is robust to non-normality, small sample sizes, and missing data. PLS-SEM is also a two-stage approach that involves estimating the measurement model and the structural model separately.

In PLS-SEM, the latent variables are estimated using a set of weighted linear combinations of the observed variables, rather than through a set of regression equations as in CB-SEM. The weights are estimated using a method called partial least squares, which involves finding the linear combinations of the observed variables that are most strongly associated with the latent variables. The latent variables are typically represented as circles in SEM diagrams, and the observed variables as rectangles.

In the measurement model of PLS, the latent variables are estimated using a set of indicators, which are typically multiple observed variables that measure the same construct. The measurement model specifies how the indicators are related to the latent variables through a set of factor loadings. These factor loadings represent the weights of the observed variables in the linear combinations used to estimate the latent variables.

In the structural model, the relationships between the latent variables are specified through a set of path coefficients, which represent the strength and direction of the relationships. These path coefficients are typically estimated using regression equations, as in CB-SEM.

Once the measurement and structural models have been specified, the next step is to estimate the model parameters. The most common method for estimating PLS-SEM models is partial least squares regression, which involves finding the parameter estimates that maximize the variance explained in the latent variables. After the model has been estimated, it is evaluated for goodness of fit using various fit indices, such as the goodness-of-fit index (GoF) and the root mean square error (RMSE) of approximation (RMSEA). These fit indices provide information about how well the model fits the data, with higher values indicating better fit.

6.2.3 Bayesian SEM

Bayesian structural equation modeling (Bayesian SEM) is a statistical approach that combines the principles of Bayesian statistics with SEM. In Bayesian SEM, prior distributions are specified for all model parameters, including the path coefficients, variances, and covariances. These prior distributions represent the researcher's beliefs about the values of these parameters before the data are collected. Once the prior distributions have been specified, the likelihood of the observed data is calculated given the model and the parameter values. This likelihood is then combined with the prior distributions using Bayes' theorem to obtain the posterior distribution of the parameters. The posterior distribution represents the researcher's updated beliefs about the values of the parameters after observing the data.

The posterior distribution can be used to estimate the model parameters, and to make inferences about the model and the data. In Bayesian SEM, the posterior distribution is typically estimated using Markov chain Monte Carlo (MCMC) methods, which involve generating a large number of random samples from the posterior distribution using a computer algorithm.

Bayesian SEM has several advantages over other approaches to SEM. For example, Bayesian SEM allows researchers to incorporate prior knowledge about the parameters into the analysis, which can lead to more accurate estimates and better inferences. Bayesian SEM is also flexible and can handle complex models with non-normal data and missing data. However, Bayesian SEM also has some limitations. For example, Bayesian SEM requires the specification of prior distributions for all model parameters, which can be difficult for researchers who are not familiar with Bayesian statistics. Bayesian SEM can also be computationally intensive and time-consuming, especially for large and complex models.

6.2.4 Exploratory SEM (ESEM)

Exploratory structural equation modeling (ESEM) is a statistical technique that combines the principles of exploratory factor analysis (EFA) and structural equation modeling (SEM) to analyze complex data structures. ESEM is used to explore the relationships among observed variables and latent factors, and to identify the underlying factors that explain the observed data. ESEM allows for the identification of cross-loadings between observed variables and latent factors, which means that an observed variable can load on more than one latent factor. ESEM also allows for the estimation of factor correlations, which are often used to identify higher-order latent factors.

ESEM is particularly useful in situations where the number and nature of latent factors are not clear, or when there is a high degree of overlap between different constructs. ESEM can help researchers identify and separate distinct latent factors, even in cases where these factors may overlap or have complex relationships with each other.

To perform ESEM, researchers first specify a hypothesized model that represents the relationships among the observed variables and latent factors. Next, the researcher estimates the model parameters using a variety of methods, including maximum likelihood estimation or Bayesian estimation. Once the model has been estimated, researchers evaluate the model fit using a variety of fit indices, including traditional indices such as the root mean square error of approximation (RMSEA) and comparative fit index (CFI), as well as newer indices such as the exploratory factor analysis fit index (EFA-FI). Good model fit indicates that the hypothesized model is a good representation of the data.

ESEM has several advantages over traditional EFA and SEM methods. For example, ESEM allows for the identification of complex relationships between observed variables and latent factors, and it can help researchers identify new factors that may not have been included in the original model. ESEM is also more flexible than traditional SEM, as it allows for cross-loadings and the estimation of factor correlations. Despite these advantages, ESEM can be more computationally intensive than traditional EFA and SEM methods, and may require larger sample sizes to obtain accurate estimates. Additionally, ESEM can be more difficult to interpret than traditional SEM methods, as it allows for more complex relationships between observed variables and latent factors.

6.2.5 Multilevel SEM

Multilevel structural equation modeling (MSEM) is a statistical technique that is used to analyze data that have a hierarchical or nested structure, such as data from multiple individuals who are nested within groups or from multiple time points that are nested within individuals.

In MSEM, the analysis is performed at multiple levels, with the lower level representing the individual or time point level, and the higher level representing the group or cluster level. The relationships between variables are modeled at each level, as well as the relationships between the variables across levels.

MSEM is often used in fields such as psychology, education, and public health to analyze data from clustered or longitudinal studies. For example, MSEM can be used to examine the relationship between individual-level variables such as personality traits and group-level variables such as team performance, or to examine the effect of individual-level interventions on group-level outcomes.

To perform MSEM, researchers first specify a model that represents the relationships among the observed variables and latent factors at each level, as well as the relationships between the levels. The model is then estimated using a variety of methods, including maximum likelihood estimation or Bayesian estimation. Once the model has been estimated, researchers evaluate the model fit using a variety of fit indices, including traditional indices such as the root mean square error of approximation (RMSEA) and comparative fit index (CFI), as well as newer indices such as the multilevel model fit index (MLM-FI). Good model fit indicates that the hypothesized model is a good representation of the data at both the individual and group levels.

MSEM has several advantages over traditional single-level SEM methods. For example, MSEM allows for the analysis of data that have a hierarchical or nested structure, which is common in many fields. MSEM can also help to identify the sources of variation in the data, and can provide insights into the relationships between variables at different levels.

Despite these advantages, MSEM can be more computationally intensive than traditional SEM methods, and may require larger sample sizes to obtain accurate estimates. Additionally, MSEM can be more difficult to interpret than traditional SEM methods, as it involves modeling relationships at multiple levels.

6.3 *Fitness Indices*

Structural equation modeling (SEM) involves testing a hypothesized model against the data to determine how well the model fits the data. There are several criteria that can be used to evaluate the fit of a structural equation model. Henseler et al. [10] proposed a comprehensive set of criteria for evaluating the fit of structural equation models, which includes the following:

- Chi-square goodness of fit test: This test assesses the difference between the observed and expected covariance matrices. A significant chi-square value indicates a poor fit between the model and the data. However, this test is sensitive to sample size, and a large sample can result in a significant chi-square value even for a well-fitting model.
- Root mean square error of approximation (RMSEA): This is a measure of the discrepancy between the model and the data, adjusted for the degrees of freedom. A smaller RMSEA value indicates a better fit between the model and the data. A commonly used guideline is that an RMSEA value of less than 0.05 indicates a good fit, and a value between 0.05 and 0.08 indicates an acceptable fit.
- Comparative fit index (CFI): This index compares the fit of the hypothesized model to the fit of a null model that assumes no relationships between the variables. A CFI value close to 1 indicates a good fit between the model and the data, while a value below 0.90 indicates a poor fit.
- Tucker-Lewis Index (TLI): This is a similar index to CFI that also compares the fit of the hypothesized model to the fit of a null model. A TLI value close to 1 indicates a good fit between the model and the data, while a value below 0.90 indicates a poor fit.
- Standardized Root Mean Square Residual (SRMR): This is a measure of the difference between the observed and predicted correlations in the model, adjusted for the number of variables in the model. A smaller SRMR value indicates a better fit between the model and the data.

- Coefficient of determination (R2): This is a measure of the amount of variance in the endogenous variables explained by the exogenous variables in the model. A higher R2 indicates a better model fit.
- Path coefficients: The strength and significance of the estimated path coefficients should be examined to determine whether they are consistent with the research hypotheses.
- Standardized Root Mean Square Residual (SRMR): This is a measure of the difference between the observed and predicted correlations in the model, adjusted for the number of variables in the model. A smaller SRMR value indicates a better fit between the model and the data.
- Root Mean Square Error of Approximation (RMSEA): This is a measure of the discrepancy between the model and the data, adjusted for the degrees of freedom. A smaller RMSEA value indicates a better fit between the model and the data. A commonly used guideline is that an RMSEA value of less than 0.05 indicates a good fit, and a value between 0.05 and 0.08 indicates an acceptable fit.
- Goodness-of-Fit Index (GFI): This is a measure of the proportion of covariance in the observed data that is accounted for by the model. A higher GFI indicates a better fit between the model and the data.
- Adjusted Goodness-of-Fit Index (AGFI): This is a modification of GFI that adjusts for the number of degrees of freedom in the model. A higher AGFI indicates a better fit between the model and the data.
- Comparative Fit Index (CFI): This index compares the fit of the hypothesized model to the fit of a null model that assumes no relationships between the variables. A CFI value close to 1 indicates a good fit between the model and the data, while a value below 0.90 indicates a poor fit.
- Tucker-Lewis Index (TLI): This is a similar index to CFI that also compares the fit of the hypothesized model to the fit of a null model. A TLI value close to 1 indicates a good fit between the model and the data, while a value below 0.90 indicates a poor fit.
- Parsimony: A good model should be parsimonious, meaning that it should have the fewest number of parameters necessary to adequately explain the data.

These criteria provide a comprehensive set of guidelines for evaluating the fit of structural equation models and should be used in conjunction with each other to determine the overall fit of the model. No single index provides a complete picture of model fit. Additionally, researchers should consider the theoretical implications of the model, the plausibility of the parameter estimates, and the practical implications of the model when interpreting the results of a structural equation modeling analysis.

6.4 SEM Softwares

SEM software, their conditions of use, and their strengths and weaknesses are presented in Table 12.2:

Table 2 SEM software

Software	Condition of use	Strengths	Weaknesses
AMOS	Widely used in social sciences, normality	User-friendly interface, good for beginners, intuitive graphical interface, Best for small to medium-sized models	Limited capability for advanced models, may not handle complex datasets
Mplus	Widely used in large and complex models	Wide range of statistical analyses, good for complex models and large datasets, handles missing data well	Steep learning curve, requires advanced statistical knowledge, expensive
LISREL	Widely used in social sciences, normality	Handles complex models well, extensive documentation and support	Limited ability to handle non-normal data distributions, expensive
EQS	Widely used in behavioral and social sciences	Extensive documentation and support, handles large and complex models well	Steep learning curve, expensive
Lavaan	widely used in R environment	Open-source, free, good for small to medium-sized models	Limited capability for advanced models, may not handle complex datasets
Stata	Widely used in social sciences	Handles complex models well, extensive documentation and support	Steep learning curve, expensive, may not handle large datasets as well as some other software
SAS	Widely used in social sciences and business research	Handles complex models well, widely used in social sciences and business research, extensive documentation and support	Steep learning curve, expensive, may not handle large datasets as well as some other software
SmartPLS	Widely used in social sciences and business research	User-friendly interface, good for beginners, handles small to medium-sized models well, runs any type of distribution	Limited capability for advanced models, may not handle complex datasets
OpenMx	Widely used in R environment	Open-source, free, handles complex models well, good for large and complex models	Steep learning curve, may not handle small datasets as well as some other software
MPLUS automation	Automation of Mplus analyses	User-friendly interface, good for small to medium-sized models	Limited capability for advanced models, requires Mplus software
Reticulate	Integration of Python-based SEM tools with R environment	Good for large and complex models	Steep learning curve, requires knowledge of both R and Python

(continued)

Table 2 (continued)

Software	Condition of use	Strengths	Weaknesses
G*Power	Power analysis for SEM and other statistical analyses	Free, handles power analysis well	Limited to power analysis, does not perform SEM analysis
WarpPLS	Focus on small sample sizes and non-normal data distributions	Handles non-normal data distributions well, good for small sample sizes	Limited to small sample sizes, may not handle large datasets as well as some other software

It should be noted that the best software option depends on the specific needs of a researcher or practitioner. The strengths and weaknesses of each software should be considered when selecting the appropriate tool for the task at hand.

6.5 SEM Application in Health

In this section, an empirical example for application of structural equation modeling in health sector is implemented. Consider the following model about people's preventive behavior and its influential factors. It this model, preventive behavior as the dependent variable, consists of three main variables (personal protection behavior, social distancing behavior and social responsibility awareness), while independent variable, namely contextual variables, includes three variables of health literacy, social norms and information sources. In this model, COVID-19 knowledge and risk perception are intermediate variables between contextual factors and preventive behaviors. Finally, among the different variables who have moderating effect on the relationship between risk perception with preventive behaviors, material status and education were selected as moderators (Fig. 12.2).

According to the above relationships, the following hypotheses could be developed:

H1: Health Literacy has a direct relationship with COVID-19 knowledge.
H2: Social norms has a direct relationship with COVID-19 knowledge.
H3: Information sources has a direct relationship with COVID-19 knowledge.
H4: Health Literacy has a direct relationship with risk perception.
H5: Social norms has a direct relationship with risk perception.
H6: Information sources has a direct relationship with risk perception.
H7: COVID-19 knowledge has a direct relationship with risk perception.
H8: COVID-19 knowledge has a direct relationship with personal protection behavior.
H9: COVID-19 knowledge has a direct relationship with social distancing behavior.

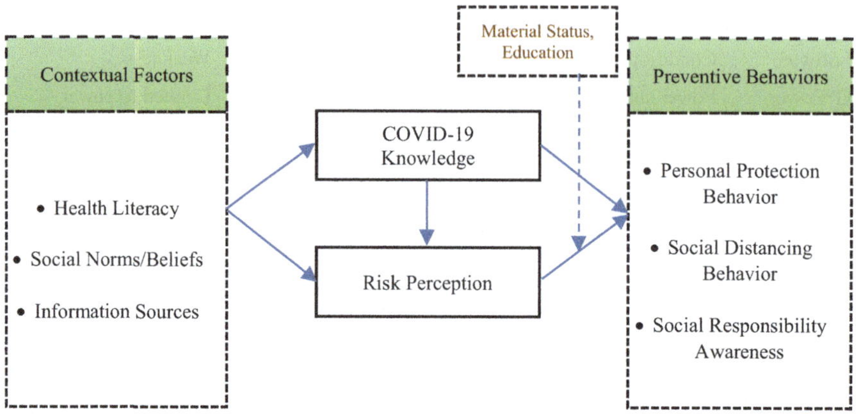

Fig. 12.2 Conceptual model

H10: COVID-19 knowledge has a direct relationship with social responsibility awareness.
H11: Risk perception has a direct relationship with personal protection behavior.
H12: Risk perception has a direct relationship with social distancing behavior.
H13: Risk perception has a direct relationship with social responsibility awareness.
H14: Material status moderates the relationship between risk perception and personal protection behavior.
H15: Material status moderates the relationship between risk perception and social distancing behavior.
H16: Material status moderates the relationship between risk perception and social responsibility awareness.
H17: Education moderates the relationship between risk perception and personal protection behavior.
H18: Education moderates the relationship between risk perception and social distancing behavior.
H19: Education moderates the relationship between risk perception and social responsibility awareness.

6.5.1 Data Collection

This research is a descriptive and correlational study conducted in one of the northern cities of Iran. The statistical population of the study includes the people who are potentially exposed to the risk of getting infected with COVID-19 during the winter of 2022. Subsequently, a sample of 140 people with the age of 18 years and older, were selected to participate in the research. To measure the path coefficients of the proposed model, and testing the hypothesis, first the authors designed a questionnaire for gathering data from the respondents based on the 5-point scale from 1 (very low) to 5 (very high) and distributed troughs social networking applications (WhatsApp and Telegram). After collecting questionnaires, data were analyzed using SPSS 26 and Smart PLS 4 software. The research questionnaire is provided in the Table 12.3.

6.5.2 Data Analysis

The analysis of collected data is composed of two main stages: (a) confirmatory factor analysis (CFA) to assess the measurement model, and (b) structural equation analysis to evaluate the path relationship among the constructs. To assess the reliability among items of each construct, the Cronbach's alpha (CA) is used, which has a recommended value of 0.7. The construct validity is evaluated through convergent and discriminant validity. Convergent validity includes factor loadings (FL), composite reliability (CR), and average variance extracted (AVE). Discriminant validity was assessed by comparing the square root values of the AVE across constructs. We used the R-squared to measure the explained variance of the endogenous variables. Finally, the direct, indirect and total effects of variables are analyzed to accept or reject the hypotheses.

- Implementation of the SEM Model

To implement the proposed model, the collected data through the questionnaire must be entered to a Microsoft excel sheet as CSV format. Obviously, table rows indicate the respondents and columns show the questions. After creating the model in workspace of the SMART PLS 4, the data file was imported for estimating the final research model. Figures 12.3 and 12.4 illustrate the model in the path coefficients and T value diagrams, respectively.

As mentioned in previous sections, in order to use the results of SEM, the measurement model must first be evaluated in terms of validity and reliability indicators. After confirming the model, decisions can be made regarding the acceptance or rejection of hypotheses, using path coefficients and t-values. The status of the measurement model is mentioned in the Table 12.4.

- Reliability of Measurement Model

According to the Table 12.4, the coefficient of Cronbach's alpha is greater than 0.7. Therefore, it can be concluded that the research questionnaire has appropriate reliability. As a result, the reliability of the measurement model is also confirmed.

- Validity of the Measurement Model

- Convergent Validity

Factor loading coefficients are calculated by measuring the correlation between a structure's indicators and the structure itself. The outputs of factor loadings revealed high loadings of all items compared to threshold (0.6). Composite reliability (CR) represents the variance ratio between each structure and its indicators to the total

Table 3 Research questionnaire

Variable	Sym	Questions	Source
Health literacy	HeL_1	To what extent do you have ability to find information on how to protect yourself from illness, how to get healthier or manage mental health problems?	[11]
	HeL_2	How much can you understand the leaflets that come with your medicine?	
	HeL_3	To what extent can you judge the advantages and disadvantages of different treatment options?	
	HeL_4	How much are you familiar to need for health screenings?	
	HeL_5	To what extent can you judge which everyday behavior is related to your health?	
Social norms	SoN_1	Most people who are important to me are personally doing something to help reduce coronavirus risk and slow down Its infection?	[12, 13]
	SoN_2	The people who are important to me are expected me to do my best to help reduce coronavirus risk and slow down Its infection?	
	SoN_3	The people who are important to me would support me if I decided to help reduce the risk of coronavirus?	
	SoN_4	The people whose opinion I value, think I should act personally to reduce the risk of coronavirus?	
Information sources	InS_2	How much information do you receive from talk to, family, friends, co-workers and etc. about COVID 19?	[14]
	InS_2	How much information do you receive from traditional/social media, web surfing, books, magazines and etc. about COVID 19?	
	InS_3	How much information do you receive from consult doctors and medical staff and etc. about COVID 19?	

(continued)

Table 3 (continued)

Variable	Sym	Questions	Source
	InS_4	How much information do you receive from other sources about COVID 19?	
COVID-19 knowledge	COK_1	How much do you know about COVID 19, its family and origins?	[15]
	COK_2	How much do you know about common symptoms of COVID 19, diagnosed tests and incubation period?	
	COK_3	How much do you know about COVID 19 transmission ways?	
	COK_4	How much do you know about COVID 19 prevention ways?	
	COK_5	How much do you know about COVID 19 treatment procedure?	
Risk perception	RiP_1	When you think about COVID-19, to what extent do you feel fearful?	[16, 17, 12]
	RiP_2	How risky do you consider COVID-19 to be to your society?	
	RiP_3	How much risk do you believe that Coronavirus poses to human health, safety or prosperity?	
	RiP_4	How likely do you think it is that you will get Coronavirus?	
	RiP_5	To what extent do you feel vulnerable to Coronavirus?	
	RiP_6	How much do you think it would be likely for you to contract the Coronavirus, if you did not follow the recommendations?	
Personal protection behavior	PPB_1	To what extent do you undertake handwashing?	[18, 19]
	PPB_2	To what extent do you undertake cough etiquette?	
	PPB_3	To what extent do you disinfect things around you?	
	PPB_4	To what extent do you avoid going out when you have a cold?	
	PPB_5	To what extent do you avoid going to clinic even when having a cold symptom?	
	PPB_6	To what extent do you prepare consultation and transportation methods for when you feel ill?	

(continued)

Table 3 (continued)

Variable	Sym	Questions	Source
	PPB_7	To what extent do you wear a surgical-style mask when going out?	
Social distancing behavior	SDB_1	How much do you avoid from poorly ventilated closed space?	
	SDB_2	How much do you avoid from large gatherings?	
	SDB_3	How much do you avoid from conversations or shouting in proximity?	
	SDB_4	How much do you participate in virtual events using online tools?	
Social responsibility awareness	SRA_1	To what extent do you stockpile surgical-style mask?	
	SRA_2	To what extent do you stockpile food, toilet paper, tissue paper, etc.?	
	SRA_3	To what extent do you avoid contact with other people?	
	SRA_4	To what extent do you get enough rest and sleep?	
	SRA_5	To what extent do you eat a nutritious diet and do exercise?	

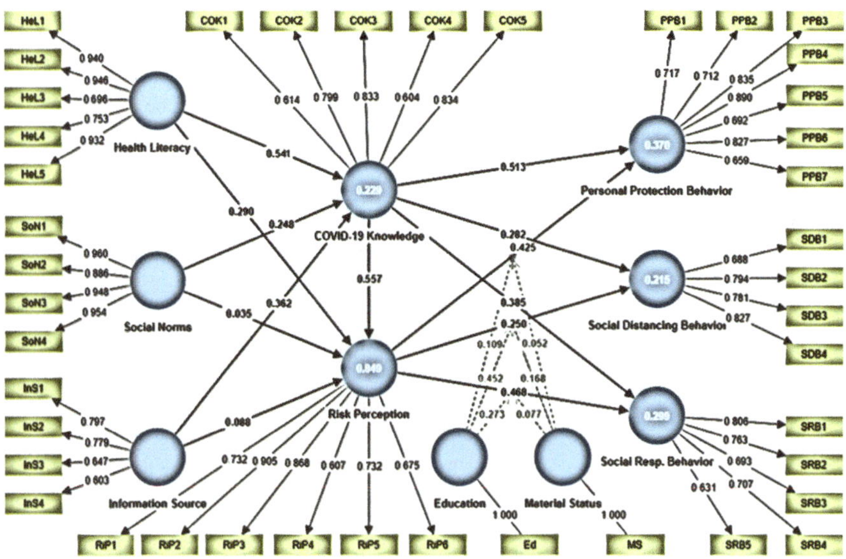

Fig. 12.3 Path coefficients diagram

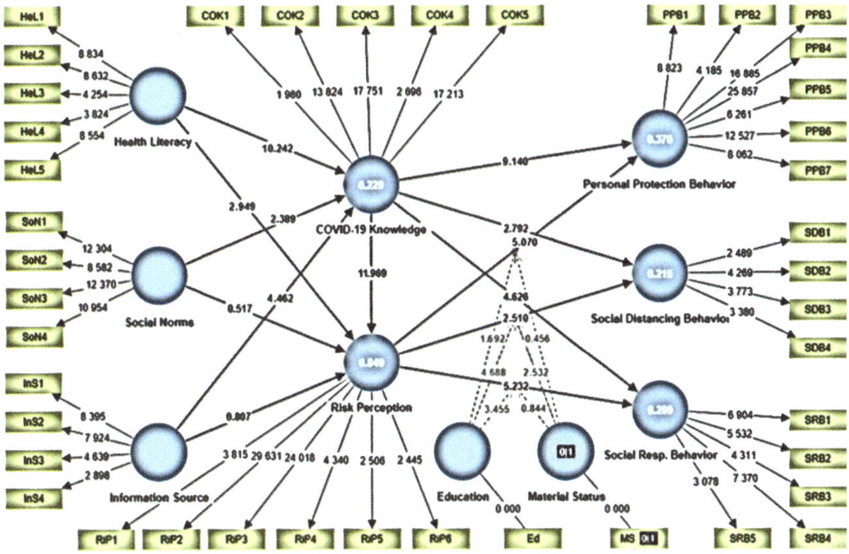

Fig. 12.4 T values diagram

variance of the structure. According to the results presented in Table 12.4, all variables have acceptable composite reliability coefficients.

In the present study, the average variance extracted (AVE) index was used to examine the convergent validity. For the latent variables, values greater than 0.5 indicate an acceptable convergent validity. According to the AVE index in Table 12.4, the AVE value for all the model constructs, the convergent validity of the model in confirmed.

- Discriminant Validity

To evaluate discriminant validity, the square root values of the AVE (numbers on the main diagonal) across constructs are compared. The value for each construct was greater than its correlation with other constructs suggesting that discriminant validity is satisfied (see Table 12.5).

- Structural Model Fit

According to the data analysis algorithm in the PLS method, after fitting the measurement models, it's time to fit the structural model. In this section, the R Squares criterion is used to show the effect of exogenous variables on an endogenous variable. The values of 0.19, 0.33, and 0.67 are introduced as weak, moderate, and strong R^2, respectively. The results of examining this criterion are presented in Table 12.4. It should be noted that this value could not calculated for exogenous variables (Health Literacy, Social Norms and Information Sources).

Table 12.4 Factor loading of confirmatory factor analysis

Variable	Questions	Loading Factor	Cronbach α	AVE	CR	R^2
Health literacy	Health information	0.940	0.858	0.662	0.898	–
	Leaflets	0.946				
	Treatment options	0.696				
	Health screenings	0.753				
	Health behaviors	0.932				
Social norms	Performance of important people	0.960	0.954	0.879	0.971	–
	Expectance of important people	0.886				
	Support of important people	0.948				
	Think of valuable people	0.954				
Information sources	People	0.797	0.781	0.603	0.717	–
	Media, web, books, magazines	0.779				
	Consult doctors and medical	0.647				
	Other sources	0.603				
COVID-19 knowledge	COVID 19, its family and origins	0.614	0.799	0.572	0.787	0.229
	Symptoms, tests, incubation period	0.799				
	COVID 19 transmission	0.833				
	Prevention ways	0.604				
	Treatment procedure	0.834				
Risk perception	Fear	0.732	0.743	0.510	0.807	0.849
	Risk for society	0.905				
	Risk for human	0.868				
	possibility of infection	0.607				
	Vulnerability	0.732				
	To follow recommendations	0.675				
Personal protection behavior	Handwashing	0.717	0.861	0.652	0.900	0.370
	Cough etiquette	0.712				
	disinfect things around you	0.835				

(continued)

Table 12.4 (continued)

Variable	Questions	Loading Factor	Cronbach α	AVE	CR	R^2
	Avoid going out	0.890				
	Avoid going to clinic	0.692				
	Transportation methods	0.827				
	Wearing surgical-style mask	0.659				
Social distancing behavior	Ventilated closed space	0.688	0.785	0.599	0.794	0.215
	Large gatherings	0.794				
	Close conversations	0.781				
	Online participation in virtual events	0.827				
Social responsibility awareness	Stockpile surgical-style mask	0.806	0.708	0.608	0.823	0.299
	Stockpile food, toilet/tissue paper	0.763				
	Avoid contact with other people	0.693				
	Get enough rest and sleep	0.707				
	Eat a nutritious diet and do exercise	0.631				

- Overall Model Fit

In this section, the overall model fit is examined based on the goodness of fit index (GFI). Considering the average values of the first-order construct loadings and the average of R^2 values for all the endogenous variables, the GFI index for the proposed model is measured as following:

$$GFI = \sqrt{\overline{Communalities} \times \overline{R^2}} = \sqrt{0.636 \times 0.392} = 0.499$$

Same as R^2 index, GFI also compare with 0.19, 0.33, and 0.67 values, which are known as weak, moderate, and strong overall model fit, respectively. Therefore, the overall model fit is moderate to strong.

Table 5 Discriminant validity

	HeL	SoN	InS	COK	RiP	PPB	SDB	SRA
Health literacy (HeL)	**0.814**							
Social norms (SoN)	0.564	**0.937**						
Information sources (InS)	0.685	0.751	**0.846**					
COVID-19 knowledge (COK)	0.574	0.425	0.633	**0.756**				
Risk perception (RiP)	0.688	0.466	0.678	0.515	**0.714**			
Personal protection behavior (PPB)	0.352	0.177	0.438	0.298	0.311	**0.807**		
Social distancing behavior (SDB)	0.34	0.485	0.454	0.354	0.432	0.355	**0.774**	
Social responsibility awareness (SRA)	0.472	0.413	0.517	0.641	0.528	0.481	0.525	**0.780**

- Hypothesis Testing

After examining the fit of measurement, structural, and overall models it's allowed to test the research hypotheses. This section consists of two parts:

(a) Examination of the t-values related to each hypothesis.
(b) Examination of path coefficients related to each hypothesis.

The path coefficients determine the significance of variable effects and accept/reject research hypotheses, while path coefficients determine the strength of the variable effects on the other variable(s). Based on the Figs. 12.3 and 12.4, the research hypotheses are examined as follows:

- Hypotheses 1 to 3

According to the Fig. 12.3, t-value between the health literacy and COVID-19 knowledge (10.242) lies outside the range of ±1.96, which confirm the significance of the H1, so, the hypothesis H1 is accepted. The strength of the relationship between health literacy and COVID-19 knowledge is equal to 0.541. This coefficient indicates the relative strong relationship between two variables. Similarly, t-value between the social norms and COVID-19 knowledge (2.389), and Information sources and COVID-19 knowledge (4.462), lies outside the range of ±1.96, which confirm the significance of the H2 and H3 so, both hypotheses are accepted. The strength of the relationship between health literacy and COVID-19 knowledge, and information sources and COVID-19 knowledge are equal to 0.248 (weak) and 0.362 (weak to moderate), respectively.

- Hypotheses 4 to 6

According to the Fig. 12.3, t-value between the health literacy and risk perception (2.949) lies outside the range of ±1.96, which confirm the significance of the H4, so, the hypothesis H4 is accepted. The strength of the relationship between health literacy and risk perception is equal to 0.290 which indicates the weak relationship between two variables. But for hypothesis H5 and H6, t-value between the social norms and risk perception (0.517), and information sources and risk perception (0.807), lies inside the range of ±1.96, which indicated the hypotheses H5 and H6 are rejected.

- Hypotheses 7 to 10

According to the Fig. 12.3, t-values between the COVID-19 knowledge and risk perception (11.969), COVID-19 knowledge and personal protection behavior (9.140), COVID-19 knowledge and social distancing behavior (2.792) and COVID-19 knowledge and social responsibility awareness (4.626), all lie outside the range of ±1.96, which confirm the significance of the H7 to H10 hypotheses. The strengths of the relationship between COVID-19 knowledge and Risk Perception is equal to 0.557. This coefficient indicates the moderate to strong relationship between two variables. In addition, the path coefficients between COVID-19 knowledge and personal protection behavior, COVID-19 knowledge and social distancing behavior and COVID-19 knowledge and social responsibility awareness are equal to 0.513 (moderate to strong), 0.282 (weak) and 0.385 (weak to moderate), respectively.

- Hypotheses 11 to 13

According to the Fig. 12.3, t-values between the risk perception and personal protection behavior (9.140), risk perception and social distancing behavior (2.792) and risk perception and social responsibility awareness (4.626), all lie outside the range of ±1.96, which confirm the significance of the H11 to H13 hypotheses. The strengths of the relationship between risk perception and social responsibility awareness is equal to 0.425 which indicates the weak to moderate relationship between two variables. In addition, the path coefficients between risk perception and personal protection behavior and risk perception and social distancing behavior are equal to 0.250 (weak) and 0.468 (weak to moderate), respectively.

- Hypotheses 14 to 16

Hypotheses H14 to H16 are related to moderating effect of education on the relationship between risk perception and components of preventive behaviors variable, namely personal protection behavior, social distancing behavior and social responsibility awareness. According to the Fig. 12.3, t-values of the education are 1.692, 4.688 and 3.455, respectively. Therefore, education does not moderate the relationship between risk perception and personal protection behavior, but has positive effect on relationships between the risk perception and social distancing behavior as well the relationship between risk perception and social responsibility awareness.

- Hypotheses 17 to 19

Hypotheses H17 to H19 are related to moderating effect of material status on the relationship between risk perception and components of preventive behaviors variable, namely personal protection behavior, social distancing behavior and social responsibility awareness. According to the Fig. 12.3, t-values of the material status are 0.456, 2.532 and 0.844, respectively. Therefore, material status does not moderate the relationship between risk perception and personal protection behavior, and risk perception and social responsibility awareness, but has positive effect on relationships between the risk perception and social distancing behavior. Table 12.6 summarized the standardized direct, indirect and total effects of variables along with hypothesis testing.

In conclusion, health literacy was found to have a direct relationship with COVID-19 knowledge and risk perception. Social norms has direct relationship with COVID-19 knowledge, but non-significant relationship with risk perception. Furthermore, information sources had direct relationship with COVID-19 knowledge, but was found to have no significant relationship with risk perception. COVID-19 knowledge. COVID-19 knowledge, however, was found to have a significant relationship with risk perception, personal protection behavior, social distancing behavior and social responsibility awareness. Risk perception also have a significant relationship, personal protection behavior, social distancing and responsibility awareness. Finally, education moderates the relationship between the risk perception and social distancing behavior, and risk perception and social responsibility awareness, but does not moderate the relationship between risk perception and personal protection behavior. Material status, does not moderate the relationship between risk perception and personal protection behavior, and risk perception and social responsibility awareness, but has positive effect on relationships between the risk perception and social distancing behavior.

6.6 Modification Indices

If the fit of a model is not adequate, it has become common practice to modify the model, by deleting parameters that are not significant, and adding parameters that improve the fit. To assist in this process, most SEM software can compute modification indices for each fixed parameter. (The statistical test used is called a Lagrange multiplier test, and the program EQS calls it by its proper statistical name. However, most programs use the term "modification index".) The value of a given modification index is the minimum amount that the chi-square statistic is expected to decrease if the corresponding parameter is freed. Researchers often use this information to conduct a sequence of model modifications. At each step a parameter is freed that produces the largest improvement in fit, and this process is continued until an adequate fit is reached. For example, if in a confirmative factor model a loading that is fixed to zero shows a large modification index, we may free this parameter and estimate its value. This will improve the fit of the model, at the cost of one degree of freedom.

Table 12.6 Results of the testing hypotheses

Exogenous variable	Endogenous variable	Direct effect (β)	Indirect effect (β)	Total effect (β)	Result
Health literacy	COVID-19 knowledge	0.541		0.541	Accept
	Risk perception	0.290	0.301	0.591	Accept
	Personal protection behavior		0.529	0.529	–
	Social distancing behavior		0.300	0.300	–
	Social responsibility awareness		0.485	0.485	
Social norms	COVID-19 knowledge	0.248		0.248	Accept
	Risk perception	0.035		0.035	Reject
	Personal protection behavior		0.248	0.248	–
	Social distancing behavior		0.035	0.035	–
	Social responsibility awareness		0.248	0.248	–
Information sources	COVID-19 knowledge	0.362		0.362	Accept
	Risk perception	0.088		0.088	Reject
	Personal protection behavior		0.271	0.271	–
	Social distancing behavior		0.152	0.152	–
	Social responsibility awareness		0.234	0.234	–
COVID-19 knowledge	Risk perception	0.557		0.557	Accept

(continued)

Table 12.6 (continued)

Exogenous variable	Endogenous variable	Direct effect (β)	Indirect effect (β)	Total effect (β)	Result
	Personal protection behavior	0.513	0.237	0.750	Accept
	Social distancing behavior	0.282	0.139	0.421	Accept
	Social responsibility awareness	0.385	0.261	0.646	Accept
Risk perception	Personal protection behavior	0.425		0.425	Accept
	Social distancing behavior	0.250		0.250	Accept
	Social responsibility awareness	0.468		0.468	Accept

References

1. Munro, B.H.: Statistical methods for health care research, 6th edn. Lippincott Williams & Wilkins, Philadelphia, PA (2005)
2. Abbasbandy, S., Viranloo, T.A.: Numerical solution of fuzzy differential equation. Math. Comput. Appl. **7**(1), 41–52 (2002)
3. Allahviranloo, T., Abbasbandy, S., Rouhparvar, H.: The exact solutions of fuzzy wave-like equations with variable coefficients by a variational iteration method. Appl. Soft Comput. **11**(2), 2186–2192 (2011)
4. Allahviranloo, T., Lotfi, F.H., Kiasari, M.K., Khezerloo, M.: On the fuzzy solution of LR fuzzy linear systems. Appl. Math. Model. **37**(3), 1170–1176 (2013)
5. Chehlabi, M., Allahviranloo, T.: Concreted solutions to fuzzy linear fractional differential equations. Appl. Soft Comput. **44**, 108–116 (2016)
6. Mahmoodirad, A., Allahviranloo, T., Niroomand, S.: A new effective solution method for fully intuitionistic fuzzy transportation problem. Soft. Comput. **23**(12), 4521–4530 (2019)
7. Allahviranloo, T., Ezadi, S.: Z-Advanced numbers processes. Inf. Sci. **480**, 130–143 (2019)
8. Moloudzadeh, S., Allahviranloo, T., Darabi, P.: A new method for solving an arbitrary fully fuzzy linear system. Soft. Comput. **17**(9), 1725–1731 (2013)
9. Rahmani, A., Lotfi, F.H., Rostamy-Malkhalifeh, M., Allahviranloo, T.: A new method for defuzzification and ranking of fuzzy numbers based on the statistical beta distribution. Adv. Fuzzy Syst. **2016**, 1–8 (2016)
10. Henseler, J., Ringle, C.M., Sinkovics, R.R.: The use of partial least squares path modeling in international marketing. Adv. Int. Mark. **20**, 277–319 (2009)
11. Homayounfar, M., Zargar, S.M., Danaei, A.: The mediating effect of self-care measures on the relationship between health literacy and quality of life of patients after open heart surgery. J Health Manag. **10**(3), 43-53 (2019)
12. Savadori, L., Lauriola, M.: Risk perceptions and COVID-19 protective behaviors: a two-wave longitudinal study of epidemic and post-epidemic periods. Soc. Sci. Med. **301**, 114949 (2022)

13. van der Linden, S.: The social-psychological determinants of climate change risk perceptions: towards a comprehensive model. J. Environ. Psychol. **41**, 112–124 (2015)
14. Li, Y., Hu, L., Mao, X., Shen, Y., Xue, H., Hou, P., Liu, Y.: Health literacy, social support, and care ability for caregivers of dementia patients: structural equation modeling. Geriatr. Nurs. **41**(5), 600–607 (2020)
15. Taghrir, M.H., Borazjani, R., Shiraly, R.: COVID-19 and Iranian medical students; a survey on their related knowledge, preventive behaviors and risk perception. Arch. Iran. Med. **23**(4), 249–254 (2020)
16. Ferrer, R.A., Klein, W.M.P., Persoskie, A., Avishai-Yitshak, A., Sheeran, P.: The tripartite model of risk perception (TRIRISK): distinguishing deliberative, affective, and experiential components of perceived risk. Ann. Behav. Med. **50**(5), 653–663 (2016)
17. Kaufman, A.R., Twesten, J.E., Suls, J., McCaul, K.D., Ostroff, J.S., Ferrer, R.A., Brewer, N.T., Cameron, L.D., Halpern-Felsher, B., Hay, J.L., Park, E.R., Peters, E., Strong, D.R., Waters, E.A., Weinstein, N.D., Windschitl, P.D., Klein, W.M.P.: Measuring cigarette smoking risk perceptions. Nicotine Tob. Res. **22**(11), 1937–1945 (2020)
18. Uddin, S., Imam, T., Khushi, M., Khan, A., Moni, M.A.: How did socio-demographic status and personal attributes influence compliance to COVID-19 preventive behaviours during the early outbreak in Japan? Lessons for pandemic management. J. Public Health **29**(1), 89–97 (2021)
19. He, J., Yang, W., He, Q., Tang, Y., Wang, Y., Wang, G., Jiang, X., Ren, J.: Chinese pregnant women's knowledge, attitude, and practice of self-protection against coronavirus disease 2019 during the post-pandemic period: a structural equation modeling-based survey. Int. J. Disaster Risk Red. **87**, 103559 (2023)

Boosting Facial Action Unit Detection with CGAN-Based Data Augmentation

Duygu Cakir, Gorkem Yilmaz, and Nafiz Arica

Abstract Contraction of the facial muscle movements is the key aspect of facial expression recognition tasks. The Facial Action Coding System (FACS) is the most widely used and accepted standard that provides a description of all major and minor visual changes in terms of action units (AUs) representing facial muscle movements. With the advancements of deep networks, the main problem shifted from detection or classification to finding sufficient amounts of data, especially when it comes to minor muscle movements on the face. This study employs Generative Adversarial Networks (GANs) as a data augmentation method for the task of AU detection on two spontaneous datasets (DISFA, BP4D) and one in-the-wild dataset (EmotioNet). Results show that AU detection scores increase using GANs when compared to using only traditional augmentation methods.

Keywords Facial action unit detection · Generative adversarial networks · Data · Augmentation

1 Introduction and Motivation

Facial expressions generated by the movement of facial muscles are mostly defined in Facial Action Units (AUs). The research on facial analysis is mostly hampered by the lack of data, which should be annotated frame by frame by experts. Facial expression research has been limited by the availability as well as the quality of

---

The original version of the chapter has been revised: The second author "Gorkem Yilmaz" has been included in the author list. A correction to the chapter can be found at https://doi.org/10.1007/978-3-031-46735-6_21

D. Cakir (✉) · G. Yilmaz
Software Engineering, Bahcesehir University, Istanbul, Turkey
e-mail: duygu.cakir@bau.edu.tr

N. Arica
Information Systems Engineering, Piri Reis University, Istanbul, Turkey

T. Allahviranloo et al. (eds.), *Decision Making in Healthcare Systems*, Studies in Systems, Decision and Control 513,
https://doi.org/10.1007/978-3-031-46735-6_13

data, which has often been limited to acted or posed images rather than genuine expressions in naturalistic settings. Labeling such data can be time-consuming and requires expert input, and the use of crowd-sourced labeling has been proposed as a solution. However, even in the case of data collected in naturalistic settings, the authenticity of expressions may be compromised if subjects are aware they are being recorded [1]. The ethical concerns around the use of facial images and the potential for misuse of facial analysis technologies must also be carefully considered, particularly in the context of privacy and security. These make it inevitable to heavily use data augmentation methods to create large, diverse, balanced datasets and to combat overfitting.

The concept of creating synthetic data from an already-annotated dataset has been used for many years and for many different tasks. One of the earliest studies that uses augmentation in the context of computer vision is the work of LeCun et al. [2] in the Fig. 1.

LeCun et al. [2] in the late 1980s, which used data augmentation techniques such as rotation and scaling to improve the recognition of handwritten digits using Convolutional Neural Networks (CNNs). Their research has dramatically increased

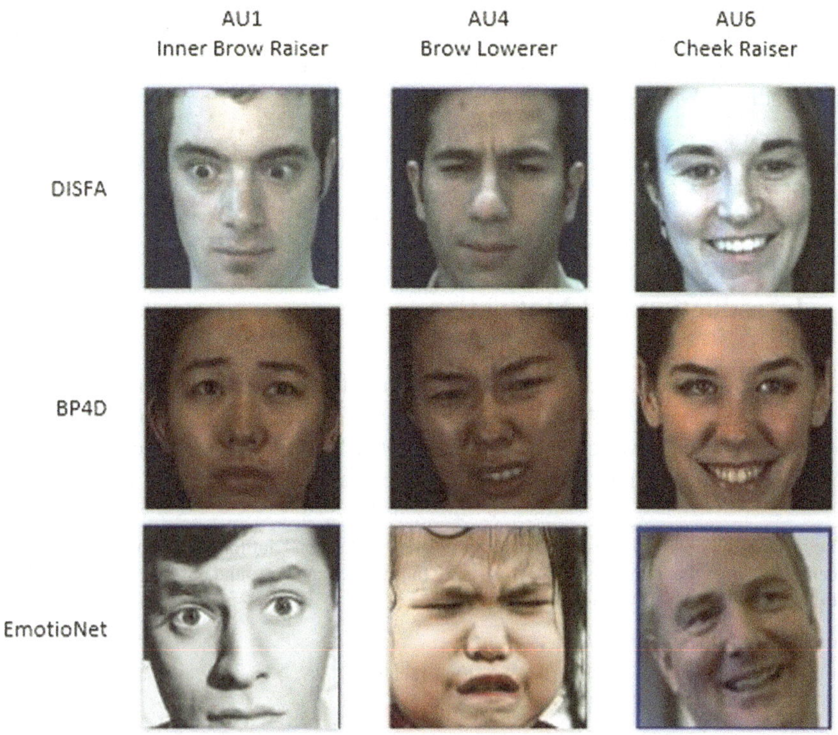

Fig. 1 Three different Action Unit (AU) categories' positively labeled samples belonging to the three datasets that are examined in this study

since it has been seen that CNNs work with any image dataset with any type of occlusion or alignment as long as the dataset is large and diverse enough while not being biased, resulting in reducing overfitting and generalizing the model.

Since the problem shifted from image alignment to data augmentation, many studies have been devoted to developing new and more advanced data augmentation techniques for specific tasks, such as facial expression recognition, where the availability of labeled training data is often limited. These techniques include methods for generating synthetic data, such as generative adversarial networks (GANs) and autoencoders, as well as more traditional techniques such as rotation, translation, scaling, flipping, and adding noise.

One of the most used datasets in computer vision is the ImageNet [3], in which two steps of traditional data augmentation is applied: flipping and then altering the intensities of the color channels. In a future study, researchers aim to find the most appropriate approach of data augmentation depending on the most famous image datasets [4] using one or more traditional augmentation techniques. Their work differs since they aim to find the best suiting augmentation method using Reinforcement Learning (RL) on a search table. Although it is practical to use traditional methods, it is just as natural to try to discover new methods for the task of augmentation. Besides using simple techniques, [5] uses an improved geometrical modification on images to randomly mask out square regions to improve the robustness of the network.

With the advancement of new technologies in deep neural networks, researchers have adapted the augmentation methods from simple techniques to more advanced ones. In their research, authors have used Long short-term memory (LSTM) and autoencoders to increase training samples [6] and use Recurrent Neural Networks (RNN) to classify electrocardiogram (ECG) signals for anomaly detection. In another research using autoencoders, they extract the decoding weights of the same class then they are linearly combined with original images from different categories [7]. Their proposed method can be used on images as well as tabular data which makes it a more generalized model.

Although simple techniques, supported by deep networks have been proven to be successful, recent studies have advanced the task of augmentation by synthesizing images with Generative Adversarial Networks (GAN) on the domains of facial expression recognition [8, 9], handwritten text datasets [8], medical studies such as covid19 detection [10], liver lesion classification [11], skin lesion detection [12]. Apart from detection/classification tasks, GANs are also used in semantic segmentation [13] in the task of augmentation. GANs have also been utilized in AU detection tasks, however they have either been analyzed in 3D domains [14] or the simplest datasets [15] in which the data is already balanced, and the classification scores are already as high as 99.9% without any complex classifiers.

In this paper, a Conditional GAN (CGAN) [16] is applied for augmenting three different AU-annotated datasets differing from the least challenging (lab-controlled) to in-the wild: DISFA, BP4D, and EmotioNet, which is, to our knowledge, the most broad study in 2D Facial Action Units. Results indicate that using traditional augmentation methods can be improved by adding synthetic images to the training set by

0.9% in average in all three datasets used in the experiments when compared to training with simple geometrical augmentation.

2 Methodology

As almost all computer vision studies suffer, the scarcity and imbalance of data forces AU detection research to use data augmentation methods as a pre-processing must. This research aims to investigate the traditional data augmentation methods and how using a CGAN to increase the data improves the AU detection accuracies.

For each face in each dataset, faces are cropped using the Viola Jones algorithm [17] which are then resized to 224×224 preserving all three channels in all datasets. In order to achieve the goal of increasing data and its diversity but at the same time preserve the shape of the facial image, only a horizontal flip is applied for augmentation as also employed by [18] both before and after using CGAN. The general pipeline of the proposed system can be found in Fig. 2.

This section outlines the details of the two spontaneous datasets (DISFA, BP4D) and one in-the-wild dataset (EmotioNet) followed by the details of how the CGAN is used as an augmentation method for improving the accuracy of AU detection. Finally, the results that are used to assess the performance on plain classification with only traditional augmentation methods as well as results after CGAN is used in addition to the traditional methods.

2.1 Database Setup

Each experimental setup has been tested on two lab-controlled datasets: Dynamic Facial Expression and Spontaneous Facial Action (DISFA) [19], BP4D [20] and one

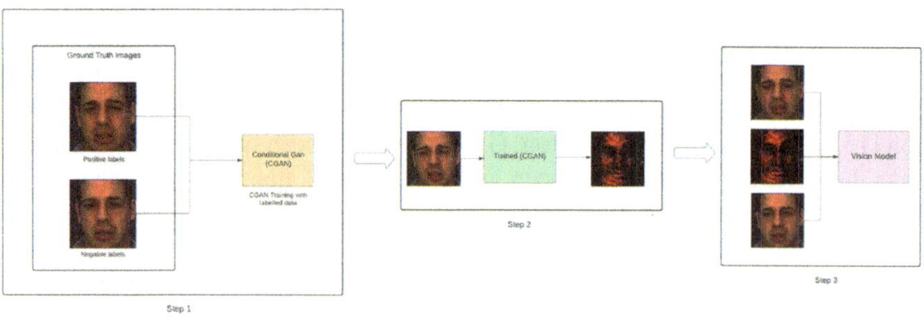

Fig. 2 The pipeline of the proposed system where (step 1) the ground truth images that are labeled are used to train the CGAN, (step 2) synthetic images are generated using the trained CGAN, and (step 3) ground truth and synthesized images are used in a CNN-based vision classification model to examine if the classifier scores increase or not

in-the-wild dataset: EmotioNet [21]. Each of these datasets are manually labelled by experts and contain frame level labelling on 2D RGB frames. The details and experimental settings of the datasets that are used in the experiments are as follows:

- **DISFA** is a collection of facial expression videos recorded from 27 participants. The dataset consists of videos of participants displaying different facial expressions and spontaneous facial actions in a controlled environment. Each video has been annotated with the presence and intensity of a set of AUs as well as the overall facial expression being displayed. The DISFA dataset has been widely used in research on facial expression recognition and analysis and has been particularly useful for studying spontaneous and dynamic facial expressions. It has also been used to evaluate the performance of various facial expression recognition algorithms and techniques. Following the experiments of [22, 23], frames with intensities greater than 2 are considered as positive. DISFA is a dataset that has severe imbalance, hence AUs with occurrence rates more than 10% have been employed in the experiments which resulted in the following AUs: 1, 2, 4, 6, 9, 12, 25, 26 as suggested by [18, 22, 24]. Subject-exclusive three-fold cross validation is employed.
- **BP4D** is a dataset that includes recordings of spontaneous facial expressions from 41 participants under 8 sessions who were asked to watch a series of videos while their facial expressions were recorded using a high resolution 3D camera. The dataset includes a total of 4,454 videos with a duration of around 3 min each, and it is annotated with the AUs, their intensities, and emotion labels according to FACS. With this dataset, AUs 1, 2, 4, 6, 7, 10, 12, 15, 17, 23, and 24 have been evaluated using the same experimental settings as DISFA.
- **EmotioNet** was created by collecting images from different sources, including public datasets, online platforms, and personal collections. The images were annotated with the corresponding emotional labels by human annotators, and the annotation process was carefully designed to ensure the quality and consistency of the labels. The EmotioNet dataset contains a total of over 1.3 million images, making it one of the largest datasets for facial expression recognition. The images in the dataset are captured under various conditions, including different lighting, poses, and backgrounds, and are representative of the variability and complexity of real-world facial expressions. It contains labels of 23 AUs as well as 16 different facial expressions, which are the six basic emotions and their combinations. Distinctively, it does not contain any subject information, hence following [25], regular three-fold cross validation has been employed and AUs 1, 2, 4, 6, 9, 12, 17, 25, 26 have been experimented.

As stated in the experimental details of [18] and [22], 800 positive and 1600 negative random frames have been taken for the settings to be consistent with all three datasets. Figure 1 contains samples of three different AUs on these three datasets.

2.2 Implementation Details

Implementation before and after using CGAN algorithm has been carried on a consistent environment to be able to compare the results fairly. The only augmentation before applying CGAN is a horizontal flip on the facial images to double the positive and negative samples, which makes 1600 positive and 3200 negative images in total to be trained using different TL techniques before applying CGAN.

CGAN has been applied on the positive images to generate synthetic positives to enlarge the dataset by 500 synthetic images (making a total of 1300) and randomly flipping 300 of the original positive images to make a total of 1600 on the positive labels. 3200 negative labels have been gathered using the same settings.

The details on the applied CGAN algorithm and TL methods before and after CGAN augmentation are as follows.

2.2.1 CGAN Generator and Discriminator

The generator of the CGAN network consists of four transposed convolutional layers, with each layer followed by a batch normalization and ReLU activation. The generator was trained using the Adam optimizer with a learning rate of 0.0002 and a beta1 value of 0.5. On the other hand, the discriminator network comprised of four convolutional layers, each followed by ReLU activation and dropout regularization. Such as the generator, the discriminator also utilized the Adam optimizer with a learning rate of 0.0002 and a beta1 value of 0.5. Both the generator and discriminator were trained with a binary cross-entropy loss (1). The training involved alternating updates between the generator and discriminator, with a batch size of 64. The CGAN has been trained for 100 epochs, monitoring the generator and discriminator losses to assess convergence. Figure 3 contains some synthetically produced AU samples on the three datasets.

The Binary Cross Entropy loss function that is used to train the CGAN model is formulated as follows:

$$\mathrm{L} = -\frac{1}{N}\sum_{i=1}^{N} y_i \cdot \log(p(y_i)) + (1 - y_i) \cdot \log(1 - p(y_i)) \tag{1}$$

For each AU, there are N samples where each sample $i \in N$ is represented as:

- N is the number of images on the dataset
- y_i is the label of the ith image
- $p(y_i)$ is the probability of the ith point being positive.

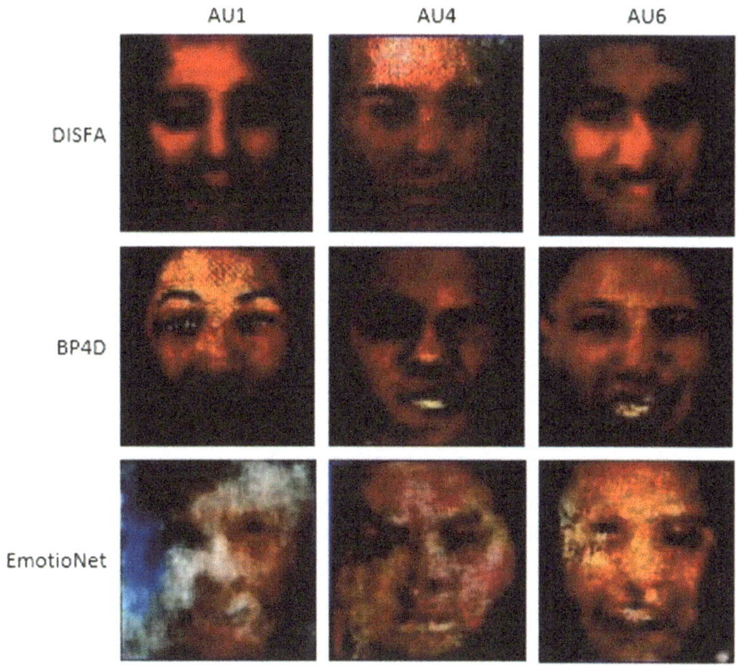

Fig. 3 Three different Action Unit (AU) categories' generated samples using CGAN belonging to the three datasets that are examined in this study

2.2.2 Transfer Learning Backbones

To investigate the AU detection scores with different techniques, some Transfer Learning (TL) models have also been examined as the base model. The most important advantage in machine learning is to start the training process with pre-trained weights. There are many architectures that are proven to be robust for many different classification tasks. To compare the proposed method's results with well-known and robust TL algorithms, a few of these models were trained with ImageNet weights. The experimented TL methods are: Xception [26], InceptionV3 [27], VGG16 and VGG19 [28], MobileNet [29], DenseNet201 [30], ResNet101V2 [31] respectively. To increase the diversity but at the same time preserve the shape of the facial image, only a horizontal flip is applied for augmentation as also employed by [18] both before and after using CGAN.

To be consistent with the experimental settings of the proposed method, three-fold subject-exclusive cross validation is employed on DISFA and BP4D and regular three-fold cross validation is employed on EmotioNet, all having a batch size of 32 and 150 epochs. No early stopping is applied.

Table 1 Comparison of the SOTA studies', popular TL methods and the proposed technique's F_1 scores and their averages on DISFA. Bolds indicate the increasing scores when compared to regular TL, underlined scores indicate the best ones

Method	1	2	4	6	9	12	25	26	Avg.
iCPM [32]	29.5	24.8	56.8	41.7	31.5	71.9	81.6	51.3	48.6
DRML [18]	17.3	17.7	37.4	29.0	10.7	37.7	38.5	20.1	26.0
wGPDE [33]	41.2	52.9	61.7	60.9	32.8	58.8	77.6	65.2	56.4
EAC-NET [24]	41.5	26.4	66.4	50.7	80.5	89.3	88.9	15.6	57.4
R-T1 [34]	42.6	27.2	65.5	55.5	22.8	82.9	88.3	51.3	54.5
GARN-1 [35]	46.6	90.9	38.8	41.3	39.4	93.8	81.4	45.1	59.7
AU-GCN [22]	32.3	19.5	55.7	57.9	61.4	62.7	90.9	60.0	55.1
DSIN [36]	44.4	43.6	64.8	33.1	43.1	72.2	88.0	41.3	53.8
res-L18M1 [37]	83.2	80.1	78.4	82.3	74.7	83.8	88.2	76.6	80.9
Transformers [38]	46.1	48.6	72.8	56.7	50.0	72.1	90.8	55.4	61.5
Xception	88.9	93.4	90.0	93.1	**95.6**	95.1	91.1	88.8	92.0
CGAN + Xception	88.9	93.1	**93.3**	**93.9**	93.9	94.5	**92.2**	**93.7**	**93.0**
InceptionV3	90.4	95.2	92.0	93.0	93.6	93.5	89.6	87.8	91.9
CGAN + InceptionV3	<u>**92.0**</u>	<u>**96.4**</u>	**93.8**	<u>**95.5**</u>	**94.6**	**94.6**	**89.7**	85.3	**92.7**
VGG16	86.9	93.4	91.1	92.8	89.7	92.7	83.5	90.9	90.1
CGAN + VGG16	**88.3**	91.1	**94.0**	90.5	**92.1**	91.5	**86.2**	89.8	**90.4**
VGG19	85.8	92.1	86.9	89.5	86.2	88.9	82.9	88.1	87.6
CGAN + VGG19	82.9	90.4	**90.0**	**91.8**	**90.2**	**92.0**	**84.7**	84.3	**88.3**
MobileNet	90.0	94.1	91.0	94.4	92.5	<u>95.9</u>	91.2	90.6	92.5
CGAN + MobileNet	**91.3**	93.7	**93.3**	**94.7**	<u>**95.6**</u>	95.1	<u>**93.6**</u>	<u>**94.3**</u>	<u>**94.0**</u>
DenseNet201	87.4	92.3	90.5	92.8	93.4	91.4	90.3	92.4	91.3
CGAN + DenseNet201	**90.4**	**93.4**	<u>**95.9**</u>	**93.8**	**95.4**	**95.0**	**92.1**	92.1	**93.5**
ResNet101V2	87.6	91.4	93.3	89.3	90.9	90.1	91.0	91.2	90.6
CGAN + ResNet101V2	**89.6**	90.6	92.0	**91.1**	**93.3**	**94.9**	**92.1**	**92.8**	**92.1**

3 Experimental Results

Tables 1, 2, and 3 show the state-of-the-art (SOTA) studies' F1 scores and their averages as well as the applied TL algorithms before augmenting faces with CGAN and after the augmentation. Results on three datasets indicate that using CGAN as an augmentation method increases the AU detection scores in all three datasets. All AU scores have increased on the DISFA dataset, 5 out of 7, and 6 out of 7 TL F1 scores have increased on the BP4D and EmotioNet datasets respectively. It is observed that the more challenging the dataset gets, the harder the scores increase since it is harder to get a clear synthetic image on in-the-wild datasets.

Table 2 Comparison of the SOTA studies', popular TL methods and the proposed technique's F_1 scores and their averages on BP4D. Bolds indicate the increasing scores when compared to regular TL, underlined scores indicate the best ones

Method	1	2	4	6	7	10	12	15	17	23	24	Avg.
JPML [39]	32.6	25.6	37.4	42.3	50.5	72.2	74.1	38.1	40.0	30.4	42.3	44.1
DRML [18]	36.4	41.8	43.0	55.0	67.0	66.3	65.8	33.2	48.0	31.7	30.0	47.1
JAA-Net [23]	53.8	47.6	58.2	78.5	75.8	82.7	88.2	43.3	61.8	45.6	49.9	62.3
DSIN [40]	51.7	40.4	56.0	76.1	73.5	79.9	85.4	37.3	62.9	38.8	41.6	58.5
ARL [41]	45.8	39.8	55.1	75.7	77.2	82.3	86.6	47.6	62.1	47.4	55.4	61.4
Transformers [38]	51.7	49.3	61.0	77.8	79.5	82.9	86.3	51.9	63.0	43.7	56.3	63.9
Xception	76.9	78.9	78.5	82.7	77.9	82.4	89.3	78.7	75.7	73.8	82.9	79.8
CGAN + Xception	**78.2**	**79.0**	**82.5**	**82.8**	76.3	80.6	88.4	77.7	71.0	**76.9**	**87.0**	**80.0**
InceptionV3	74.7	75.8	79.7	82.1	75.9	83.1	86.7	76.6	71.1	69.2	84.6	78.1
CGAN + InceptionV3	**76.7**	75.3	**83.3**	**82.5**	**77.1**	**83.3**	**88.2**	**75.5**	**75.7**	**73.6**	**85.3**	**79.7**
VGG16	76.0	80.2	73.9	82.4	79.2	84.1	86.5	79.1	76.3	71.1	82.1	79.2
CGAN + VGG16	75.7	76.8	**75.1**	78.7	77.7	81.4	86.3	74.6	69.2	**74.4**	80.8	77.3
VGG19	73.5	74.3	77.0	79.4	77.6	79.4	86.2	72.1	69.0	66.3	78.7	75.8
CGAN + VGG19	**73.6**	73.5	73.2	75.1	76.1	**79.7**	84.7	72.0	**71.4**	**73.8**	72.7	75.1
MobileNet	76.4	74.6	78.9	79.4	77.9	80.5	87.3	73.2	74.0	76.6	80.6	78.1
CGAN + MobileNet	**77.9**	**76.6**	78.6	**81.1**	**78.9**	**84.6**	86.8	**78.8**	**74.7**	75.2	**86.1**	**79.9**
DenseNet201	74.8	79.5	78.8	81.2	76.0	84.0	85.2	77.4	76.4	72.9	84.1	79.1
CGAN + DenseNet201	**78.1**	79.4	**78.9**	78.3	**80.3**	**85.9**	**87.2**	**77.7**	73.8	**77.2**	**86.6**	**80.3**
ResNet101V2	78.1	76.4	80.5	78.2	76.3	84.6	86.2	74.6	72.7	74.2	83.3	78.6
CGAN + ResNet101V2	**79.4**	**78.3**	**81.1**	**79.5**	**77.9**	**84.9**	**88.5**	74.1	**73.9**	72.8	**85.1**	**79.6**

Table 3 Comparison of the SOTA studies', popular TL methods' and the proposed technique's F_1 scores and their averages on EmotioNet. Bolds indicate the increasing scores when compared to regular TL, underlined scores indicate the best ones

Method	1	2	4	6	9	12	17	25	26	Avg.
DRML [18]	26.3	–	35.5	78.7	–	88.1	–	88.9	49.1	63.5
GL-CNN [42]]	59.0	50.0	60.0	84.0	50.0	92.0	43.0	93.0	66.0	66.3
ADLD [43]	19.8	25.2	31.0	58.2	–	78.3	8.6	–	–	36.9
MLCR [25]	61.4	49.3	75.9	83.5	68.3	92.0	50.8	95.2	65.1	71.3
Mean Teachers [44]	55.5	46.3	71.1	81.6	61.7	91.0	46.7	94.7	60.2	67.6
Xception	65.1	65.3	69.4	76.2	76.8	79.3	70.1	68.6	57.9	69.9
CGAN + Xception	**69.1**	**66.3**	**74.2**	**77.7**	**76.9**	**80.4**	68.9	**70.5**	**66.2**	**72.2**
InceptionV3	64.3	64.4	67.2	74.0	73.6	77.7	71.5	66.3	63.1	69.1
CGAN + InceptionV3	**66.3**	**68.2**	**67.6**	**74.5**	**76.9**	74.4	**73.8**	65.5	60.4	**69.7**
VGG16	67.2	73.2	66.1	71.9	75.7	74.4	63.9	67.5	62.6	69.2
CGAN + VGG16	**70.4**	64.8	58.5	**76.6**	**77.3**	78.3	**67.7**	**69.0**	**63.6**	**69.6**
VGG19	66.4	67.7	58.8	67.9	76.4	77.6	67.6	64.9	60.3	67.5
CGAN + VGG19	64.3	66.6	**62.4**	**70.2**	71.8	71.9	67.2	64.5	**64.6**	67.1
MobileNet	64.5	68.6	65.3	71.8	81.5	76.8	67.6	63.3	63.4	69.2
CGAN + MobileNet	**71.3**	63.6	**69.6**	**74.7**	79.7	**82.0**	**69.7**	**68.3**	**65.4**	**71.6**
DenseNet201	62.5	66.9	60.7	71.8	78.8	76.3	69.9	65.2	62.9	68.3
CGAN + DenseNet201	**64.2**	66.0	**68.8**	**76.0**	**79.4**	**78.2**	**73.3**	**69.4**	**63.9**	**71.0**
ResNet101V2	68.4	63.7	70.1	77.3	78.0	81.9	70.8	66.9	61.4	70.9
CGAN + ResNet101V2	67.4	**65.4**	68.2	**79.0**	78.0	81.0	70.7	**72.7**	**62.6**	**71.7**

4 Conclusion

In this study, the use of conditional generative adversarial networks (CGANs) as an augmentation method for improving the accuracy of automated facial action unit (AU) detection has been investigated. The results demonstrate that using CGANs to generate synthetic facial images as an augmentation technique can significantly improve the performance of AU detection systems.

It has been found that the performance improvement varied across the three datasets we tested, with the DISFA dataset (being the least challenging) showing the most significant improvement and the EmotioNet dataset (being the most challenging) showing the least, however still being improved. As previously foreseen, the effectiveness of CGAN-based augmentation depends on the characteristics of the dataset, such as the degree of variation in facial muscle movements and the spontaneous nature of the recorded face.

However, there is still room for improvement, particularly when it comes to applying this technique to in-the-wild datasets where real-world variability and noise can present a challenge. Future studies could focus on exploring the potential of other generative models or developing hybrid approaches that combine different techniques for data augmentation. Additionally, it would be valuable to investigate the transferability of the models trained with CGANgenerated data to other domains or tasks, as well as the impact of this technique on the generalization and fairness of the resulting models.

References

1. Bettadapura, V.: Face expression recognition and analysis: the state of the art. arXiv preprint arXiv:1203.6722 (2012)
2. LeCun, Y., Boser, B., Denker, J.S., Henderson, D., Howard, R.E.; Hubbard, W., Jackel, L.D.: Backpropagation applied to handwritten zip code recognition. Neural Comput. **1**, 541–551 (1989)
3. Krizhevsky, A., Sutskever, I., Hinton, G.E.: Imagenet classification with deep convolutional neural networks. Adv. Neural. Inf. Process. Syst. **25**, 1097–1105 (2012)
4. Cubuk, E.D., Zoph, B., Mane, D., Vasudevan, V., Le, Q.V.: Autoaugment: learning augmentation policies from data. In: Proceedings of the IEEE Conference on Computer Vision and Pattern Recognition, pp. 113–123 (2019)
5. DeVries, T., Taylor, G.W.: Improved regularization of convolutional neural networks with cutout. In: International Conference on Learning Representations (2018)
6. Al Nazi, Z., Biswas, A., Rayhan, M.A., Abir, T. A. (2019). Classification of ECG signals by dot residual lstm network with data augmentation for anomaly detection. In: 2019 22nd International Conference on Computer and Information Technology (ICCIT). IEEE, pp. 1–5 (2019)
7. Feng, X., Wu, Q.J., Yang, Y., Cao, L.: An autuencoder-based data augmentation strategy for generalization improvement of dcnns. Neurocomputing **402**, 283–297 (2020)
8. Antoniou, A., Storkey, A., Edwards, H.: Data augmentation generative adversarial networks. arXiv preprint arXiv:1711.04340 (2017)
9. Zhu, X., Liu, Y., Li, J., Wan, T., Qin, Z.: Emotion classification with data augmentation using generative adversarial networks. In: Advances in Knowledge Discovery and Data Mining: 22nd Pacific-Asia Conference, PAKDD 2018, Melbourne, VIC, Australia, June 3–6, 2018, Proceedings, Part III 22. Springer, pp. 349–360 (2018)
10. Waheed, A., Goyal, M., Gupta, D., Khanna, A., Al-Turjman, F., Pinheiro, P.R.: Covidgan: data augmentation using auxiliary classifier gan for improved covid-19 detection. IEEE Access **8**, 91916–91923 (2020)
11. Frid-Adar, M., Klang, E., Amitai, M., Goldberger, J., Greenspan, H.: Synthetic data augmentation using gan for improved liver lesion classification. In: 2018 IEEE 15th International Symposium on Biomedical Imaging (ISBI 2018). IEEE, pp. 289–293 (2018)
12. Bissoto, A., Valle, E., Avila, S.: Gan-based data augmentation and anonymization for skin-lesion analysis: a critical review. In: Proceedings of the IEEE/CVF Conference on Computer Vision and Pattern Recognition, pp. 1847–1856 (2021)
13. Choi, J., Kim, T., Kim, C.: Self-ensembling with gan-based data augmentation for domain adaptation in semantic segmentation. In: Proceedings of the IEEE/CVF International Conference on Computer Vision, pp. 6830–6840 (2019)

14. Niinuma, K., Ertugrul, I.O., Cohn, J.F., Jeni, L.A.: Synthetic expressions are better than real for learning to detect facial actions. In: Proceedings of the IEEE/CVF Winter Conference on Applications of Computer Vision, pp. 1248–1257 (2021)
15. Huang, Q., Pei, L., Wang, Y., Zeng, L.: AU data augmentation method based on generative adversarial networks. In: Proceedings of the 2nd International Conference on Artificial Intelligence and Advanced Manufacture, pp. 243–246 (2020)
16. Mirza, M., Osindero, S.: Conditional generative adversarial nets. arXiv preprint arXiv:1411.1784 (2014)
17. Viola, P., Jones, M.J.: Robust real-time face detection. Int. J. Comput. Vision **57**, 137–154 (2004)
18. Zhao, K., Chu, W.-S., Zhang, H.: Deep region and multi-label learning for facial action unit detection. In: Proceedings of the IEEE Conference on Computer Vision and Pattern Recognition, pp. 3391–3399 (2016)
19. Mavadati, S.M., Mahoor, M.H., Bartlett, K., Trinh, P., Cohn, J.F.: Disfa: a spontaneous facial action intensity database. IEEE Trans. Affect. Comput. **4**, 151–160 (2013)
20. Zhang, X., Yin, L., Cohn, J.F., Canavan, S., Reale, M., Horowitz, A., Liu, P., Girard, J.M.: Bp4d-spontaneous: a high-resolution spontaneous 3d dynamic facial expression database. Image Vis. Comput. **32**, 692–706 (2014)
21. Fabian Benitez-Quiroz, C., Srinivasan, R., Martinez, A.M.: Emotionet: an accurate, real-time algorithm for the automatic annotation of a million facial expressions in the wild. In: Proceedings of the IEEE Conference on Computer Vision and Pattern Recognition, pp. 5562–5570 (2016)
22. Liu, Z., Dong, J., Zhang, C., Wang, L., Dang, J.: Relation modeling with graph convolutional networks for facial action unit detection. In: International Conference on Multimedia Modeling. Springer, pp. 489–501 (2020)
23. Shao, Z., Liu, Z., Cai, J., Ma, L.: Deep adaptive attention for joint facial action unit detection and face alignment. In: Proceedings of the European Conference on Computer Vision (ECCV), pp. 705–720. (2018).
24. Li, W., Abtahi, F., Zhu, Z., Yin, L.: Eac-net: a region-based deep enhancing and cropping approach for facial action unit detection. In: 2017 12th IEEE International Conference on Automatic Face & Gesture Recognition (FG 2017). IEEE, pp. 103–110 (2017b)
25. Niu, X., Han, H., Shan, S., Chen, X.: Multi-label co-regularization for semi-supervised facial action unit recognition. arXiv preprint arXiv:1910.11012 (2019)
26. Chollet, F.: Xception: Deep learning with depthwise separable convolutions. In: Proceedings of the IEEE Conference on Computer Vision and Pattern Recognition, pp. 1251–1258 (2020)
27. Szegedy, C., Vanhoucke, V., Ioffe, S., Shlens, J., Wojna, Z.: Rethinking the inception architecture for computer vision. In: Proceedings of the IEEE conference on computer vision and pattern recognition, pp. 2818–2826. (2016)
28. Simonyan, K., Zisserman, A.: Very deep convolutional networks for large-scale image recognition. arXiv preprint arXiv:1409.1556. (2014)
29. Howard, A.G., Zhu, M., Chen, B., Maleficence, D., Wang, W., Weyand, T., Andreetto, M., Adam, H.: Mobilenets: Efficient convolutional neural networks for mobile vision applications. arXiv preprint arXiv:1704.04861 (2017)
30. Huang, G., Liu, Z., Van Der Maaten, L., Weinberger, K.Q.: Densely connected convolutional networks. In: Proceedings of the IEEE Conference on Computer Vision and Pattern Recognition, pp. 4700–4708. (2017)
31. He, K., Zhang, X., Ren, S., Sun, J.: Deep residual learning for image recognition. In: Proceedings of the IEEE Conference on Computer Vision and Pattern Recognition, pp. 770–778 (2016)
32. Zeng, J., Chu, W.-S., De la Torre, F., Cohn, J.F., Xiong, Z.: Confidence preserving machine for facial action unit detection. In: Proceedings of the IEEE international conference on computer vision, pp. 3622–3630 (2015)
33. Eleftheriadis, S., Rudovic, O., Deisenroth, M.P., Pantic, M.: Gaussian process domain experts for modeling of facial affect. IEEE Trans. Image Process. **26**, 4697–4711 (2017)

34. Li, W., Abtahi, F., Zhu, Z.: Action unit detection with region adaptation, multi-labeling learning and optimal temporal fusing. In: Proceedings of the IEEE Conference on Computer Vision and Pattern Recognition, pp. 1841–1850 (2017a)
35. Wang, C., Wang, S.: Personalized multiple facial action unit recognition through generative adversarial recognition network. In: Proceedings of the 26th ACM international conference on Multimedia, pp. 302–310 (2018)
36. Corneanu, C., Madadi, M., Escalera, S., Martinez, A.: Explainable early stopping for action unit recognition. In: 2020 15th IEEE International Conference on Automatic Face and Gesture Recognition (FG 2020). IEEE, pp. 693–699 (2020)
37. Chen, J., Wang, C., Wang, K., Liu, M.: Computational efficient deep neural network with differential attention maps for facial action unit detection. arXiv preprint arXiv:2011.12082 (2020)
38. Jacob, G.M., Stenger, B.: Facial action unit detection with transformers. In: Proceedings of the IEEE/CVF Conference on Computer Vision and Pattern Recognition, pp. 7680–7689 (2021)
39. Zhao, K., Chu, W.-S., De la Torre, F., Cohn, J. F., Zhang, H.: Joint patch and multi-label learning for facial action unit detection. In: Proceedings of the IEEE Conference on Computer Vision and Pattern Recognition, pp. 2207–2216 (2015)
40. Corneanu, C., Madadi, M., Escalera, S.: Deep structure inference network for facial action unit recognition. In: Proceedings of the European Conference on Computer Vision (ECCV), pp. 298–313 (2018)
41. Shao, Z., Liu, Z., Cai, J., Wu, Y., Ma, L.: Facial action unit detection using attention and relation learning. In: IEEE transactions on affective computing. (2019b)
42. Benitez-Quiroz, C.F., Wang, Y., Martinez, A.M.: Recognition of action units in the wild with deep nets and a new global-local loss. In ICCV, pp. 3990–3999 (2017)
43. Shao, Z., Cai, J., Cham, T.-J., Lu, X., Ma, L.: Semi-supervised unconstrained action unit detection via latent feature domain. arXiv preprint arXiv:1903.10143 (2019a)
44. Tarvainen, A., Valpola, H.: Mean teachers are better role models: weight-averaged consistency targets improve semi-supervised deep learning results. arXiv preprint arXiv:1703.01780 (2017)

Resiliency in Green Supply Chains of Pharmaceuticals

Saliha Karadayi-Usta

Abstract The pharmaceutical industry, a vital stakeholder in the global market, places a high priority on research and development, and the COVID-19 pandemic led to concerns in April 2020 about possible disruptions in the supply chain of medicines. The pharmaceutical industry must prioritize resilient green supply chain operations in order to mitigate potential disruptions, as indicated in industrial reports. As per the literature, green supply chain management involves the incorporation of the reduce, reuse, recycle, reclaim, and degradable principle into green supply chains, beginning from manufacturing to operations and culminating with end-of-life management. Thus, the purpose of this study is to extract the concepts to achieve the green supply chain for pharmaceutical industry, and to obtain a conceptual framework via cognitive mapping process. The findings of the analysis reveal that biodiversity and corporate social responsibility together provide a basis for the green chemistry and green pharmaceutical production. In case the medical institutions adopt recycling, reverse logistics and waste management operations, a green supply chain can be achieved. Moreover, by adding the digitalization and risk management practices, finally the resiliency in green supply chain of medicine can be attained. As a result, this paper contributes to the literature by extracting the concepts to be green in pharmaceutical supply chain and by analyzing these cognitive maps for these defined concepts. As of the knowledge of the author, this is the first paper conducting a cognitive map for green pharmaceutical supply chains. In addition, practitioner can benefit from this research findings to determine the tactical and strategical plans for their institutions. Accordingly, risk management and digitalization applications plus the green pharmaceutical supply chain brings resiliency.

Keywords Sustainability · Green supply chain · Supply chain · Pharmaceutical · Drug · Medication · Medicine · Healthcare

S. Karadayi-Usta (✉)
Industrial Engineering Department, Istinye University, Istanbul, Turkey
e-mail: saliha.usta@istinye.edu.tr

T. Allahviranloo et al. (eds.), *Decision Making in Healthcare Systems*,
Studies in Systems, Decision and Control 513,
https://doi.org/10.1007/978-3-031-46735-6_14

1 Introduction and Motivation

Pharmaceutical industry is an important stakeholder of the global market that primarily relies on research and development with the investments more than twenty percent of total sales on it. Both new small biotech and large pharmaceutical companies were drawn attention during the pandemics with their innovative sides. Besides, medications' research, development, manufacture, and distribution are all handled by the pharmaceutical sector. The industry has grown significantly over the last 20 years, and in 2022, global pharma revenues reached 1.48 trillion dollars [1]. As of April 2020, the concern about potential medicine supply chain disruptions caused by the COVID-19 pandemic has been raised. Approximately 66 percent of the pharma companies were worried that COVID-19 would cause a probable interruption in the supply chain for pharmaceutical items [2].

As the industrial reports address the potential disruption problems, the green supply chain with a resiliency is a must to maintain the supply chain operations in pharmaceutical industry [3]. Indeed, the literature reveals that green supply chain management (GSCM) comprises integrating the 4R1D (reduce, reuse, recycle, reclaim, and degradable) principle into traditional supply chains from manufacturing to operations through end-of-life management [4]. Reducing the environmental impact of factors including pollution, deforestation, ozone depletion, and global warming is the aim of supply chain sustainability. Utilizing the proper-sized packing boxes, avoiding utilizing large boxes for smaller shipments, and substituting recyclable paper pads for plastic packaging are all examples of intelligent packaging strategies [5].

The supply chain members of a pharmaceutical industry can be listed as chemical industry, warehouses, cold chain providers, logistics providers, green materials/packaging vendors, hospitals/health institutions/patients and veterinary/pets as customers [6, 7].

The green/sustainable pharmaceutical supply chain studies mainly grounds on cold chain [8], reverse logistics [9], recycling [10], waste management [11], life cycle assessment [12], circular economy [13], energy efficiency [14], corporate social responsibility [15], biodiversity [16], green chemistry [17], biorefinery [18], risk management [19], Industry 4.0/digital transformation/digitalization concepts with traceability [20], blockchain [21], information sharing [22], coordination [23], cooperation [24], and collaboration [25], and finally resilience [6].

The methodologies of these reviewed green pharmaceutical supply chain studies are multi-criteria decision making techniques [26] are the ones mostly in use. Furthermore, machine learning [27, 28], optimization [29], system dynamics [30] publications exist in the literature for the green pharmaceutical supply chain management.

The frameworks within this field of study includes assessment of health care system performance [31], environmentally sustainable pharmaceutical supply chain network design [32, 33], establishing impactful global health programs [34], blockchain-based traceability to tackle drug-counterfeiting [35].

Therefore, the motivation of this book chapter grounds on the fact that there is limited research handling green supply chain in medicine with a comprehensive framework.

There is a gap in literature dealing with supplying raw materials for drug production and distribution and finally selling it to consumers according to the type of product forms a supply chain.

Hence, the purpose of this study is to extract the concepts to achieve the green supply chain for pharmaceutical industry, and to obtain a conceptual framework via cognitive mapping process.

A cognitive map as a visual model that illustrates the concepts that individuals utilize in order to understand any event/problem, as well as the relationships between these concepts with their cause-and-effect directions [36]. Although there several types of cognitive maps as [37], this study adopts simple cognitive mapping due to the criticisms [38, 39] for fuzzy cognitive maps which are not sensitive to different initial conditions, in other words, the same result is obtained regardless of the initial vector.

The findings of the analysis reveal that biodiversity and corporate social responsibility together provide a basis for the green chemistry and green pharmaceutical production. In case the medical institutions adopt recycling, reverse logistics and waste management operations, a green supply chain can be achieved. Moreover, by adding the digitalization and risk management practices, finally the resiliency in green supply chain of medicine can be attained.

This paper contributes to the literature by extracting the concepts to be green in pharmaceutical supply chain and by analyzing these cognitive maps for these defined concepts. As of the knowledge of the author, this is the first paper conducting a cognitive map for green pharmaceutical supply chains. In addition, practitioner can benefit from this research findings to determine the tactical and strategical plans for their institutions. Accordingly, risk management and digitalization applications plus the green pharmaceutical supply chain brings resiliency.

In the following sections, the literature review, methodology, application and findings, and conclusion section are provided.

2 Literature Review

Green supply chain management (GSCM) entails introducing sustainable environmental procedures into traditional supply chains from production to operations to end-of-life management by incorporating the 4R1D (reduce, reuse, recycle, reclaim, and degradable) principle [4]. The goal of supply chain sustainability is to lessen the environmental effect of variables such as pollution, deforestation, ozone depletion, and global warming. Intelligent packaging solutions might include employing right-sized packing boxes, avoiding big boxes for smaller consignments, and using recyclable paper pads in place of plastic packaging [5].

A literature review on 15th June 2023 was conducted to reach the recent document via Scopus database with "medicine/drug/pharmaceutical/medication" and "supply chain/service network/supply network/value chain/value network" and "green/sustainable/sustainability" keywords in article title, abstract and keywords sections, and finally 751 documents found. Accordingly, there is an obvious increasing trend in the number of publications by 2010 with 20 to 30 papers per year, while beginning with the 2017, this numbers reach to a hundred by 2021, and so on. This is clear that many researchers will be dealing with this topic.

The major journals publishing this issue most frequently are Sustainability, Journal of Cleaner Production, Resources Conservation and Recycling, and Vaccine. Moreover, the countries/territories of these papers' authors are mostly from United States, United Kingdom, India, China, Iran and Germany. In addition, while 65% of these papers are articles, 13% of them are reviews, 9% of them are conference papers, 6% of them are book chapters, and the remaining part covers conference reviews, books, notes, short surveys, editorials, and letters. While engineering discipline contributes to this field of study by 11.5%, it is 11% for the environmental science, 11% for the business and management studies, 10% for medicine, 6% for the computer science, 5% for the social sciences, 5% for the agriculture, 5% for the decision science, 5% for the energy, etc. As it can be clearly inferred from these percentages, green pharmaceutical supply chain is an umbrella term including many fields.

By applying a systematic bibliometric analysis approach via VosViewer software [40], a visual graph is generated to highlight the important keywords with their interrelations (See Fig. 1). In this analysis, minimum number of occurrences of w keyword was taken as 7, and for the 2353 keywords, 22 of them meet this threshold.

The pharmaceutical supply chain includes the steps of obtaining the raw materials, producing, distributing, and delivering pharmaceuticals to patients. Because the pharma supply chain network is made up of many different stakeholders, careful coordination and compliance to regulatory criteria is required at every level to guarantee patients get safe and effective medicines [41]. Both providers and customers face risks and problems in the pharmaceutical supply chain. However, in a health-conscious culture, managing pharmaceutical supply chains offers various complications since it requires many critical components and stakeholders in order to efficiently provide life-saving drugs to patients [42].

Moreover, *cold chain* is a must for the medications' delivery that should be conformed with the requirements of the World Health Organization [8] to enable the safety and security of these perishable products. Cold chain medical items must be held at a specific temperature in order to retain their safety and quality. These items might be vaccinations, cell components, gene treatments, or biologics within the scope of pharmaceutical supply chain [43].

In addition, *reverse logistics* in the pharmaceutical industry involves acquiring items from customers and categorizing the various components to either dispose of or recover them at various stages in the supply chain and remanufacturing process [9].

Recycling in the pharmaceutical industry is a difficult process, especially for the unused and waste pharmaceuticals, and out-of-use packages, government has

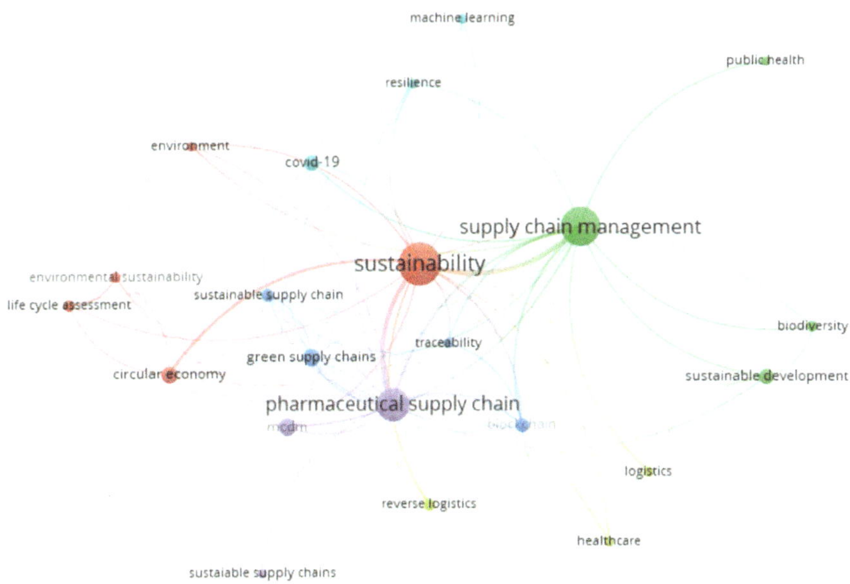

Fig. 1 Keywords' bibliometric analysis for green pharmaceutical supply chain field of study

placed strict constraints on this business. Recycling is challenging, but not impossible. There are many successful examples implemented by local authorities, municipalities, medical institutions, and individuals [10]. Indeed, it is known that drugs that are thrown into the trash or spilled into the sink return to the human body through agricultural products by mixing with nature and cause negative effects [44]. Antimicrobial resistance is also another important issue as a result of waste medications [45]. Since the agriculture is directed affected by the waste drugs, the recycling becomes an even more important issue [46].

Pharmaceutical *waste management* is critical due to the technical ability to regional counterparts to minimize the indirect or direct effects resulting from inadequately handled medication waste. While leftover drugs might aid those who need them but have no access to them with adequate planning, massive drug wastes in many pharmaceutical supply chains result in major financial losses and environmental/ social problems [11].

For example, owing to hygiene concerns during the COVID-19 pandemics, single-use packaging, non-timber forest products, and plastics were demanded at the highest level as numerous wastes as a hazard to public health [47]. Pharmaceutical waste management is an important concern in medical management, as the current pandemic has proven. Furthermore, due to the daily entry of a substantial volume of pharmaceutical waste into the ecosystem, the ecological and social implications of pharmaceutical waste management are obvious [48].

Accordingly, *life cycle assessment* is an effective method for identifying potential environmental implications across the pharmaceutical supply network [49]. During the travel of the drugs in the cold chain, it is difficult to create and put into use pharmaceuticals rapidly since a medication's life cycle is often long and complicated, taking approximately a maximum of fifteen years for a treatment to be approved and commercialized. The process of developing pharmaceuticals can be difficult with obstacles, including the identification of viable pharmacological targets, diminishing market approval success rates, rising development costs, and reimbursement constraints. As a result, it is critical that biotechnology and pharmaceutical companies work together to improve the drug life cycle and speed the approval process while still delivering safe and effective medications [12].

The continually growing levels of pollution and waste generation have forced enterprises all over the world to adopt the *circular economy* idea into their supply chains. *Circular supply chain management* is the combination of the circular economy strategy with supply chain management. Among other businesses, the pharmaceutical industry contributes to environmental degradation. As a result, an effective framework for the implementation of circular supply chain management in a certain industry is critical [13].

As pharmaceutical producers confront an increasingly competitive conditions, they are seeking for ways to cut manufacturing costs while maintaining *productivity* or *quality* of the drug. Volatility in energy prices can have a detrimental impact on financial performance. Investing in *energy-efficient technology and techniques* can help to meet the challenge of maintaining good product quality while lowering manufacturing costs. Energy-efficient technology may provide additional benefits such as enhanced quality, greater output, and enhanced process efficiency, all of which can contribute to increased productivity. *Energy efficiency* additionally serves as an essential component of a company's ecological approach since advances in energy efficiency can lead to lower pollution emissions [14].

Corporate social responsibility is being explored from a variety of angles and has achieved remarkable attention in recent years, particularly in emerging markets. Pharmaceutical businesses, via their corporate social responsibility and corporate governance requirements play a critical role in the well-being and health of people worldwide. It is an approach to strategic planning that pharmaceutical firms employ as a chance for pharmaceutical businesses to decide how to proceed and to advertise their position [15].

In addition to these industrial management concepts, there is a link between pharmaceutical industry and *biodiversity*. The main steps of the pharmaceutical supply chain for *biodiversity* include extraction of the plants, processing, logistics, utilization and waste generation processes [16].

Biodiversity establishes the necessary foundations for the pharmaceutical industry's development of new medications. To reduce supply risk, it is important to invest in operations that benefit biodiversity rather than harm it. Inaction might result in the loss of at least one significant undiscovered medication every two years. *Green chemistry* principles also help biodiversity by lowering the amount of hazardous chemicals and active medicinal components released into the environment [17].

The pharmaceutical sector was among the first to embrace *green chemistry*, with several pharma corporations establishing green chemistry teams and utilizing metrics, tools, and educating people relating to green medicine design and production [7]. Green chemistry is a vital concept for the green supply chain of medicine as the major vendor of the supply chain. For future sustainable development, *biorefinery* is a possible alternative source of renewable materials, minerals, energy, and fuels [18].

Along with the whole pharmaceutical supply chain, *risk management* plays an important role to overcome the challenges. It is critical, for example, to evaluate COVID-19 effects on delivery security as well as enterprises' readiness and actions. The investigations center on supply networks, which were vital for ensuring the delivery of basic items while vast segments of the businesses shut down in the pandemics. This is also valid for the pharmaceutical supply chain by encompassing imports, exports, domestic distribution, and home-delivery services. Hence, supply chain risk management, resilience, dependability, assessments of strengths and weaknesses in enterprises', recognizing linkages, overlaps are all important within the scope of *pharmaceutical supply chain risk management* to be green [19].

In addition to the aforementioned industrial management concepts, biodiversity and green chemistry, and risk management requirements to have a green supply chains in pharmaceutical industry, *Industry 4.0/digital transformation/digitalization* concepts are a must to enable the *traceability* [20]. *Blockchain* [21], *information sharing* [22], *coordination* [23], *cooperation* [24], and *collaboration* [25] are remarkable points for daily operational activities from a medicinal plant to distribution of these perishable goods to the customers.

Hence, *resilience* in green pharmaceutical supply chains can be achieved by implementing the whole aforementioned concepts and applications [6].

In order to investigate the methodologies applied in these green pharmaceutical supply chain studies, the literature review is extended, and find out that Multi-Criteria Decision Making (MCDM) techniques [26, 50–52] are the ones mostly used. In these papers, uncertainty [53, 54] and supplier selection [55–57] topics are mostly discussed. Additionally, machine learning [27, 28], optimization [29, 58, 59], system dynamics [30, 60] publications exist in the literature for the green pharmaceutical supply chain management.

The following section covers the preliminaries of cognitive mapping as the methodology part.

3 Methodology

Swan [36] defines a cognitive map as a visual model that depicts the concepts that individuals utilize in order to understand any event/problem, as well as the relationships between these concepts with their cause-and-effect directions. The cognitive mapping approach is an efficient way for revealing individuals' hidden ideas and revealing specific directed relationships concerning the issue. There are three forms of cognitive maps: concept maps, semantic maps, and cause-effect maps [37].

Concepts, relationships, and the strength of relationships are specified as cognitive map *elements* [61]. These maps can be represented as neighborhood matrices that display both concepts and relationships, or as an accessibility matrix that additionally reveals relationships that impact the concept indirectly [62].

There are also *simple*, *weighted*, and *fuzzy* cognitive maps (CM) in the literature. In particular, criticisms [38, 63] draw attention that classical fuzzy cognitive maps are not sensitive to different initial conditions, that is, the same result is obtained regardless of the initial vector. Therefore, the first proposed simple cognitive mapping technique is applied in this study.

In simple CM, relationships between concepts take values of $+$, $-$, and 0. A positive relationship indicates that the two concepts increase or decrease in the same direction; on the other hand, the negative relationship indicates that the two concepts increase/decrease in the opposite direction; 0 means that there is no relationship between these two concepts [64].

Expert opinions can be gathered through surveys, data extraction from documents, or interviews [62]. Especially in the analysis of complex systems, questionnaires and data analysis are used. Since the number of criteria discussed in this study is low, in-depth interviews were preferred.

The cognitive mapping process includes the following steps: determination of causal relationships, concepts, conceptual maps, coding of concepts and structures, updating concept schemes in line with expert opinions, creation, verification and analysis of cognitive maps [65].

Following the determination of the concepts and the relationships between the concepts, the CM is drawn visually. Nodes and the directed arrows connecting these nodes are clarified, and indirect relationships are visualized. For example, if there is a relationship from a variable x to the variable y, and from the variable y to the variable z, it also means that there is a relationship from the variable x to the variable z. This operation is called "multiplication" and the following rules apply: a positive value multiplied by the corresponding value is equal to that value again; multiplication by zero equals to zero; the product of two opposite signs is negative; a negative value multiplied by a negative value is positive; the multiplication operation is dispersive and symmetrical. Also, if more than two directed relationships start from the same point and end at the same point, the effect of the first point is added to the "total effect" on the second point and the operation is called the "addition" operation, the rules of addition apply [62].

Visually represented cognitive maps can be converted into matrix form, called "valency matrix" or "value matrix" or "adjacency matrix" [66]. The value matrix is an $n \times n$ square matrix with concepts in rows and columns. In the cells (v_{ij}) in the matrix, the strength of the relations between the related concepts (1, -1 or 0) is located. All elements in the diagonal take the value 0.

The sum of the absolute values of the elements of a row i in the neighborhood matrix gives the "outdegree—od" of the concept i, in other words, the number of other concepts affected by the concept i. Similarly, the sum of the absolute values of the elements in the column represents the "indegree—id", that is, the level of influence. The sum of in- and out- degrees gives the total degree (td) [67].

When the value matrix is expressed mathematically,

$$id_i = \sum_{j=1}^{n} v_{ij} \tag{1}$$

$$od_i = \sum_{j=1}^{n} v_{ji} \tag{2}$$

$$td_i = od_i + id_i \tag{3}$$

equations are obtained.

The contribution of a CM variable can be understood by calculating the centrality of that variable. A map can be considered as the total number of "receiver" variables and the "index of complexity". Many "transmitter" variables show the flatness of the cognitive map, but the causal explanations are not detailed enough. Also, passing variables can be called forcing functions that cannot be controlled by any other variable in the map. An acceptor variable can be viewed as a variable that has no effect on other variables in the system.

The neighborhood matrix has a form suitable for the "reachability matrix R" calculations. By squaring the $n \times n$ square matrix, in other words, multiplying the matrix with itself (second power), the reachability matrix is obtained. Thus, indirect relationships can also be detected. The reachability matrix can be calculated as $\mathrm{R} = \mathrm{k} + \mathrm{k}^2 + \mathrm{k}^3 + \ldots + \mathrm{k}^{\mathrm{n}-1}$.

Computation can be terminated at the mth point where m prime is zero, usually without needing to take the (n-1)th power. At this point the calculation can be terminated. Similar to the adjacency matrix, row sum shows which other concepts can be reached from the determined concept, while column totals reveal from which concepts the determined concept is reached.

After obtaining the reachability matrix, the connection index (CI) value between the concepts is calculated. The maximum number of links in the cognitive map is $\frac{n^2-n}{2}$. Here n represents the number of concepts. The connection index is found with $\mathrm{CI} = = \frac{2(n-1)}{n^2-n}$. CI takes a value in the range of [0, 1], its value approaches 1 as the level of interaction between concepts gets stronger, and gets closer to 0 as it gets weaker. The lowest acceptable CI values are given in Table 1.

Next, the hierarchy index $\mathrm{h} = \frac{\sigma^2_{od_i}}{n^2-1}$ is calculated [53, 68–70]. Here, od_i is the sum of the rows of the adjacency matrix, and $\sigma^2_{od_i}$ is the variance value of the corresponding vector. The hierarchy index takes a value in the closed range of [0, 1], and if it is

Table 1 Lowest acceptable connectivity index values

n	3	4	5	6	7	8	9	10	11	12	12	14
CI	0.67	0.50	0.40	0.33	0.29	0.25	0.22	0.20	0.18	0.17	0.15	0.14

close to 1, the cognitive map is called "fully hierarchical", if it is close to 0, it is described as "fully democratic" [66].

The degree of centralization is determined by the sum of the variables od_i and id_i [68]. The adjacency matrix, in other words, the sum of the elements in each row and each column of the pairwise comparison square matrix, and the vector cd_i, which expresses the degrees of centrality of the concepts, is calculated. The concept with the most interaction gets the highest value in this vector, while the concept with the least interaction gets the lowest value as expected [66]. The concept with the highest degree of centrality has a weight in the cognitive map as it will be the factor with the most interaction [71].

In the following section, the concepts defined will be analyzed with cognitive maps.

4 Analysis and Findings

By following the detailed literature review, the concept list is determined as follows: (1) Biodiversity, (2) Green chemistry and production, (3) Corporate social responsibility, (4) Recycling, waste management, reverse logistics, (5) Green supply chain of pharmaceuticals, (6) Risk management, (7) Industry 4.0/Digitalization, (8) Resiliency in green pharmaceuticals supply chain.

These defined concepts have been evaluated by MLP Care experts including digital transformation manager, business development manager, procurement manager, assistant general manager for processes, and assistant general manager for procurement via a short in-depth interview. MLP Care is one of the largest medical institution groups in Türkiye with 28 hospitals spread over 14 cities from Bursa to Ankara, Antalya to Baku. These experts' judgements were gathered through a Delphi technique to gather their mutual opinions on this issue to create the adjacency matrix (See Table 2). Table 2 indicates the how these concepts affect each other positively/negatively.

These relationships are visualized in Fig. 2. According to the expert opinions, biodiversity and corporate social responsibility together triggers the green chemistry and green pharmaceutical production. In case the medical institutions here include the recycling, reverse logistics and waste management activities, a green supply chain is possible. Furthermore, by adding the digitalization instruments and risk management practices, finally the resiliency in green supply chain of medicine can be achieved.

The adjacency matrix shows the direct relationship between concepts. The sum of the absolute values of the row elements gives the outdegree–*od*, that is, the sum of the other concepts affected by the concept *i*. Similarly, the sum of the absolute values of the column elements represents the indegree–*id*, that is, the level of influence. Indirect relations with the reachability matrix R are revealed.

In order to indicate the indirect relationships, the reachability matrix R is calculated by $R = k + k^2 + k^3$, and reach to the zero matrix by third power, thus, the

Table 2 Adjacency matrix

Concept no	1	2	3	4	5	6	7	8	*od*	Centrality ($od_i + id_i$)
1	0	1	0	0	0	0	0	0	1	1
2	0	0	0	0	1	0	0	0	1	3
3	0	1	0	0	0	0	0	0	1	1
4	0	0	0	0	1	0	0	0	1	1
5	0	0	0	0	0	0	0	1	1	3
6	0	0	0	0	0	0	0	1	1	1
7	0	0	0	0	0	0	0	1	1	1
8	0	0	0	0	0	0	0	0	0	3
id	0	2	0	0	2	0	0	3		

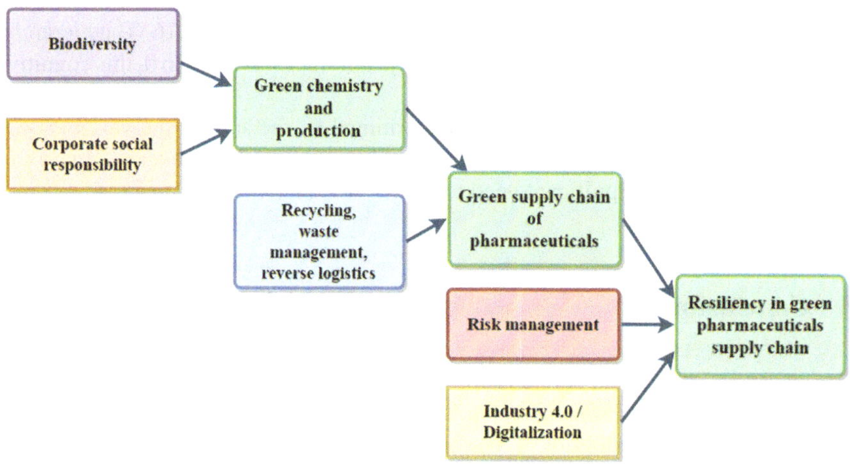

Fig. 2 The initial cognitive map including only direct relationships

multiplication process is terminated. The matrices obtained at each force taking were summed up and the R matrix (Table 3) is obtained.

After obtaining the reachability matrix, the connection index (CI) value between the concepts is calculated. The maximum number of links in the cognitive map is $\frac{n^2-n}{2} = \frac{8^2-8}{2} = 28$ in this situation. Here n represents the number of concepts. The connection index is found with $\mathrm{CI} = \frac{2(n-1)}{n^2-n} = \frac{2(8-1)}{8^2-8} = 0{,}25$.

CI takes a value in the range of [0, 1], its value approaches 1 as the level of interaction between concepts gets stronger, and gets closer to 0 as it gets weaker.

By examining the Table 1 that illustrates the lowest acceptable CI values, one can infer that this case study is within the acceptable connection levels.

Table 3 Reachability matrix

Concept no	1	2	3	4	5	6	7	8	*od*	Centrality ($od_i + id_i$)
1	0	1	0	0	1	0	0	1	3	3
2	0	0	0	0	1	0	0	1	2	4
3	0	1	0	0	1	0	0	1	3	3
4	0	0	0	0	1	0	0	1	2	2
5	0	0	0	0	0	0	0	1	1	5
6	0	0	0	0	0	0	0	1	1	1
7	0	0	0	0	0	0	0	1	1	1
8	0	0	0	0	0	0	0	0	0	7
id	0	2	0	0	4	0	0	7		

Next, the hierarchy index is calculated as $h = \frac{\sigma_{od_i}^2}{n^2-1} = \frac{1}{8^2-1} = 0{,}16$. The hierarchy index takes a value in the closed range of [0, 1], and since it is close to 0, this cognitive map is called fully democratic.

The degree of centralization can be determined by the sum of the variables od_i and id_i with reachability matrix. however, since it is a fully democratic matrix in hierarchy, there is no significant need to address the indirect relationships.

5 Conclusion

The pharmaceutical industry requires a resilient green supply chain to continue supply chain operations as industry publications discuss possible disruption possibilities. According to the literature, green supply chain management entails incorporating the "reduce, reuse, recycle, reclaim, and degradable" principle across traditional supply chains, from production to operations to end-of-life management. The goal of supply chain sustainability is to minimize the environmental effects of variables including pollution, deforestation, ozone depletion, and global warming. Intelligent packaging techniques include using the right-sized packing boxes, avoiding using huge boxes for smaller shipments, and replacing plastic wrapping with recyclable paper pads. Since there is a gap in literature dealing with supplying raw materials for drug production and distribution and finally selling it to consumers according to the type of product forms a supply chain, the purpose of this study is to extract the concepts to achieve the green supply chain for pharmaceutical industry, and to obtain a conceptual framework via cognitive mapping process.

The analysis's findings show that corporate social responsibility and biodiversity work together to support green chemistry and green pharmaceutical development. A green supply chain may be achieved if the medical institutions use recycling, reverse logistics, and waste management practices. Additionally, the resilience in the green supply chain of medication can eventually be accomplished by using digitalization and risk management techniques.

The concepts to be green in the pharmaceutical supply chain are extracted in this research, and the cognitive mappings for these specified concepts are examined as a theoretical contribution. As of the knowledge of the author, this is the first research to undertake a cognitive map for eco-friendly pharmaceutical supply chains. The results of this research may also be utilized by practitioners to decide on the tactical and strategic plans for their organizations. As a result, risk management and digitalization applications plus the green pharmaceutical supply chain brings resiliency.

As a limitation of this paper, the expert opinions are just illustrated by a private hospital's representatives. More industry experts from the supply chain members of a pharmaceutical industry such as chemical industry, warehouses, cold chain providers, logistics providers, green materials/packaging vendors, hospitals/health institutions/ patients and veterinary/pets as customers could bring more insights for the research topic.

Further research might include more industry experts, or might apply different cognitive mapping techniques like weighted or fuzzy cognitive maps, and indeed, fuzzy cognitive maps might be extended with different fuzzy sets. Moreover, instead of in-depth interviews, data gathering process van be enriched by conducting a questionnaire, and several time series analysis and machine learning methodologies might be implemented.

References

1. Mikulic, M.: Global Pharmaceutical Industry. Statista (2023). https://www.statista.com/topics/1764/global-pharmaceutical-industry/
2. Mikulic, M.: COVID-19 Caused Possible Drug Supply Chain Disruptions 2020. Statista (2020). https://www.statista.com/statistics/1110180/concern-on-drug-supply-chain-disruption-due-to-covid-19/
3. Silva, A.C., Marques, C.M., de Sousa, J.P.: A simulation approach for the design of more sustainable and resilient supply chains in the pharmaceutical industry. Sustainability **15**(9), 9 (2023). https://doi.org/10.3390/su15097254
4. Le, T.T.: The association of corporate social responsibility and sustainable consumption and production patterns: the mediating role of green supply chain management. J. Clean. Prod. **414**, 137435 (2023). https://doi.org/10.1016/j.jclepro.2023.137435
5. Karadayi-Usta, S.: A novel neutrosophical approach in stakeholder analysis for sustainable fashion supply chains. J. Fash. Market. Manag. Int. J. **27**(2), 370–394 (2023). https://doi.org/10.1108/JFMM-03-2022-0044
6. Vann Yaroson, E., Breen, L., Hou, J., Sowter, J.: The role of power-based behaviours on pharmaceutical supply chain resilience. Supply Chain Manag. Int. J. **28**(4), 738–759 (2023). https://doi.org/10.1108/SCM-08-2021-0369
7. Veleva, V.R., Cue, B.W., Todorova, S.: Benchmarking green chemistry adoption by the global pharmaceutical supply chain. ACS Sustain. Chem. Eng. **6**(1), 2–14 (2018). https://doi.org/10.1021/acssuschemeng.7b02277
8. Nyirimanzi, J.D., Ngenzi, J., Kagisha, V., Bizimana, T., Kayitare, E.: Assessment of medicines cold chain storage conformity with the requirements of the World Health Organization in health

facilities of the Eastern Province of Rwanda. J. Pharm. Policy Pract. **16**(1) (2023). https://doi.org/10.1186/s40545-023-00534-3
9. Lima, P.A.B., Delgado, F.C.M., dos Santos, T.L., Florentino, A.P.: Medications reverse logistics: a systematic literature review and a method for improving the Brazilian case. Clean. Logist. Supply Chain **3**, 100024 (2022). https://doi.org/10.1016/j.clscn.2021.100024
10. Karadayi-Usta, S.: Kullanılmayan ve atik ilaçlarin tersine lojistik faaliyetleri ile toplanmasina tüketicinin bakiş açisinin değerlendirilmesi. Int. J. Adv. Eng. Pure Sci. **34**(4), 4 (2022a)
11. Tat, R., Heydari, J.: Avoiding medicine wastes: Introducing a sustainable approach in the pharmaceutical supply chain. J. Clean. Prod. **320**, 128698 (2021). https://doi.org/10.1016/j.jclepro.2021.128698
12. Martin, N.L., Kononova, N., Cerdas, F., Herrmann, C.: LCA-based framework to support planning of centralized vs. Decentralized production of solid pharmaceuticals. Procedia CIRP **105**, 128–133 (2022). https://doi.org/10.1016/j.procir.2022.02.022
13. Khan, F., Ali, Y.: Implementation of the circular supply chain management in the pharmaceutical industry. Environ. Dev. Sustain. **24**(12), 13705–13731 (2022). https://doi.org/10.1007/s10668-021-02007-6
14. Shamkishore, L., Manmadha Reddy, K., Pathy, A.P.: Energy conservation in pharmaceutical manufacturing. Pharm. Technol. Sourc. Manag. **7**(11) (2011). https://www.pharmtech.com/view/energy-conservation-pharmaceutical-manufacturing
15. Demir, M., Min, M.: Consistencies and discrepancies in corporate social responsibility reporting in the pharmaceutical industry. Sustain. Account. Manag. Policy J. **10**(2), 333–364 (2019). https://doi.org/10.1108/SAMPJ-03-2018-0094
16. Giuliani, A., Undurraga, J.T., Dunkel, T., Aung, S.M.: Access and benefit sharing and the sustainable trade of biodiversity in Myanmar: the case of Thanakha. Sustainability (Switzerland) **13**(22) (2021). https://doi.org/10.3390/su132212372
17. Brown, L.: Nature's Medicine: The Link Between The Pharmaceutical Industry and Biodiversity. Nature Positive (2022). https://naturepositive.com/natures-medicine-the-link-between-the-pharmaceutical-industry-and-biodiversity/
18. Clark, J.H.: Green chemistry for the second generation biorefinery—sustainable chemical manufacturing based on biomass. J. Chem. Technol. Biotechnol. **82**(7), 603–609 (2007). https://doi.org/10.1002/jctb.1710
19. Bø, E., Hovi, I.B., Pinchasik, D.R.: COVID-19 disruptions and Norwegian food and pharmaceutical supply chains: Insights into supply chain risk management, resilience, and reliability. Sustain. Fut. **5** (2023). https://doi.org/10.1016/j.sftr.2022.100102
20. Ding, B.: Pharma industry 4.0: literature review and research opportunities in sustainable pharmaceutical supply chains. Process Saf. Environ. Prot. **119**, 115–130 (2018). https://doi.org/10.1016/j.psep.2018.06.031
21. Babu, E.S., Kavati, I., Nayak, S.R., Ghosh, U., Al Numay, W.: Secure and transparent pharmaceutical supply chain using permissioned blockchain network. Int J Log Res Appl **1**, 28 (2022). https://doi.org/10.1080/13675567.2022.2045578
22. Ma, J.-Y., Shi, L., Kang, T.-W.: The effect of digital transformation on the pharmaceutical sustainable supply chain performance: the mediating role of information sharing and traceability using structural equation modeling. Sustainability **15**(1), 1 (2023). https://doi.org/10.3390/su15010649
23. Song, Z., He, S., Wang, Y., An, J.: Green pharmaceutical supply chain coordination considering green investment, green logistics, and government intervention. Environ. Sci. Pollut. Res. **29**(42), 63321–63343 (2022). https://doi.org/10.1007/s11356-021-18275-8
24. Santos, J.A.M., Sousa, J.M.C., Vieira, S.M., Ferreira, A.F.: Many-objective optimization of a three-echelon supply chain: a case study in the pharmaceutical industry. Comput. Ind. Eng. **173**, 108729 (2022). https://doi.org/10.1016/j.cie.2022.108729
25. Nematollahi, M., Hosseini-Motlagh, S.-M.: A collaborative decision-making model for collecting unused medications in an environmentally responsible pharmaceutical supply chain. Int. J. Environ. Sci. Technol. **19**(3), 1907–1924 (2022). https://doi.org/10.1007/s13762-021-03332-z

26. Hossain, M.K., Thakur, V.: Drivers of sustainable healthcare supply chain performance: multi-criteria decision-making approach under grey environment. Int. J. Qual. Reliab. Manag. **39**(3), 859–880 (2022). https://doi.org/10.1108/IJQRM-03-2021-0075
27. Sharma, V., Tsai, M-L., Chen, C-W., Sun, P-P., Nargotra, P., Dong, C-D.: Advances in machine learning technology for sustainable biofuel production systems in lignocellulosic biorefineries. Sci. Total Environ. **886** (2023) https://doi.org/10.1016/j.scitotenv.2023.163972
28. Wang, H.S.-H., Yao, Y.: Machine learning for sustainable development and applications of biomass and biomass-derived carbonaceous materials in water and agricultural systems: a review. Resour. Conserv. Recycl. **190** (2023). https://doi.org/10.1016/j.resconrec.2022.106847
29. Mawengkang, T.A.H.: An optimization model for hospitals inventory management in pharmaceutical supply chain. Syst. Rev. Pharm. **11**(3), 324–332 (2020). https://doi.org/10.5530/srp.2020.3.38
30. Harpring, R., Maghsoudi, A., Fikar, C., Piotrowicz, W.D., Heaslip, G.: An analysis of compounding factors of epidemics in complex emergencies: a system dynamics approach. J. Human. Log. Supply Chain Manag. **11**(2), 198–226 (2021). https://doi.org/10.1108/JHLSCM-07-2020-0063
31. Kress, D.H., Su, Y., Wang, H.: Assessment of primary health care system performance in Nigeria: using the primary health care performance indicator conceptual framework. Health Syst. Reform **2**(4), 302–318 (2016). https://doi.org/10.1080/23288604.2016.1234861
32. Halim, I., Ang, P., Adhitya, A.: A decision support framework and system for design of sustainable pharmaceutical supply chain network. Clean Technol. Environ. Policy **21**(2), 431–446 (2019). https://doi.org/10.1007/s10098-018-1646-8
33. Low, Y.S., Halim, I., Adhitya, A., Chew, W., Sharratt, P.: Systematic framework for design of environmentally sustainable pharmaceutical supply chain network. J. Pharm. Innov. **11**(3), 250–263 (2016). https://doi.org/10.1007/s12247-016-9255-8
34. Pastakia, S.D., Tran, D.N., Manji, I., Schellhase, E., Karwa, R., Miller, M.L., Aruasa, W., Khan, Z.M.: Framework and case study for establishing impactful global health programs through academia—biopharmaceutical industry partnerships. Res. Soc. Adm. Pharm. **16**(11), 1519–1525 (2020). https://doi.org/10.1016/j.sapharm.2020.07.018
35. Nitsche, B., Straube, F., Kämper, T-L., Zarnitz, S.: Implementation framework for blockchain-based traceability to tackle drug-counterfeiting: embracing sustainable pharma logistics networks. Lect. Notes Mech. Eng. 630–637 (2023). https://doi.org/10.1007/978-3-031-28839-5_71
36. Swan, J.A.: Exploring knowledge and cognitions in decisions about technological innovation: mapping managerial cognitions. Hum. Relat. **48**(11), 1241–1270 (1995). https://doi.org/10.1177/001872679504801101
37. Siau, K., Tan, X.: Improving the quality of conceptual modeling using cognitive mapping techniques. Data Knowl. Eng. **55**(3), 343–365 (2005). https://doi.org/10.1016/j.datak.2004.12.006
38. Asan, U., Kadaifçi, Ç.: A new product positioning approach based on fuzzy cognitive mapping. J. Fac. Eng. Arch. Gazi University **35**(2) (2020). https://doi.org/10.17341/gazimmfd.528766
39. Rahmani, A., Lotfi, F.H., Rostamy-Malkhalifeh, M., Allahviranloo, T.: A new method for defuzzification and ranking of fuzzy numbers based on the statistical beta distribution. Adv. Fuzzy Syst. **2016**, 1–8 (2016). https://doi.org/10.1155/2016/6945184
40. van Eck, N.J., Waltman, L.: VOSviewer—Visualizing Scientific Landscapes [English; VOSviewer]. Leiden University's Centre for Science and Technology Studies (2023). https://www.vosviewer.com
41. Seddigh, M.R., Targholizadeh, A., Shokouhyar, S., Shokoohyar, S.: Social media and expert analysis cast light on the mechanisms of underlying problems in pharmaceutical supply chain: an exploratory approach. Technol. Forecast. Soc. Chang. **191**, 122533 (2023). https://doi.org/10.1016/j.techfore.2023.122533
42. Pathy, S.R., Rahimian, H.: A resilient inventory management of pharmaceutical supply chains under demand disruption. Comput. Ind. Eng. **180**, 109243 (2023). https://doi.org/10.1016/j.cie.2023.109243

43. Wang, Z., Wang, X., Guo, J.: Research on collaborative optimization of pharmaceutical cold chain logistics inventory and distribution. In: ACM International Conference Proceeding Series, Par F180470 (2022). https://doi.org/10.1145/3529299.3530205
44. Alhomoud, F.: "Don't let medicines go to waste"—a survey-based cross-sectional study of pharmacists' waste-reducing activities across gulf cooperation council countries. Front. Pharmacol. **11**, 1334 (2020). https://doi.org/10.3389/fphar.2020.01334
45. Ahmad, A., Patel, I., Khan, M.U., Babar, Z.: Pharmaceutical waste and antimicrobial resistance. Lancet. Infect. Dis. **17**(6), 578–579 (2017). https://doi.org/10.1016/S1473-3099(17)30268-2
46. Abbas, H., Farooquie, J.A.: Reverse logistics practices in Indian pharmaceutical supply chains: a study of manufacturers. Int. J. Logist. Syst. Manag. **35**(1), 72–89 (2020). https://doi.org/10.1504/IJLSM.2020.103863
47. Parashar, N., Hait, S.: Plastics in the time of COVID-19 pandemic: protector or polluter? Sci. Total Environ. **759**, 144274 (2021). https://doi.org/10.1016/j.scitotenv.2020.144274
48. Sazvar, Z., Zokaee, M., Tavakkoli-Moghaddam, R., Salari, S.A., Nayeri, S.: Designing a sustainable closed-loop pharmaceutical supply chain in a competitive market considering demand uncertainty, manufacturer's brand and waste management. Ann. Oper. Res. **315**(2), 2057–2088 (2022). https://doi.org/10.1007/s10479-021-03961-0
49. Siegert, M., Lehmann, A., Emara, Y., Finkbeiner, M.: Harmonized rules for future LCAs on pharmaceutical products and processes. Int. J. Life Cycle Assess. 24 (2019). https://doi.org/10.1007/s11367-018-1549-2
50. Kayani, S.A., Warsi, S.S., Liaqait, R.A.: A smart decision support framework for sustainable and resilient supplier selection and order allocation in the pharmaceutical industry. Sustainability (Switzerland) **15**(7) (2023). https://doi.org/10.3390/su15075962
51. Lotfi, A., Shakouri, M., Abazari, S.R., Aghsami, A., Rabbani, M.: A multi-objective optimization for a closed-loop sustainable pharmaceutical supply chain network design: a case study. J. Adv. Manag. Res. (2023). https://doi.org/10.1108/JAMR-05-2022-0100
52. Moosivand, A., Rangchian, M., Zarei, L., Peiravian, F., Mehralian, G., Sharifnia, H.: An application of multi-criteria decision-making approach to sustainable drug shortages management: evidence from a developing country. J. Pharm. Health Care Sci. **7**(1) (2021). https://doi.org/10.1186/s40780-021-00200-3
53. Karadayi-Usta, S.: Sustainable digital servicization: conceptual modeling of the car sharing business model. J. Yasar University **17**(67), 754–775 (2022b)
54. Ziya-Gorabi, F., Ghodratnama, A., Tavakkoli-Moghaddam, R., Asadi-Lari, M.S.: A new fuzzy tri-objective model for a home health care problem with green ambulance routing and congestion under uncertainty. Expert Syst. Appl. 201 (2022). https://doi.org/10.1016/j.eswa.2022.117093
55. Hosny, H., El-Henawey, I., Abo-Elhadid, S.: Selection a suitable supplier for enhancing supply chain management under neutrosophic environment. Neutrosoph. Sets Syst. **47**, 332–450 (2021)
56. Ishizaka, A., Khan, S.A., Kheybari, S., Zaman, S.I.: Supplier selection in closed loop pharma supply chain: a novel BWM–GAIA framework. Ann. Oper. Res. **324**(1–2), 13–36 (2023). https://doi.org/10.1007/s10479-022-04710-7
57. Khan, M.M., Bashar, I., Minhaj, G.M., Wasi, A.I., Hossain, N.U.I.: Resilient and sustainable supplier selection: an integration of SCOR 4.0 and machine learning approach. Sustain. Resilient Infrast. (2023). https://doi.org/10.1080/23789689.2023.2165782
58. Taleizadeh, A.A., Haji-Sami, E., Noori-daryan, M.: A robust optimization model for coordinating pharmaceutical reverse supply chains under return strategies. Ann. Oper. Res. **291**(1–2), 875–896 (2020). https://doi.org/10.1007/s10479-019-03200-7
59. Wang, S., He, L., Cheng, G.: Energy consumption optimization management mechanism based on drug green crowd data in biological pharmaceutical cloud environment. Eurasip J. Embed. Syst. **2017**(1) (2017). https://doi.org/10.1186/s13639-017-0071-0
60. Tsolakis, N., Srai, J.S.: Mapping supply dynamics in renewable feedstock enabled industries: a systems theory perspective on 'green' pharmaceuticals. Oper. Manag. Res. **11**(3–4), 83–104 (2018). https://doi.org/10.1007/s12063-018-0134-y

61. Nadkarni, S., Nah, F.F.-H.: Aggregated causal maps: an approach to elicit and aggregate the knowledge of multiple experts. Commun. Assoc. Inform. Syst. **12**(1) (2003). https://doi.org/10.17705/1CAIS.01225
62. Axelrod, R.: Structure of Decision: The Cognitive Maps of Political Elites. Princeton University Press (1976). https://www.jstor.org/stable/j.ctt13x0vw3
63. Mahmoodirad, A., Allahviranloo, T., Niroomand, S.: A new effective solution method for fully intuitionistic fuzzy transportation problem. Soft Comp. **23**(12), 4521–4530 (2019). https://doi.org/10.1007/s00500-018-3115-z
64. Eden, C.: Analyzing cognitive maps to help structure issues or problems. Eur. J. Oper. Res. **159**(3), 673–686 (2004). https://doi.org/10.1016/S0377-2217(03)00431-4
65. Nakayama, V.K., Armstrong, D.J.: Causal Mapping for Research in Information Technology. Idea Group Publishing (2005)
66. Özesmi, U., Özesmi, S.L.: Ecological models based on people's knowledge: a multi-step fuzzy cognitive mapping approach. Ecol. Model. **176**(1), 43–64 (2004). https://doi.org/10.1016/j.ecolmodel.2003.10.027
67. Shapiro, M.J., Bonham, G.M.: Cognitive process and foreign policy decision-making. Int. Stud. Quart. **17**(2), 147–174 (1973). https://doi.org/10.2307/2600226
68. Çoban, O., Seçme, G.: Prediction of socio-economical consequences of privatization at the firm level with fuzzy cognitive mapping. Inf. Sci. **169**(1), 131–154 (2005). https://doi.org/10.1016/j.ins.2004.02.009
69. Kandasamy, W.B.V., Smarandache, F.: Fuzzy Cognitive Maps and Neutrosophic Cognitive Maps. Xiquan, (2003)
70. Karadayi-Usta, S.: The role of the paper packaging industry in the circular economy: the causal relationship analysis via neutrosophic cognitive maps. In: Broumi, S. (ed.) Handbook of research on advances and applications of fuzzy sets and logic, pp. 605–618. IGI Global, Hershey, PA (2022c). https://doi.org/10.4018/978-1-7998-7979-4
71. Emel, G.G., Saraç, M., Kabak, C.: A two-phase model for strategic decision making: activation of scenarios with cognitive maps and an application on automotive industry. Anadolu Üniversitesi Sosyal Bilimler Dergisi **12**(4), 85–99 (2012)

Exploring Congestion in Fuzzy DEA by Solving One Model; Case Study: Hospitals in Tehran

Saber Saati, Maryam Shadab, and Sajedeh Mohamadniaahmadi

Abstract In recent decades, the number of private hospitals has increased in many countries, leading to an oversupply of drugs in the country's medical industry. This leads to hospital congestion and a decline in hospital profits, efficiency, and performance. One of the appropriate methods to detect congestion is Data Envelopment Analysis (DEA). In this study, we identified congested Tehran hospitals with fuzzy and vague data. For this purpose, we developed for the first time the methods proposed by Shadab et al. (Shadab, M., Saati, S., Farzipoor Saen, R., Mostafaee. (2021). Detecting congestion in DEA by solving one model. Operations Research and Decisions. 77–97.) and presented a novel fuzzy nonlinear DEA model for identifying congested hospitals as Decision Making Units (DMUs). We improved the method suggested by Saati et al. (Saati et al. in Fuzzy Optimization Decision making. 1:255–267, 2002) and transformed our proposed possibilistic model into a crisp nonlinear DEA model. The type of congestion (weak and strong) and its magnitude are also determined. Finally, the proposed model is used in an empirical example to identify 15 congested hospitals in Tehran (the capital of Iran) and measure the role of congestion and its magnitude to improve their performance. The result showed that congestion occurred in 39.9% of 15 hospitals.

Keywords Medical industry · Congestion · Fuzzy data envelopment analysis · Possibilistic model · Crisp non-linear DEA model

1 Introduction and Motivation

Calculating the efficiency and assessing the performance of a Decision-Making Unit (DMU) is so noticeable topic for managers in the real world. One of the appropriate methods to measure the relative efficiency of peer DMUs is Data Envelopment Analysis (DEA). DEA is a non-parametric method based on Linear Programming (LP) to

S. Saati (✉) · M. Shadab · S. Mohamadniaahmadi
Departement of Mathematics, North Tehran Branch, Islamic Azad University, Tehran, Iran
e-mail: s_saatim@iau-tnb.ac.ir

T. Allahviranloo et al. (eds.), *Decision Making in Healthcare Systems*,
Studies in Systems, Decision and Control 513,
https://doi.org/10.1007/978-3-031-46735-6_15

determine efficient and inefficient DMUs and compare their efficiencies. DEA model was first proposed by Charnes et al. [1] and named CCR model relying on Constant Returns to Scale (CRS). Then, Banker et al. [2] proposed BCC model with Variable Returns to Scale (VRS) assumption.

Some studies have been conducted using DEA to assess DMUs and measure the efficiency score of systems; for example see; Banker et al [3], Amirteimoori et al. [4, 5], Mahmoodirad et al. [6]. The presence of congestion in inputs is one of the factors that decrement the efficiency of DMUs. Congestion is a phenomenon in the production processes where the increase in one or more inputs does not increase output. The elimination of congestion results in an improvement in the performance and efficiency of DMUs. In other words, congestion is a wasteful stage of the production process where outputs are reduced due to excessive amounts of inputs.

The study of congestion commenced with Fare and Svensson in 1980 [7]. Many studies have been carried out to detect congestion in the field of DEA. For instance: Fare and Grosskopf [8], Jahanshahloo et al. [9], Khodabakhshi [10], Noura et al. [11], and Wei and Yan [12]. The detecting congestion issue was seriously investigated by the efforts of Cooper et al. [13]. They have been at the forefront of DEA-based congestion: see, for instance, [14, 15]. Afterward, detecting congestion based on DEA models was followed by Tone and Sahoo [16]. They introduced a novel Production Possibility Set (PPS) with convexity and strong output disposability assumption and omitted input possibility postulate. Also, new concepts of "strong congestion" and "weak congestion" were suggested by them. For determining congested inefficient units, some previous studies encountered problems. According to their method, the congested inefficient unit is defined as its efficient projection. Sometimes multiple projections occur, and one of them is chosen arbitrarily, whereas choosing any of the efficient projections leads to changes in their congestion status. To tackle this issue, further studies have been done on this crucial issue. For instance, Sueyoshi and Sekitiani [17], Mehdiloozad et al. [18], Ebrahimzade Adimi et al. [19], Kerstens and Van de Woestyne [20] and Shadab et al. [21]. One of the techniques for decision making is Data Envelopment Analysis (DEA), and many researchers have conducted research on this topic. Several recent papers have been cited to mention their research area.

Shadab et al. [22] proposed a novel LP model to obtain congested DMU. In their method, the DMU under evaluation was removed from the production technology. Afterwards, the omitted DMU was compared with other DMUs of the production technology. If there exists a unit belongs to the production technology with less input and more output, we declare that this evaluated unit has congestion in inputs.

Noticeable that eliminating the congestion leads to improved performance and efficiency. Determining the amount and type of congestion in a system is economically valuable because the change in inputs directly affects the output of the system.

One of the fields that is receiving a lot of attention is the health field, and evaluating the efficiency and performance of hospitals plays an important role in this regard.

There have been many studies on the efficiency of hospitals because competition between hospitals has an important effect on their productivity.

Optimizing resources and their proper allocation can be associated with reducing congestion in hospitals. Hospital congestion is a pervasive problem that causes care delays, frustration for patients and stressed staffs. This could reduce the quality of care and ruin a hospital's reputation. Also, due to the increasing the number of patients, congestion in hospitals has become an important concern in the modern era.

Bloom et al. [23], did a study on the impact of competition on the management quality and performance of English public hospitals in the UK. Cooper et al. [24] achieved that the efficiency and performance of the public hospitals improved compared to private hospitals in UK. Park and Kim [25] in year 2015, investigated the congestion in the field of nursing in different hospitals and found that there is congestion in this area in 54% of all 159 hospitals.

Simõs and Marques [26] investigated the presence of congestion in Portugal hospitals and showed that there was congestion in more than half of the hospitals.

Park et al. [27], used the model suggested by Cooper et al. [28] and investigated the impact of hospital specialization on congestion and efficiency of hospitals in Korea. They found that there is 72% of hospital faced with congestion and hospital specialization had a negative effect on congestion.

Besancenot et al. [29] asessed the congestion in hospital of developing countries. They stated that congestion is the result of the interaction between doctors who refers patients to the hospitals and hospitals that mus diagnose the severity of the disease of the referring patients. They presented the two equilibria of the game theory to assess the interaction among physicians in their referral role, patienta and hospitals.

Hou et al. [30] assessed less disruptive interventions based on hospital simulation model and suggested objective reasoning to support hospital management decisions. They showed that reducing the extra hospital beds compared to discharging patients is a suitable solution to decrease congestion.

In the mentioned studies, the data were considered accurate, but we know that in the real word, we encounter imprecise data. Also, in conventional DEA models, the information of all inputs and outputs data is crisp and precise. It means the measurement of inputs and outputs are sometimes imprecise or vague. Imprecise or vague evaluations maybe are the result of unquantifiable and incomplete information. Nowadays, various fuzzy DEA methods have been presented to deal with this impreciseness and ambiguity in DEA. Fuzzy sets were suggested by Zadeh [31] has been applied to determine DMUs' efficiency in presence of imprecise data. Then, studies in this area were developed and raised; for instance, see; Zhou and Xu [32], Ahmadvand and Pishvaee [33], Saati et al. [34], Esfandiari and Saati [35], Saati et al. [36], Amirteimoori et al. [37], Rahimi et al. [38], Allahviranloo and Ezadi [39]. In general, fuzzy DEA methods can be classified into four categories.

(i) the tolerance approach (ii) α-cut based approach (iii) fuzzy ranking approach (iv) possibility approach.

The best of our knowledge, there is no research to identify congested DMUs and its amount with fuzzy data via solving solely one model. For the first time, in this study, we developed the model proposed by Shadab et al. [22] for fuzzy data and then by utilizing the method suggested by Saati et al. [36], we detect the amount and type of congestion via solving one non-linear Fuzzy DEA (NLFD) model. Eventually, we applied our proposed model for determining congested hospitals in Tehran the Capital of Iran. We found out the congested hospitals with fuzzy data for the first time.

The novel contributions of the research are listed as under:

- To identify congested units with fuzzy data with solving one (NLFD) model
- To determine the amount of congestion in fuzzy inputs of DMUs for improving performance of them
- To investigate congestion in Iranian hospitals with fuzzy data through applying one model

The rest of this paper is organized as follows:

Some essential preliminaries and basic definitions are included in Sect. 2. In Sect. 3, a novel NLP model is proposed to identify the congestion and its amount with fuzzy triangular number. In Sect. 4, the proposed models are utilized in a real the case study are provided. Eventually, some conclusions are provided in Sect. 5.

2 Preliminaries

2.1 DEA Models

Consider a set of peers observed DMUs, (DMUj, $j = 1, \ldots, n$) such that each DMUj produces multiple non-negative outputs y_{rj} $(r = 1, \ldots, s)$ utilizing multiple non-negative inputs x_{ij} $(i = 1, \ldots, m)$. It is supposed that $x_j = (x_{1j}, \ldots, x_{mj})^T \neq 0_m$ and $y_j = (y_{1j}, \ldots, y_{sj})^T \neq 0_s$ for each j. Moreover, assume that $D_j = (x_j, y_j)^T$ expresses input and output vectors of each DMUj, $j \in J = \{1, \ldots, n\}$.

The PPS is defined as the set of all possible input–output vectors as follow:

PPS = {(x, y): x can produce by **y**}.

After presenting the CCR model [1], Banker et al. [2] proposed the new PPS under VRS assumption as below:

$$T_v = \left\{(x, y)\,\middle|\,x\lambda \leq x, y\lambda \geq y, 1^T\lambda = 1, \lambda \geq 0\right\}$$

T_v satisfies the postulates of inclusion of observations, convexity, input possibility postulate, output possibility postulate and minimum extrapolation.

Depending on the input possibility postulate, the next relationship is maintained:

$$(x, y) \in T_v, \overline{x} \geq x \Leftrightarrow (\overline{x}, y) \in T_v$$

Due to a lack of input disposability postulates, Tone and Sahoo [16] presented a novel production technology with VRS assumption as follows and called it T_{convex}.

$$T_{convex} = \{(x, y) | x = \lambda x, y\lambda \leq y, 1^T\lambda = 1, \lambda \geq 0\}$$

T_{convex} is a bounded convex set, which is satisfies the postulates of inclusion observations, convexity, output possibility postulate and minimum extrapolation.

Definition 1 (Efficiency) Consider the output-oriented Model (1) to evaluate efficiency of $DMU_o = (x_o, y_o)$ under a set of T_{convex} and ε as a non-Archimedean number. DMU_o is called efficient if and only if $\beta^* = 1$ and $s^{+*} = 0_s$ in model (1). Otherwise, DMU_o is called inefficient.

$$\begin{aligned}
& Max\ \beta + \varepsilon\left(\sum_{r=1}^{s} s_r^+\right) \\
& s.t \quad \sum_{j=1}^{n} \lambda_j x_{ij} = x_{io} && \forall i \\
& \sum_{j=1}^{n} \lambda_j y_{ir} - s_r^+ = \beta\, y_{ro} && \forall r \\
& \sum_{j=1}^{n} \lambda_j = 1 \\
& \lambda_j, s_r^+ \geq 0 && \forall j, r \\
& \beta : URS
\end{aligned} \tag{1}$$

2.2 Congestion

Generally, a DMU is confronted with congestion if an increase in one or some input decreases one or some output with no worsening the rest of inputs or outputs.

Many methods have been used to investigate congestion by presenting the conventional DEA models. One of these studies was done by Tone and Sahoo [16]. They proposed an algorithm to detect congested DMUs and proposed the concept of "strong congestion" and "weak congestion" as follows:

Definition 2 (Strong congestion) $DMU_o = (x_o, y_o)$ has strong congestion if it is efficient with respect to T_{convex} and there exists an activity $(\overline{x}, \overline{y}) \in T_{convex}$ such that $\overline{x} = \alpha\, x_o (0 < \alpha < 1)$ and $\overline{y} \geq \beta\, y_o (\beta > 1)$. In other words, strong congestion occurs in DMU_o if proportional decrement in all inputs of DMU_o results an increment in all outputs.

Definition 3 (Weak congestion) $DMU_o = (x_o, y_o)$ has weak congestion if there exists an activity $(\overline{x}, \overline{y}) \in T_{convex}$ that consumes fewer resources in one or more inputs to obtain more products in one or more outputs, it means; $\overline{x} \leq x_o, \overline{y} \geq y_o$ and $\overline{y} \neq y_o$.

Shadab et al. [22] proposed a new one LP DEA model to determine the role and amount of congested DMUs. According their method, evaluated DMU is omitted from the T_{convex} and the removed unit is depicted onto the new efficiency frontier. Then, the unit is compared with the rest of units belong to T_{convex}. If there is a DMU with less or equal input consumption produces more output, the evaluated unit has congestion.

They proposed the following definition to find the status of input congestion for DMUs:

Definition 4 (Congestion in the DEA) Let $\text{DMU}_o = (\text{x}_\text{o}, \text{y}_\text{o})$ belongs to T_{convex}. The next two statements defined the weak and strong congestion, respectively.

(i) $\text{DMU}_o = (\text{x}_\text{o}, \text{y}_\text{o})$ evidences weak congestion if there exists some $(\hat{x},\ \hat{y}) \in T_{convex\backslash o}$ such that $\hat{x} \leq \text{x}_\text{o}$ and $\hat{y} \geq \text{y}_\text{o}, \hat{y} \neq \text{y}_\text{o}$.
(ii) $\text{DMU}_o = (\text{x}_\text{o}, \text{y}_\text{o})$ evidences strong congestion if there exists some $(\hat{x},\ \hat{y}) \in T_{convex\backslash o}$ such that $\hat{x} < \text{x}_\text{o}$ and $\hat{y} > \text{y}_\text{o}$.

By the following definition, the applied method to determine congested units was introduced.

Definition 5 Let $\text{DMU}_o = (\text{x}_\text{o}, \text{y}_\text{o})$ be an extreme efficient unit of T_{convex}. It is facing strong (weak) congestion if and only if in Model (2) $\phi^* > 1$ and $s_i^{-*} > 0$ ($s_i^{-*} \geq 0$ and $s_i^{-*} \neq 0$) for $i \in \{1, ..., m\}$ in any alternative optimal solution of Model (2).

$$
\begin{aligned}
&Max\ \varphi + \varepsilon \sum_{i=1}^{m} s_i^- \\
&s.t \qquad \sum_{\substack{j=1 \\ j\neq o}}^{n} \lambda_j x_{ij} = x_{io} - s_i^- \qquad \forall i \\
&\qquad\quad \sum_{\substack{j=1 \\ j\neq o}}^{n} \lambda_j y_{rj} \geq \varphi y_{ro} \qquad \forall r \\
&\qquad\quad \sum_{\substack{j=1 \\ j\neq o}}^{n} \lambda_j = 1 \\
&\qquad\quad \lambda_j, s_i^- \geq 0 \qquad \forall i, j, j \neq o
\end{aligned}
\tag{2}
$$

Also, Shadab et al. [22] proved that definition (2.4) and (2.5) are equivalent.

2.3 Fuzzy Numbers

Fuzzy sets were introduced by Zadeh [31] to represent imprecise and inaccurate data associated with human cognition processes with fuzzy numbers. Also, Sengupta [40] proposed a fuzzy mathematical program approach and used fuzziness in the DEA model.

Now, we review some of the basic definitions of fuzzy sets Dubois and Prade [41], Kauffman and Gupta [42], Zimmermann [43].

Definition 6 (Fuzzy sets) Suppose X is an un-empty set. The fuzzy set $\tilde{A}$ in X is specified by its membership function:

$$\mu_{\tilde{A}} : X \to [0, 1]$$

where $\mu_{\tilde{A}}(x)$ is named the degree of membership of element x belongs to fuzzy set $\tilde{A}$ for each $x \in X$. Obviously, $\tilde{A}$ is a set of ordered pairs which can be written as bellow:

$$\tilde{A} = \left\{(x, \mu_{\tilde{A}}(x)) | x \in X\right\}$$

Definition 7 (α-cut) An α-cut set a fuzzy set $\tilde{A}$ is a crisp set demonstrated by A_α and is defined as follow:

$$A_\alpha = \left\{x \in X \middle| \mu_{\tilde{A}}(x) \geq \alpha\right\}$$

Each member of the A_α set has a membership degree greater than or equal to value α.

One of the most popular and widely used fuzzy DEA methods is α-cut approach.

Definition 8 (Fuzzy number) A fuzzy set $\tilde{A}$ of real set $\mathbb{R}$ is called a fuzzy number if following conditions be hold:

(i) $\mu_{\tilde{A}}(x)$ is piece wise continues.
(ii) There exists exactly one $x \in R$ with $\mu_{\tilde{A}}(x) = 1$.
(iii) The fuzzy set $\tilde{A}$ must be normal and convex.

Definition 9 (Triangular number) A fuzzy number $\tilde{A} = (a^l, a^m, a^u)$ is named a triangular fuzzy number whose membership function $\mu_{\tilde{A}}$ satisfies the following properties; see Fig. 1.

(i) $\mu_{\tilde{A}}(x)$ is a continues mapping from $\mathbb{R}$ to the closed interval [0,1].
(ii) $\mu_{\tilde{A}}(x) = 0$ for all $x \in (-\infty, a]$.
(iii) $\mu_{\tilde{A}}(x)$ is strictly increasing on $a \leq x \leq b$.
(iv) $\mu_{\tilde{A}}(x) = 1$ for $x = b$.
(v) $\mu_{\tilde{A}}(x)$ is strictly decreasing on $b \leq x \leq c$.
(vi) $\mu_{\tilde{A}}(x) = 0$ for all $x \in [c, \infty)$.

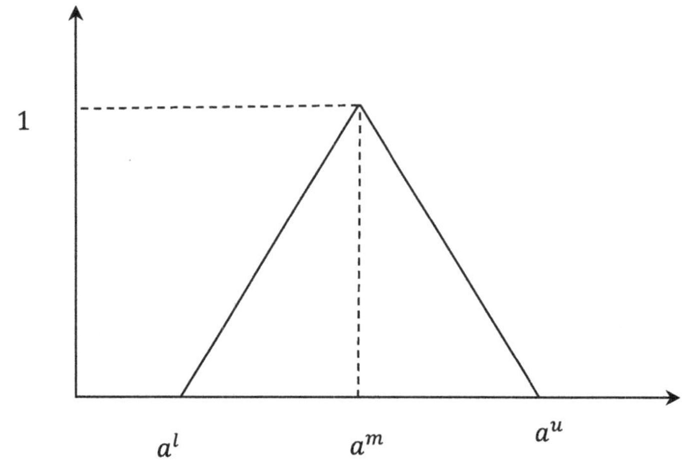

Fig. 1 Membership of a triangular fuzzy number

The membership function $\mu_{\tilde{A}}(x)$ of $\tilde{A}$ is given as bellows:

$$\mu_{\tilde{A}}(x) = \begin{cases} 0 & x < a^l \\ \dfrac{x - a^l}{a^m - a^l} & a^l \le x \le a^m \\ \dfrac{a^u - x}{a^u - a^m} & a^m \le x \le a^u \\ 0 & x > a^u \end{cases}$$

3 Proposed Method

Suppose that there are n DMUs, $\text{DMU}_j = (\tilde{x}_j, \tilde{y}_j);\ j \in \{1, ..., n\}$ with imprecise data can be represented by $\tilde{x}_j = (x_j^m, x_j^l, x_j^u)$ and $\tilde{y}_j = (y_j^m, y_j^l, y_j^u)$. To find out congested units with fuzzy data, Model (2) can be written as follow:

$$
\begin{aligned}
& Max\, \varphi + \varepsilon \sum_{i=1}^{m} s_i^- \\
& s.t \quad \sum_{\substack{j=1 \\ j \neq o}}^{n} \lambda_j \tilde{x}_{ij} = \tilde{x}_{io} \qquad \forall i \\
& \sum_{\substack{j=1 \\ j \neq o}}^{n} \lambda_j \tilde{y}_{rj} = \varphi \tilde{y}_{ro} \quad \forall r \\
& \sum_{\substack{j=1 \\ j \neq o}}^{n} \lambda_j = 1 \\
& \lambda_j, s_i^- \geq 0 \qquad \forall j, j \neq o, i
\end{aligned}
\tag{3}
$$

Model (3) is a possibilistic linear programming which there is various methods to solve it. One of the popular methods is α-cut method which has been many studies in this area, for instance; Meada et al. [44], Wang et al. [45], Arya and Yadav [39], Saati et al. [36]. In this method, the intervals in both sides of the constraints are compared with each other. Therefore, above model can be modified as below:

$$
\begin{aligned}
& Max\, \varphi + \varepsilon \sum_{i=1}^{m} s_i^- \\
& s.t \quad \sum_{\substack{j=1 \\ j \neq o}}^{n} \lambda_j (\alpha x_{ij}^m + (1-\alpha) x_{ij}^l, \alpha x_{ij}^m + (1-\alpha) x_{ij}^u) = \\
& (\alpha x_{io}^m + (1-\alpha) x_{io}^l, \alpha x_{io}^m + (1-\alpha) x_{io}^u - s_i^- \qquad \forall i \\
& \sum_{\substack{j=1 \\ j \neq o}}^{n} \lambda_j (\alpha y_{rj}^m + (1-\alpha) y_{rj}^l, \alpha y_{rj}^m + (1-\alpha) y_{rj}^u) \geq \\
& \varphi (\alpha y_{ro}^m + (1-\alpha) y_{ro}^l, \alpha y_{ro}^m + (1-\alpha) y_{ro}^u) \qquad \forall r \\
& \sum_{\substack{j=1 \\ j \neq o}}^{n} \lambda_j = 1 \\
& \lambda_j, s_i^- \geq 0 \qquad \forall j, j \neq o, \; i
\end{aligned}
\tag{4}
$$

All coefficients of Model (4) are stated as intervals and therefore we are facing an interval model. To solve this type of problem, Saati et al. [36] proposed a new approach. They defined suitable variables in the intervals not only satisfies the set of constraints, but also maximizes the efficiency value. Based on this manner, the proper variables are considered as below:

$$\hat{x}_{ij} \in [\alpha x_{ij}^{m} + (1-\alpha)x_{ij}^{l}, \alpha x_{ij}^{m} + (1-\alpha)x_{ij}^{u}]$$
$$\hat{y}_{rj} \in [\alpha y_{rj}^{m} + (1-\alpha)y_{rj}^{l}, \alpha y_{rj}^{m} + (1-\alpha)y_{rj}^{u}]$$

By substituting the new variables, Model (4) can be written as follows:

$$\begin{aligned}
& Max\ \varphi + \varepsilon \sum_{i=1}^{m} s_i^- \\
& s.t \quad \sum_{\substack{j=1\\ j\neq o}}^{n} \lambda_j \hat{x}_{ij} = \hat{x}_{io} - s_i^- \qquad \forall i \\
& \sum_{\substack{j=1\\ j\neq o}}^{n} \lambda_j \hat{y}_{rj} \geq \varphi \hat{y}_{ro} \quad \forall r \\
& \sum_{\substack{j=1\\ j\neq o}}^{n} \lambda_j = 1 \\
& \alpha x_{ij}^{m} + (1-\alpha)x_{ij}^{l} \leq \hat{x}_{ij} \leq \alpha x_{ij}^{m} + (1-\alpha)x_{ij}^{u} \\
& \alpha y_{rj}^{m} + (1-\alpha)y_{rj}^{l} \leq \hat{y}_{rj} \leq \alpha y_{rj}^{m} + (1-\alpha)y_{rj}^{u} \\
& \lambda_j, s_i^- \geq 0 \quad \forall j, i
\end{aligned} \tag{5}$$

where $\alpha \in [0, 1]$. Model (5) is a non-linear model. We put $\begin{cases} \lambda_j \hat{x}_{ij} = \overline{x}_{ij} & \forall i \\ \lambda_j \hat{y}_{rj} = \overline{y}_{rj} & \forall r \end{cases}$ for $j \in J = \{1, ..., n\}, j \neq o$ and $\begin{cases} \hat{x}_{io} = \overline{x}_{io} & \forall i \\ \hat{y}_{ro} = \overline{y}_{ro} & \forall r \end{cases}$ for $j = o$. By these substitution, above model can be modified as bellow:

$$
\begin{aligned}
& Max\,\varphi + \varepsilon \sum_{i=1}^{m} s_i^- \\
& s.t \quad \sum_{\substack{j=1\\ j\neq o}}^{n} \overline{x}_{ij} = \overline{x}_{io} - s_i^- \qquad \forall i \\
& \qquad \sum_{\substack{j=1\\ j\neq o}}^{n} \overline{y}_{rj} \geq \varphi \overline{y}_{ro} \quad \forall r \\
& \qquad \sum_{\substack{j=1\\ j\neq o}}^{n} \lambda_j = 1
\end{aligned} \tag{6}
$$

$$\lambda_j(\alpha x_{ij}^m + (1-\alpha)x_{ij}^l) \leq \overline{x}_{ij} \leq \lambda_j(\alpha x_{ij}^m + (1-\alpha)x_{ij}^u) \qquad \forall i, j, j \neq o \tag{6a}$$

$$\lambda_j(\alpha y_{rj}^m + (1-\alpha)y_{rj}^l) \leq \overline{y}_{rj} \leq \lambda_j(\alpha y_{rj}^m + (1-\alpha)y_{rj}^u) \qquad \forall r, j, j \neq o \tag{6b}$$

$$\alpha x_{io}^m + (1-\alpha)x_{io}^l \leq \overline{x}_{io} \leq \alpha x_{io}^m + (1-\alpha)x_{io}^u \qquad \forall i \tag{6c}$$

$$
\begin{aligned}
& \alpha y_{ro}^m + (1-\alpha)y_{ro}^l \leq \overline{y}_{ro} \leq \alpha y_{ro}^m + (1-\alpha)y_{ro}^u \qquad \forall r \\
& \lambda_j, s_i^- \geq 0 \qquad \forall j, i
\end{aligned} \tag{6d}
$$

where $\alpha \in [0, 1]$. Above model is a linear programming model which congestion and its amount can be achieved with triangular fuzzy number.

Definition 10 Let $\text{DMU}_o = (\tilde{x}_o, \tilde{y}_o)$ belongs to T_{convex}. The latter two statements define the congested weakly and strongly DMU_o, respectively.

1. $\text{DMU}_o = (\tilde{x}_o, \tilde{y}_o)$ faces weak congestion if there exists some $(\tilde{x}', \tilde{y}') \in T_{convex\backslash o}$ such that $\tilde{x}' \leq \tilde{x}_o$ and $\tilde{y}' \geq \tilde{y}_o$, $\tilde{y}_o \neq \tilde{y}'$.
2. $\text{DMU}_o = (\tilde{x}_o, \tilde{y}_o)$ faces strong congestion if there exists some $(\tilde{x}', \tilde{y}') \in T_{convex\backslash o}$ such that $\tilde{x}' < \tilde{x}_o$ and $\tilde{y}' > \tilde{y}_o$.

Based on above definition, the applied method is introduced as below:

Definition 11 Let $\text{DMU}_o = (\tilde{x}_o, \tilde{y}_o) \in T_{convex}$. DMU_o has strong (weak) congestion in inputs if the optimal objective function solution of Model (6) is greater than one, i.e., $\varphi^* > 1$ and $s_i^{-*} > 0\,(s_i^{-*} \geq 0)$ for $i \in \{1, ..., m\}$ in any alternative solution of Model (6) and for $0 \leq \alpha \leq 1$.

Theorem 1 Let $\text{DMU}_o = (\tilde{x}_o, \tilde{y}_o) \in T_{convex}$. DMU_o has strong (weak) congestion in inputs based on Definition 3–1 if and only if the optimal objective function solution of Model (6) is greater than one and $s_i^{-*} > 0\,(s_i^{-*} \geq 0)$ for $i \in \{1, ..., m\}$ in any alternative solution of Model (6) for $0 \leq \alpha \leq 1$. i.e., definitions 3–1 and 3–2 are equivalent to each other.

Proof Let $\text{DMU}_o = (\tilde{x}_o, \tilde{y}_o) \in T_{convex}$ and $(\varphi^*, \lambda^*, s^{-*}, \overline{x}^*, \overline{y}^*)$ be the optimal solution of model (6). Also, assume that $\varphi^* > 1$ and $s_i^{-*} > 0$ for $i \in \{1, ..., m\}$ in Model (6). Therefore, we have:

$$x' = \sum_{\substack{j=1 \\ j \neq o}}^{n} \overline{x}_{ij}^* = \overline{x}_{io}^* - s_i^{-*} < \overline{x}_o^* \tag{7}$$

$$y' = \sum_{\substack{j=1 \\ j \neq o}}^{n} \overline{y}_{rj}^* \geq \varphi^* \overline{y}_{ro}^* > \overline{y}_o^* \tag{8}$$

Therefore, there exists an activity such as $(\tilde{x}', \tilde{y}') \in T_{convex\backslash o}$ that $\begin{cases} x' < \overline{x}^* \\ x' > \overline{y}^* \end{cases}$. Since $(\tilde{x}', \tilde{y}') \in T_{convex}$ then (x', y') satisfies in constraints (6a) to (6d). So, according to the Definition 3–1, DMUo faces strong congestion in inputs.

Conversely, let $\text{DMU}_o = (\tilde{x}_o, \tilde{y}_o) \in T_{convex}$ has strong congestion in inputs based on Definition 3–1. Let $(\lambda^*, \varphi^*, \overline{x}^*, \overline{y}^*)$ is an optimal solution of model (6). According to Definition 3–1, there exist an activity such as $(\tilde{x}', \tilde{y}') \in T_{convex\backslash o}$ that $\tilde{x}' < \tilde{x}_o$ and $\tilde{y}' > \tilde{y}_o$. Also, $(\tilde{x}', \tilde{y}') \in T_{convex}$,therefore we have:

$$\sum_{\substack{j=1 \\ j \neq o}}^{n} y'_{rj} \geq y'_{ro} > y'_o > y_o$$

$$\sum_{\substack{j=1 \\ j \neq o}}^{n} x'_{ij} < x'_o < x_o$$

Therefore,

$$\sum_{\substack{j=1 \\ j \neq o}}^{n} x'_{ij} < x'_o \rightarrow \sum_{\substack{j=1 \\ j \neq o}}^{n} x'_{ij} - s_i^- = x'_o \rightarrow s_i^- > 0$$

Moreover, $\hat{\varphi} = \min\left\{ \dfrac{\sum_{\substack{j=1 \\ j \neq o}}^{n} \overline{y}_{rj}}{\overline{y}_o} \right\} \rightarrow \hat{\varphi} > 1 \rightarrow 1 < \hat{\varphi} < \varphi^*$.

4 Case Study

One of the most important service systems of any country is the health system (Hospitals). Therefore, their performance has of special importance because they prevent and improve the level of health in society. In the real world, sometimes improper allocation of resources (inputs) leads to the phenomenon of congestion in inputs and an increase in outputs. Therefore, we intend to investigate the presence of congestion in 15 private hospitals in Tehran, and by identifying the causes of congestion and eliminating them, we can contribute a lot to improving the performance and efficiency of hospitals and medical staff. Since in the real world, health data is sometimes imprecise due to security issues, all data including inputs and outputs are considered fuzzy.

In this paper, we have considered three inputs and outputs, and all of the data is fuzzy, also each of the input and output criteria has three sub-criteria which are stated below.

Inputs: number of doctors such as sub-specialty, specialist, and general practitioner, number of nurses such as special ward nurse, ward nurse, and operating room nurse, number of beds such as ICU room bed, emergency room bed, and ward bed. Outputs: Number of inpatients such as ICU inpatient, outpatient, surgery inpatient, number of outpatients such as injections, outpatient surgery, laboratory service, hospital revenue such as visits, surgical operation, and medical imaging. Table 1 shows the geometric mean of fuzzy inputs and outputs.

Using the data in Table 1 and solving model (6), we evaluate the presence of congestion in the desired units. Table 2 shows the results of solving model (6).

As mentioned before, in our method, under evaluation DMU should be removed from the production possibility set, and hence the new efficient frontier is created. Then, we depicted the removed unit on the new frontier and compare it with the rest of units on the efficiency frontier. Some units cannot be depicted on the frontier and the proposed model (6) becomes infeasible which indicates that these DMUs are not congested.

As can be seen in Table 2, DMU_1, DMU_2, DMU_3, and DMU_4 are efficient because $\varphi^* = 1,\ \ s_1^{-*}, s_2^{-*}, s_3^{-*} = 0$. According to definitions (2–3), units have weak congestion that $\varphi^* > 1$, and at least one of the scale variables is greater than zero. According to the result of Table 2, DMU_5 and DMU_7, $\forall\alpha \in [0, 1]$ are weak congestion also according to definitions (2–2) only DMU_{10}, $\forall\alpha \in [0, 1]$ is strong congestion, because $\varphi^* > 1,\ \ s_1^{-*}, s_2^{-*}, s_3^{-*} > 0$. However, Units are inefficient, if the value φ^* is less than one, so DMU_6 and DMU_{15} $\forall\alpha \in [0, 1]$, according to congestion definition (2–5) do not face congestion. On the other hand, DMU_{10} shows that there exists an observed activity belonging to PPS with more output and less input compare with DMU_{10}. It means that there exists an activity that belongs to this technology that produces more outputs, it is enough to reduce the value each of slack variable from its inputs and increase the output by giving effect φ^*, $\forall\alpha \in [0, 1]$ to each of them. Moreover, DMU_5 and DMU_7 face weak congestion $\forall\alpha \in [0, 1]$. Therefore,

Table 1 Data of 15 private hospitals

	I_1	I_2	I_3	O_1	O_2	O_3
DMU1	(55.6,67.6,84)	(103.4,115,131)	(37,49.5,66)	(10,684,10,699,10,714)	(13,273,13,287,13,301)	(12.6,15.3,18)
DMU2	(14,27.5,41)	(21.4,34.6,47)	(8,10.5,13)	(4741,4756.4,4771)	(61,178,61,192.7,61,206)	(9,18.2,27)
DMU3	(72,85.5,99)	(111.7,125.8,140)	(20.6,35.8,51)	(1955,1979.8,2003)	(12,695,12,711.4,12,727)	(5.6,14.3,23)
DMU4	(95.7,109.8,124)	(95.7,109.8,124)	(38.6,48.8,59)	(13,145,13,159,13,173)	(10,694,10,711.6,10,729)	(8.7,13.3,18)
DMU5	(95,104.7,113)	(95,104.7,113)	(41,53.5,66)	(10,906,10,922,10,938)	(12,686,12,701.5,12,717)	(6,11.5,17)
DMU6	(232,246.8,260)	(215,228.5,242)	(57.6,70.3,83)	(62,682,63,700,64,718)	(63,573,63,592.2,63,612)	(42,53.5,65)
DMU7	(7,12.5,18)	(6,9.5,13)	(3,5.4,7)	(865,883,901)	(24,258,24,274,24,290)	(2,3.8,7)
DMU8	(185,202.8,221)	(174,192.7,210)	(38,55.6,72)	(4126,4149.5,4163)	(53,374,533,938,53,412)	(27.6,38,49)
DMU9	(57,72.5,88)	(99,114.2,129)	(32,41.2,48)	(1057,1075.6,1093)	(13,686,13,700,13,714)	(7,12.7,19)
DMU10	(58,76.8,94)	(95,112.9,129)	(19,38.5,68)	(1048,1083.5,1118)	(13,582,13,601,13,620)	(7,12.7,19)
DMU11	(58,72.3,90)	(108,125.6,142)	(29,59.8,73)	(1059,1076.8,1093)	(1332,1344.5,13,620)	(6,12.5,19)
DMU12	(205,217.6,230)	(196,205.5,215)	(50,64.5,79)	(1211,1238.2,1265)	(7368,7401.5,7435)	(177,189,201)
DMU13	(249,268.5,288)	(173,190.6,207)	(29,40.5,52)	(2960,2986.7,3012)	(3254,3263.5,3273)	(122,139.4,156)
DMU14	(276,290.5,305)	(191,200.9,210)	(51,57.5,63)	(2163,2173.5,2187)	(3535,3549.5,3564)	(122,153.5,185)
DMU15	(379,407.6,432)	(94,106.7,134)	(69,82.5,96)	(1945,1977.3,2001)	(4325,4361.2,4379)	(102,123.5,165)

Table 2 Results

	$\alpha = 0$				$\alpha = 0.25$				$\alpha = 0.5$				$\alpha = 0.75$				$\alpha = 1$			
	φ^*	s_1^{-*}	s_2^{-*}	s_3^{-*}	φ^*	s_1^{-*}	s_2^{-*}	s_3^{-*}	φ^*	s_1^{-*}	s_2^{-*}	s_3^{-*}	φ^*	s_1^{-*}	s_2^{-*}	s_3^{-*}	φ^*	s_1^{-*}	s_2^{-*}	s_3^{-*}
DMU1	1.00	0	0	0	1.00	0	0	0	1.00	0	0	0	1.00	0	0	0	1.00	0	0	0
DMU2	1.00	0	0	0	1.00	0	0	0	1.00	0	0	0	1.00	0	0	0	1.00	0	0	0
DMU3	1.00	0	0	0	1.00	0	0	0	1.00	0	0	0	1.00	0	0	0	1.00	0	0	0
SMU4	1.00	0	0	0	1.00	0	0	0	1.00	0	0	0	1.00	0	0	0	1.00	0	0	0
DMU5	3.1	0	0	1.65	3.75	8.1	0	0	2.78	2.34	0	0	1.69	3.76	0	0	2.56	1.34	0	0
DMU6	0.43	0	0	0	0.89	0	0	0	0.76	0	0	3.21	0.87	2.21	1.4	0	0.76	3.7	1.5	0
DMU7	3.21	4.75	0	2.34	1.78	2.76	0	0	3.67	0	5.87	0	0.47	1.25	0	0	0.74	0	0	4.31
DMU8	4.036	1.02	0	0	1.00	0	0	0	0.97	0	0	0	2.06	1.21	0	0	0.23	0	0	0
DMU9	3.11	2.25	0	0	1.00	0	0	0	3.43	2.21	3.65	0	2.06	1.21	0	0	1.76	2.9	0	0
DMU10	2.88	0.98	0.54	2.98	3.25	2.13	1.67	3.54	1.08	0.87	0.23	2.98	1.98	1.21	5.82	3.65	4.95	0.24	0.78	0.65
DMU11	0.654	0	0	0	4.36	1.02	0	0	0.32	0	0	0	3.21	2.6	3.8	0	1.43	0	0	0
DMU12	1.00	4.3	3.25	0	0.75	0	0	0	1.87	0	0	0	0.87	0	0	0	1.43	0	0	0
DMU13	3.76	4.9	2.8	0	2.76	2.9	0.74	0	0.99	0	0	0	1.00	1.21	0	0	0.63	1.21	0	0
DMU14	0.99	0	0	0	1.56	0	0	0	4.43	8.6	00	0	3.66	0	0	0	0.51	0	0	0
DMU15	0.99	0	0	0	0.25	0.87	0	0	0.65	0	2	0	0.99	1.32	0	0	0.97	3.84	0	0

for DMU_5, if $\alpha = 0$, $\varphi^* = 3.1$ and $s_3^{-*} = 1.65$ it is enough reducing the value by 1.65 of its input to increase its output.

Therefore, DMU_5, DMU_7, and DMU_{10} can improve their efficiency and performance by reducing their demands and orders to its supplier stage by the amount of their slack variables (s_1^{-*},s_2^{-*} and s_3^{-*}). Briefly, out of 15 hospitals, only four of them and 2 of them are efficient and inefficient for each α respectively. In other words, 26.6% of units are efficient and 13.33% of units are inefficient. Therefore, only 39.9% of the efficient units should reduce their demand to the previous stage to reach higher efficiency and the rest of the efficient ones do not face congestion and do not need to change. The rest of the units, create a different nature for each α, so it is infeasible using the proposed model 6, which states that these units are not congested.

5 Conclusion

Health is one of the most effective factors in maintaining and promoting the health of society. The health sector is one of the indicators of development in social welfare. Considering the importance of investing in the development of the health system and its impact on increasing the productivity of labour and production, the allocation of resources in this area is one of the main operational units of this sector. The numbers of hospitals, their performance and the provision of their services have a great impact on the development of the community health. Sometimes, improper allocation of resources (inputs) leads to congestion in inputs and increment in outputs. Due to the importance of this issue, we presented a novel Fuzzy NLP DEA model and since in the real world the data is imprecise, our model was considered with fuzzy data. By providing the model, we obtain the type and amount of congested inputs. This leads to the improvement of the performance of the DMUs. In Iran, there has been a very well growth in health development in recent years. In this study, we have considered 15 well known hospitals in Tehran to evaluate in terms of resource allocation and presence of congestion. The main results of this study are as follows: congestion analysis showed that congestion occurred in 39.9% of hospitals (3 hospitals of 15 hospitals). Therefore, only 39.9% of the efficient units should reduce their demand to the previous stage to reach higher efficiency and the rest of the efficient ones do not face congestion and do not need to change.

References

1. Charnes, A., Cooper, W.W., Rhodes, E.: Measuring the efficiency of decision-making units. Eur. J. Oper. Res. **2**, 429–444 (1978)
2. Banker, R.D., Charnes, A., Cooper, W.W: Some models for estimating technical and scale inefficiencies in data envelopment analysis. Manag. Sci. **30**(9), 1078–1092 (1984)

3. Banker, R.D., Amirteimoori, A., Allahviranloo, T., Sinha, R.P.: Performance analysis and managerial ability in the general insurance market: a study of India and Iran. Inf. Technol. Manage. (2023). https://doi.org/10.1007/s10799-023-00405-y
4. Amirteimoori, A., Allahviranloo, T., Kordrostami, S., Bagheri, S.F.: Improving decision-making units in performance analysis methods: a data envelopment analysis approach. Math. Sci. (2023). https://doi.org/10.1007/s40096-023-00512-5
5. Amirteimoori, A., Allahviranloo, T., Zadmirzaei, M.: Scale elasticity and technical efficiency analysis in the European forest sector: a stochastic value-based approach. Eur. J. Forest Res. (2023). https://doi.org/10.1007/s10342-023-01589-2
6. Mahmoodirad, A., Allahviranloo, T., Niroomand, S.: A new effective solution method for fully intuitionistic fuzzy transportation problem. Soft Comp. **23**(12), 4521–4530 (2019)
7. Fare, R., Svensson, L.: Congestion of production factors. Econ. J. Econ. Soc. **48**, 1745–1753 (1984)
8. Fare, R., Grosskopf, S.: Measuring congestion in production. Zeitsc hrift fur National Okonomie **43**, 257–271 (1983)
9. Jahanshahloo, G.R., Khodabakhshi, M.: Suitable combination of inputs for improving outputs in DEA with determining input congestion considering textile industry of China. Appl. Math. Comp. **151**, 263–273 (2004)
10. Khodabakhshi, M.: Chance constrained additive input relaxation model in stochastic data envelopment analysis. J. Inform Syst. Sci. **6**(1), 99–112 (2010)
11. Noura, A.A., Hosseinzadeh Lotfi, F., Jahanshahloo, G.R., Fanati Rashidi, S., Parker, B.R: A new method for measuring congestion in data envelopment analysis. Socio-Econ. Plan. Sci. **44**, 240–246 (2010)
12. Wei, Q.L., Yan, H.: Congestion and returns to scale in data envelopment analysis. Eur. J. Oper. Res. **153**, 641–660 (2004)
13. Cooper, W.W., Thompson, R.G., Thrall, R.: Introduction extensions and new developments in DEA. Ann. Operat. Res. **66**, 3–45 (1996)
14. Cooper, W.W., Seiford, L.M., Zhu, J.: A unified additive model approach for evaluating inefficiency and congestion with associated measures in DEA. Socioecon. Plann. Sci. **4**, 1–25 (2000)
15. Cooper, W.W., Deng, H., Huang, Z.M., Li, S.L: A one model approach to congestion in DEA. Socio-Econ. Plan. Sci. **36**, 231–238 (2002)
16. Tone, K., Sahoo, B.K: Degree of scale economics and economics and congestion: a unified DEA approach. Eur. J. Operat. Res. **153**, 641–660 (2004)
17. Sueyoshi, T., Sekitiani, K.: DEA congestion and returns to scale under an occurrence of multiple optimal projections. Eur. J. Oper. Res. **194**, 592–607 (2009)
18. Mehdiloozad, M., Zhu, J., Sahoo, B.K: Identification of congestion in data envelopment analysis under the occurrence of multiple projections: A reliable method capable of dealing with negative data. Eur. J. Operat. Res. **265**, 644–654 (2018)
19. Ebrahimzade Adimi, M., Rostamy-Malkhalifeh, M., Hosseinzadeh Lotfi, F., Mehrjoo, R.: A new linear to find the congestion hyperplane in DEA. J. Math. Sci. **13**, 43–52 (2019)
20. Kerstens, K., Van de Woestyne, I.: The remarkable incidence of congestion in production: a review, empirical illustration, and research agenda. Data Envelop. Anal. J. **4**(2), 109–147 (2019)
21. Shadab, M., Saati, S., Farzipoor Saen, R., Mostafaee, A.: Measuring congestion by anchor points in DEA. J. Sadhana **45**(1), 37–47 (2020)
22. Shadab, M., Saati, S., Farzipoor Saen, R., Mostafaee, A.: Detecting congestion in DEA by solving one model. Operat. Res. Decis. 77–97 (2021)
23. Bloom, N., Propper, C., Seiler, S., Reenen, J.V.: The impact of competition on management quality: evidence from public hospitals. Natl. Bureau Econ. Res. **82**, 37–77 (2010)
24. Cooper, Z., Gibbons, S., Skellern, M.: Does competition from private surgical centres improve public hospitals' performance? Evidence from the english national health service. J. Public Econ. **166**, 63–80 (2018)

25. Park, S.H., Kim, D.C.: Congestion and efficiency analysis of public hospitals. Prod. Rev. **29**, 61–29 (2015)
26. Simões, P., Marques, R.C.: Performance and congestion analysis of the Portuguese hospital services centre. Eur. J. Operat. Res. **19**, 39–63 (2009)
27. Park, S., Ko, J.H., Bae, E.S., Chang, M., Kim, D.: The impact of hospital specialization on congestion and efficiency. Sustain. J. **14**, 32–46 (2019)
28. Cooper, W.W., Deng, H., Huang, Z.M., Li, S.L.: A one model approach to congestion in DEA. Socio-Econ. Plan. Sci. **36**, 231–238 (2002)
29. Besancenot, D., Sirven, N., Vranceanu, R.: A model of hospital congestion in developing countries. ESSEC Work. Paper **1804**, 72–94 (2018)
30. Hou, W., Qin, S., Thompson, C.H.: A vertual evaluation of options for managing risk of hospital congestion with minimum intervention. Sci. Rep. **12**, 34–46 (2022)
31. Zadeh, L.A.: Fuzzy sets. Inf. Control. **8**, 338–353 (1965)
32. Zhou, W., Xu, Z.: An overview of the fuzzy data envelopment analysis research and its successful applications. Int. J. Fuzzy Syst. **22**, 1037–1055 (2020)
33. Ahmadvand, S., Pishvaee, M.S.: An efficient method for kindly allocation problem: a credibility- based fuzzy common weights data envelopment analysis aproach. Health Care Manage. **21**(4), 587–603 (2018)
34. Saati, S., Hatami Marbini, A., Tavana, M., Agrell, P.J.: A fuzzy data envelopment analysis for clustring operating units with imprecies data. Int. J. Uncert. Fuzz. Knowl. Based Syst. **21**, 29–54 (2014)
35. Esfandiari, M., Saati, S.: Data Envelopment Analysis with fuzzy complex numbers with an emprical case on power plans of Iran. Rairo-Oerat. Res. 2013–2025 (2021)
36. Saati, S., Memariani, A., Jahanshahloo, G.R.: Efficiency analysis and ranking of DMUs with fuzzy data. Fuzzy Optim. Decis. Mak. **1**, 255–267 (2002)
37. Amirteimoori, A., Allahviranloo, T., Zadmirzaei, M., Hasanzadeh, F.: On the environmental performance analysis: a combined fuzzy data envelopment analysis and artificial intelligence algorithms. Expert Syst. Appl. **224**, 119953 (2023). https://doi.org/10.1016/j.eswa.2023.119953
38. Rahmani, A., Lotfi, F.H., Rostamy-Malkhalifeh, M., Allahviranloo, T.: A new method for defuzzification and ranking of fuzzy numbers based on the statistical beta distribution. Adv. Fuzzy Syst. **2016**, 1–8 (2016)
39. Arya, A., Yadav, S.P.: Development of FDEA models to measure the performance efficiencies of DMUs. Int. J. Fuzzy Syst. **20**, 163–173 (2018)
40. Sengupta, J.K.: A fuzzy systems approach in data envelopment analysis. Comput. Math. Appl. **24**(8–9), 259–266 (1992)
41. Dubois, D., Prade, H.: Possibility Theory: An Approach to Computerized Processing of Uncertainty. Plenum Press, New York (1988)
42. Kaufmann, A., Gupta, M.M.: Introduction to Fuzzy Arithmetic: Theory and Applications. Van Nostrand Reinhold, New York (1991)
43. Zimmermann, H.J.: Fuzzy Set Theory-and Its Applications, 4th edn. Kluwer Acadmic Publishers, Norwell, MA (2001)
44. Meada, Y., Entani, T., Tanaka, H.: Fuzzy DEA with interval efficiency. In: 6th European Congress on Intelligent Techniques and Soft Computing vol. 2, pp. 1067–1071 (1998)
45. Wang, Y.M., Chin, K.S., Yang, J.B.: Measuring the performance of decision-making units using geometric average efficiency. J. Operat. Res. Soc. **58**, 929–937 (2007)
46. Allahviranloo, T., Ezadi, S.: Z-Advanced numbers processes. Inf. Sci. **480**, 130–143 (2019)

Performance and Managerial Ability Analysis in Health Sector: A Data Envelopment Analysis Approach

Alireza Amirteimoori, Sharmineh Safarpour, Sohrab Kordrostami, and Leila Khoshandam

Abstract Since the healthcare system is one of the most important key sectors in a society and as health service supply is one of the personal development factors in any country, so paying heed to this sector can result in social well-being and prosperity. To ensure a better and more qualified health care, treatment and protection services, analysis of the related performance plays a major role in any health system. In so doing, proper usage of assets is an undeniable fact. This research aims at introducing an applicable case in health system sector of all hospitals in Iran where the performance analysis is measured. To do so, the data of thirty-one state hospitals are collected and after recognizing contextual variables and undesirable factor, performance analysis and managerial ability of each hospital are measured. To measure it, first, technical performance with undesirable factor, is calculated using data envelopment analysis. Then, the technical analysis logarithm of the first stage has been applied to a set of contextual variables which impact hospitals analysis. All the results are regressed later. Next, the managerial ability is measured by the remaining regression of the previous stage. Finally, a unique ranking according to managerial ability criterion is suggested. All in all, the results are analyzed in order to give practical recommendations to managers and for more efficient management of hospitals in Iran.

Keywords Data envelopment analysis · Managerial ability · Contextual variables · Efficiency · Ranking

---

A. Amirteimoori (✉)
Faculty of Engineering and Natural Sciences, Istinye University, Istanbul, Turkey
e-mail: alireza.amirteimoori@istinye.edu.tr

S. Safarpour · L. Khoshandam
Department of Applied Mathematics, Islamic Azad University, Rasht Branch, Rasht, Iran

S. Kordrostami
Department of Applied Mathematics, Islamic Azad University, Lahijan Branch, Lahijan, Iran

T. Allahviranloo et al. (eds.), *Decision Making in Healthcare Systems*,
Studies in Systems, Decision and Control 513,
https://doi.org/10.1007/978-3-031-46735-6_16

1 Introduction

It is essential for a healthcare system to deeply recognize the factors affecting health in a society for detailed plans in a country so the undesirable factors will be minimized. Equal distribution of healthcare resources for the sake of meeting overall health needs of citizens has been a long-lasting concern of policy-makers and made management and allocation of resources part and parcel of a healthcare system. To ensure a better and more qualified healthcare services necessitates analysis of healthcare system performance. So, it seems that applying efficiency-measuring and performance-improvement methods can lead to a better procedure and optimal use of resources to deliver more appropriate services. There have been several methods for measuring the efficiency of decision-making units which can be divided into two groups of parametric and non-parametric.

Farrell [1] suggested non-parametric method for the first time in 1957 and after that Charnes et al. [2] developed the first analysis of Farrell with several inputs and one output to several inputs and outputs in 1978. The result was called CCR. Then, Banker et al. [3] introduced BCC model in 1984. The non-parametric method is based on linear planning where for any decision-making unit, a linear-based solution is given. This field of research has been developed briskly and was called data envelop analysis (DEA). DEA is a mathematical planning technique for analyzing decision-making units and plays a major role in recognizing efficient borders and measuring relative efficiency units under investigation. DEA makes comparison of units possible. Since the frequent implementation of DEA in different issues, there have been many researches in this case of which those of Charnes et al. [4], Russel [5], Sueyoshi [6], Green et al. [7], Tone [8], Dyson et al. [9], Coelli and et al. [10], Zhu and Cook [11], Cooper and Seiford [12], Emrouznejad et al. [13], Zhu [14], Wu et al. [15], Chu et al. [16] can be mentioned.

Of other effective factors of healthcare is effective management in this unit which has a direct impact on performance level. So, analysis of managerial ability is of highest importance. It is because the performance analysis of such units disregarding managerial ability can ignore several contextual variables including amount of assets and number of GPs of each unit in development and non-development of each unit and as a result it can deny weak points and strong points of the managers which may be appreciated.

There have been much speculations on management quality of companies of which Castanias and Helfat [17], Barr and Siems [18], Adner and Helfat [19], Helfat and Peteraf [20] can be mentioned. Demirijian et al. [21, 22] were among those who suggested an applicable method for measuring managerial ability: First, the relative efficiency of the unit under investigation is calculated with several contextual variables including managerial ability applying data envelopment analysis and in the next step, since it is needed that management factor to be involved in managerial ability, the impact of contextual variables should be omitted. Demirijian et al. [21, 22]showed in their research that there is a direct and significant relationship between manager's ability levels with its profitability and, following that, performance improvement.

Of other researches in this field, it can be referred to Murthi et al. [23], Leverty and Grace [24], Kweh et al. [25], Banker and Park [26], Banker et al. [27] and Cvetkoska et al. [28].

Since the impact of undesirable factors such as greenhouse gases, noise, waste, tax and overdue claims in trade centres and banks, waste and sewage and the rate of death in medical centres such as hospitals and so on are ignored in performance analysis, Shephard [29] defined weak availability in 1970. Later, Fare and Grosskopf [30] developed such idea. Criticizing the former approach, Kuosmanen [31] reformulated and suggested a more general approach whose method is applied in this research paper for estimating technical performance.

It is essential to pay attention to healthcare in a society so there have been lots of researches in this case. Zhu [32] has suggested a set of DEA models for performance analysis and decision objectives. Rivera [33] has conducted valuable researches regarding performance analysis of healthcare systems from public expenditure viewpoint. Shwartz et al. [34] recommended a new method using technology for applying DEA. In this paper the focus is on healthcare quality indexes where patients are impacted with different characteristics of organisation behavior. Darabi et al. [35] took into consideration the impact of background variables on efficiency of healthcare system performance in some states when they were focused on birth results.

The innovation of that research lies in application of two environmental variables in the model. They realised that ignoring contextual factors would result in maximum performance estimation. Ortega-Díaz and Martín [36] stated that undesirable outputs have impacts on measuring performance. They also came up with instruments for increasing hospital performance. Liu et al. [37] suggests a model in his measurement. He showed that while service efficiency of child healthcare is increased annually in different provinces in China, there are geographical differences and more improvements and reasonable allocation of resources are needed. In his analysis, the healthcare system is ranked completely truly and competitively.

Choosing input and output variables are of important issues for performance analysis of healthcare units since it is different from one research to another and so it is mental. Among all the previous researches on healthcare, it is supposed that the number of inputs of each decision-making unit is used in order to produce some outputs. In this research, a mode is considered where in addition to specific inputs and outputs of each unit, contextual and descriptive variables are considered. The main question of the research is how to analyze and calculate managerial ability of units alongside specific inputs and outputs of each unit and undesirable factors in production line. Also, this paper aims at evaluating healthcare performance of Iran using data envelopment model and its ranking with managerial ability criterion. In so doing, the statistical data of thirty-one hospital of Iran are used. The conceptual framework of the research is given in Fig. 1.

Other parts of the article are as following: the next part focuses on the methodology and efficiency analysis and calculation of managerial ability considering the impact of contextual variables with undesirable factors. Part 3 the theoretical framework is provided with a set of true data regarding healthcare of Iran. Also, the impact of

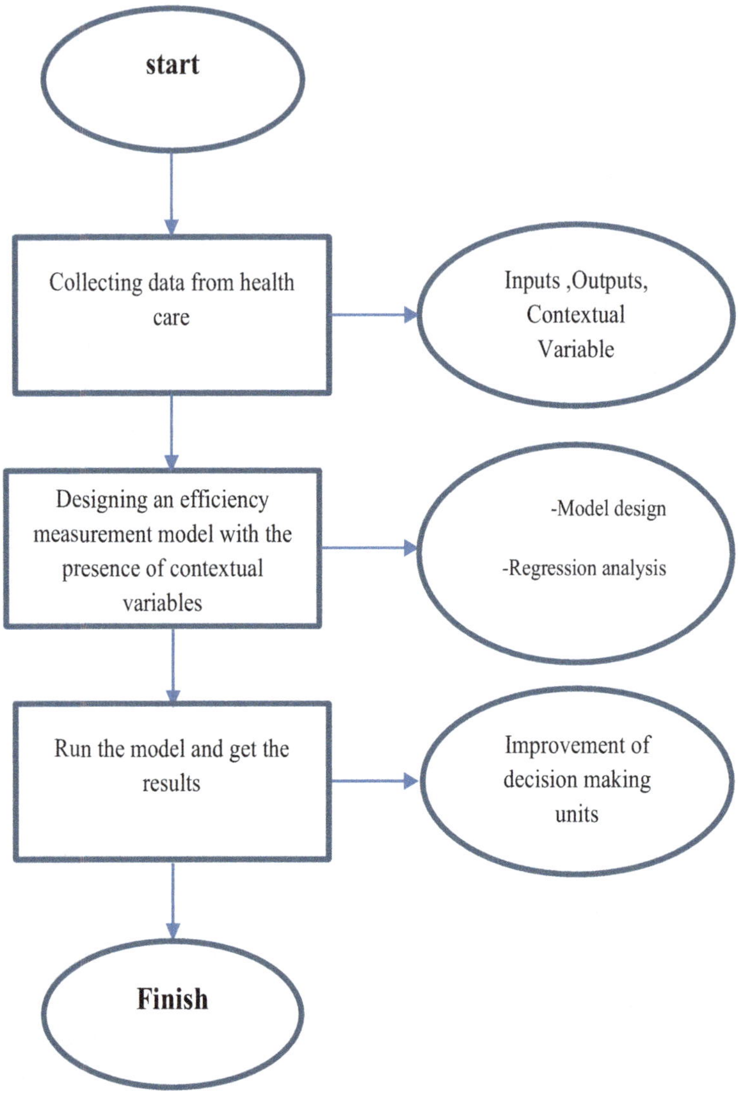

Fig. 1 Conceptual framework

background variables on thirty-one hospitals in thirty-one provinces are measured and later, a unique ranking based on management ability for each unit is given. Finally, the last part provides results and further suggestions.

2 Methodology

According to studies by Demirijian et al. [21, 22] and Banker and Park [26]formance analysis and managerial ability of thirty-one hospitals in Iran will be provided through a three-stage procedure. So, concerning undesirable factors, performance analysis of the units is carried out using efficiency measurement model suggested by Kuosmanen [28] with (3) technology. Then, applying least squares, the impact of each contextual variable, including "a set of assets", "density", and "number of doctors", on efficiency scores of the first stage will be regressed (Fig. 2).

T = {(x, y, z)| outputs (y, z) can be produced by input x}.

Accepting the weak disposability principle by Kuosmanen [31] for the presence of undesirable outputs in production procedure and also by accepting observation inclusion principle, strongdisposability, convexity and extrapolation, the technology can be defined as following:

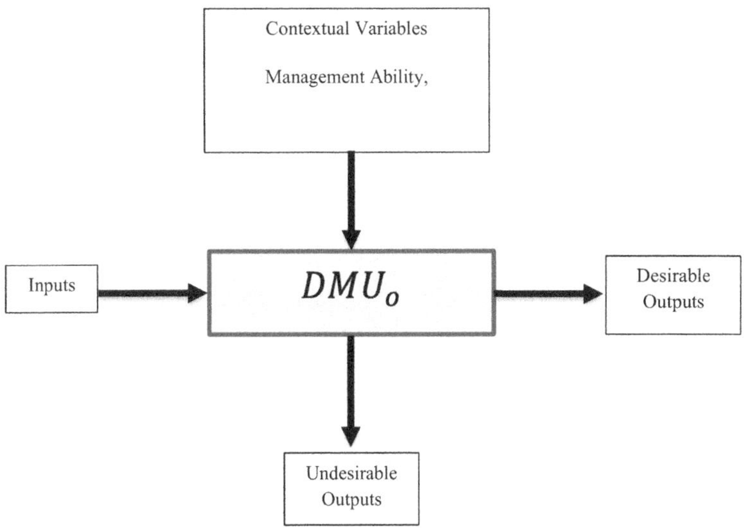

Fig. 2 A systemic view of the production process

$$
\mathrm{T}=\left\{(x,y,z): y\le\sum_{j=1}^{n}\theta_j w_j y_{rj} \quad r=1,\ldots,s,\right.
$$
$$
\begin{aligned}
z &= \sum_{j=1}^{n}\theta_j w_j z_{kj} && k=1,\ldots,K,\\
x &\ge \sum_{j=1}^{n} w_j x_{ij} && i=1,\ldots,m,\\
&\sum_{j=1}^{n} w_j = 1, && \\
&w_j \ge 0 && j=1,\ldots,n,\\
&0\le\theta_j\le 1 && j=1,\ldots,n.\}
\end{aligned}
\tag{1}
$$

The technology is non-linear. To convert this non-linear technology to a linear one, the following variable is used:

$$
\begin{aligned}
w_j &= \mu_j+\lambda_j\\
\mu_j &= (1-\theta_j)w_j\\
\theta_j &= \frac{\lambda_j}{(\mu_j+\lambda_j)},\\
\lambda_j &= \theta_j w_j.
\end{aligned}
\tag{2}
$$

The final technology can be calculated as following:

$$
\mathrm{T}=\left\{(x,y,z): y\le\sum_{j=1}^{n}\lambda_j y_{rj} \quad \mathrm{r}=1,\ldots,s,\right.
$$
$$
\begin{aligned}
x &\ge \sum_{j=1}^{n}(\mu_j+\lambda_j)x_{ij} && i=1,\ldots,m,\\
z &= \sum_{j=1}^{n}\lambda_j z_{kj} && k=1,\ldots,K,
\end{aligned}
\tag{3}
$$
$$
\sum_{j=1}^{n}(\mu_j+\lambda_j)=1,
$$
$$
\left.\mu_j,\lambda_j\ge 0\cdots\right\}
$$

In classic model of data envelopment analysis, the aim is to minimize inputs and maximize outputs but in some production procedure such as hospital, factory and so on, there are desirable factors as well as undesirable factors such as waste, death, air pollutants, pollution and so on. To analyze such units, the major aim is to use methods to minimize undesirable factors and maximize desirable factors. According to technology suggested in (the efficiency measurement model used in the first stage can be defined as following:

$$
\begin{aligned}
&\mathrm{Min}\varphi \\
&\mathrm{s.t} \\
&\quad y_{ro} \le \sum_{j=1}^{n} \lambda_j y_{rj} \qquad r = 1, \ldots s, \\
&\quad x_{io} \ge \sum_{j=1}^{n} (\mu_j + \lambda_j) x_{ij} \; i = 1, \ldots, m, \\
&\quad \varphi z_{ko} = \sum_{j=1}^{n} \lambda_j z_{kj} \quad k = 1, \ldots, K, \\
&\quad \sum_{j=1}^{n} (\mu_j + \lambda_j) = 1 \\
&\quad \mu_j, \lambda_j \ge 0 \qquad j = 1, \ldots, n
\end{aligned}
\tag{4}
$$

DMU0 is called efficient that if and only if φ^* equals 1 and corresponding covariate variables of inputs and outputs equal zero. Otherwise the DMU0 is called inefficient. Accordingly, the figure of this unit on the efficient border is as following:

$$
\begin{aligned}
\overline{x_o} &= \sum_{j=1}^{n} (\mu_j + \lambda_j) x_j \\
\overline{y_o} &= \sum_{j=1}^{n} \lambda_j y_j \\
\overline{Z_o} &= \sum_{j=1}^{n} \lambda_j Z_j
\end{aligned}
\tag{5}
$$

It can be easily proved that $\overline{DMU_o}$ unit with $(\overline{x}_0, \overline{y}_0, \overline{z}_0)$ has relative efficiency. According the formula below, the regression will be applied on contextual variables. Banker and Natarajan [38] and Banker et al. [39] suggested a statistical basis for regression analysis in this stage. For the same reason, the efficiency logarithm is described as dependent and contextual variables and considered as dependent variables and regression is applied according to the following formula.

$$
\log_{10} \theta = \beta_0 + \beta_1 t_1 + \cdots + \beta_k t_k \tag{6}
$$

where , $t_1 \ldots t_k$ are contextual variables and θ is efficiency result from model (5). $\beta_i (i = 1, 2, 3)$ shows the sensitivity of the dependent variable $\log_{10} \theta$ in comparison to independent variables $t_i (i = 1, 2, 3)$ In other words, how much difference the one-unit increase of an independent variable can bring to dependent variable.

3 A Real Application in Healthcare System

According to the importance of healthcare system in Iran and regarding the significance of treatment in government's policy making in public sphere of developed countries, it can determine the social and economic status of a country. In a sense, any kind of payment in healthcare is a type of investment so it is of highest importance. As a result, the method described above will be applied to data gathered from thirty-one hospitals in Iran. Each hospital is considered as a decision-making unit. So, each hospital uses inputs to produce outputs. There have been numerous studies on selecting input and output variables in healthcare and each has come up with various indexes for performance analysis. In the following Table 1 a few of them are given:

Although several variables can be defined in this research, five indexes as inputs, four indexes as desirable outputs and two indexes as undesirable outputs were chosen based on previous studies scholarly works. In addition, three variables are defined as contextual variables so their impacts on performance will be analysed.

Operational definition of the indexes mentioned in Table 2.

- **Number of Beds in Each Province:**
  Beds in hospitals are among the most important resources in each province and it means a number of beds of hospitals which has received a certified license from Ministry of Health Organization.
- **Operational Costs:**
  It includes all costs covered in a hospital (all personnel and non-personnel costs).
- **Healthcare Costs:**
  It includes all costs covered in healthcare system except operational costs (such as buying medicine and so on).
- **Number of MRI Scanners:**
  A number of MRI scanners active in hospitals.
- **Number of CT Scanners:**
  A number of CT scanners active in hospitals.
- **A Number of Inpatients:**
  Patients who are hospitalized half of a day (6 hours) and used healthcare and medication.
- **A Number of Outpatients:**
  Patients who are not hospitalized or used any bed in hospital and undergone medication.
- **A Number of Surgeries:**
  It is one or some surgical procedures such as removing part of body such as gallbladder, appendix or any infected or cancerous tissue. It also refers to using any device like prosthesis or valve.
- **Rate of Beds used**
  It shows a number of beds patients are hospitalized in a span of time (monthly or annually).

Table 1 Inputs and outputs introduced by other researchers

Inputs and Outputs	Journal	Publication date	Authors	References
Inputs: ✔ Number of doctors ✔ Number of beds. Number of beds used during the term for each unit **Out puts:** ✔ Weighted admissions: ✔ Consultations: (first consultations) ✔ Successive consultations number of surgical interventions	Mathematical and Computer Modelling	2010	Caballer-Tarazona et al.	[40]
Inputs: ✔ Total salary for doctors ✔ Total salary for nurses **Outputs:** ✔ No. of served patients ✔ Bed productivity ✔ Average turnover interval	International Journal of Engineering and Technology	2011	Al-Shayea	[41]
Inputs: ✔ Number of doctors ✔ Number of beds ✔ d public health expenditure as percent of GDP **Outputs:** ✔ Life expectancy at birth ✔ Health adjusted life expectancy ✔ d Infant mortality rate	Procedia Economics and Finance	2014	Asanduluia et al.	[42]
Inputs: ✔ Number of doctors ✔ Number of nurses ✔ Number of beds ✔ Number of other employees Amount of expense **Outputs:** ✔ No.of surgical operations ✔ No. of discharged patients ✔ No. of outpatient ✔ No. of inpatient ✔ No. of inpatient days	Ankara Sağlık Bilimleri Dergisi	2017	Yeşilaydin	[43]

(continued)

Table 1 (continued)

Inputs and Outputs	Journal	Publication date	Authors	References
Inputs: ✔ Number of beds ✔ Number of medical staff ✔ Number of CT ✔ Number of MR ✔ Number of medical equipment together **Outputs:** ✔ Bed occupancy rate ✔ Average nursing time in day	Health Economics Review	2018	Stefko et al.	[44]
Inputs: ✔ The sum of public and private health expenditure which covers health service provision (preventive and curative) but does not include provision of water and sanitation ✔ Hospital beds include inpatient beds available in public, private, general, and specialized hospitals and rehabilitation centers **Outputs:** ✔ Life expectancy at birth indicates the number of years a newborn infant would live if prevailing patterns of mortality at the time of its birth were to stay the same throughout its life ✔ Maternal mortality ratio is the number of women who die from pregnancy-related causes while pregnant or within 42 days of pregnancy termination ✔ Infant mortality rate is the number of infants dying before reaching one year of age ✔ Number of adults (aged 15+) and children (aged 0–14) newly infected with HIV	Journal of Healthcare Engineering	2018	Ibrahim and Daneshvar	[45]

(continued)

Table 1 (continued)

Inputs and Outputs	Journal	Publication date	Authors	References
Inputs: ✔ Average time of hospitalization (in days) ✔ Average costs of day hospital treatment **Outputs:** ✔ an Average number of patients per bed per year ✔ Share of accredited hospitals as a proportion of the number of all hospitals ✔ Net profit per physician	Business Administration and Management	2018	Kocisova et al.	[46]
Inputs: ✔ Number obstetrics & gynecologists per 1000 ✔ Number of physicians per 1000 people ✔ Number of patients' beds per 1000 people ✔ Amount of healthcare expenditure per capita ($) ✔ Number of pregnant women who smoke per 1000 people **Outputs:** ✔ Infant survival rate per 1000 live birth ✔ Number of babies with normal birthweight per 1000 live birth ✔ Number of fullterm infants per 1000 live birth	Expert Systems With Applications	2021	Darabi et al.	[35]

- **A Number of Doctors:**
  It refers to doctors who work in emergency or treatment ward of a hospital.
- **A Set of Assets:**
  It refers to a set of assets of a hospital. Assets are valuable economic items which are cost for making profit during time. Such assets are usually registered in accounting records (Some simple assets are money, stock exchange, pre-payment costs.
- **Density:**
  It refers to ratio of hospitals to the whole population of a province.
- **Death Rate:**
  It means all death rates of men, women and children.

Table 2 Introduction of indicators

Index type	Introduction of index
Input variables	1.Operating cost including personnel cost 2. Health cost 3.Number of CT 4. Number of MRI 5. The number of beds in each province
Desirable output variables	1. No. of Inpatient 2. No. of Outpatient 3. No. of Surgical Operations 4. Number of beds
Undesirable output variables	1. Number of deaths 2. Infectious waste
Contextual variables	1.Total assets 2. Density 3. Number of doctors

- **Infectious Waste:**
  It refers to waste produced in healthcare organizations such as hospitals and clinics. They are classified as dangerous waste and their disposal need special measures.

The descriptive statistics of input, output and contextual variables mentioned above which include mean, standard deviation, maximum and minimum and median are given in Tables 3, 4 and 5, respectively.

Table 3 Statistical description of input data

Indicator	Operational and health costs	Number of MRI	Number of CT	Number of beds
Average	188,602.51	11.41	8.90	3025.00
Stdev	66,970.37	1.38	5.26	612.35
Max	297,841.52	23.52	16.28	25,866.00
Min	85,492.46	4.95	3.20	7049.00
Median	203,004.54	14.92	8.58	2302.00

Table 4 Statistical description of contextual variable

Indicator	Number of physicians	Density	Total assets
Average	185.83	67,841.20	2,353,270.19
Stdev	202.27	67,761.98	148,165.43
Max	1227.08	67,786.18	2,579,830.48
Min	61.08	67,568.33	2,016,104.20
Median	148.42	66,875.18	2,361,634.36

Table 5 Statistical description of output data

Indicator	Number of inpatient	Number of outpatient	Number of surgical operation	Bed occupancy rate	Death	Infectious waste
Average	9668.94	1,016,668.01	4188.93	77.14	134.19	16.45
Stdev	1068.20	2466.59	1365.43	7.90	62.91	7.50
Max	15,731.49	1,023,578.64	8928.11	116.59	288	31.5
Min	4359.42	1,011,502.57	1910.54	13.93	14	4.12
Median	9953.16	1,017,267.81	4166.57	84.30	131	15.53

4 The Impact of Contextual Variables on Efficiency Scores

It is because the amount of calculated efficiency based on efficiency measurement model (4) from above and below is bounded set so the logarithm of base 10 of the index can be considered as a dependent variable and for the impact of contextual variables the following regression can be used:

$$Log_{10}(\theta) = \beta_0 + \beta_1 t_1 + \beta_2 t_2 + \beta_3 t_3 + \varepsilon \tag{7}$$

where $(i = 1, 2, 3)$ β_i indicates the sensitivity of dependent variable θ to independent variables $(i = 1, 2, 3)$ t_i. The numerical value of statement (7) is a normal numerical value for measuring managerial ability. The efficiency scores gained from model (4) and results from managerial ability of hospitals under investigation and also, efficiency after impact of contextual variables on this index are given in columns 2,3,4 of Table 6, respectively. As it can be seen, calculating model (4), 25 efficient units are evaluated but if contextual variables impact efficiency index, no unit will be efficient. So, it proves the high impact of such indexes on the performance of units. In addition, according to the calculations, in ranking units applying managerial ability approach, DMU_{27} has the first rank and DMU_{11},which has the weakest performance among units under consideration, is rank as the last one. The charts of efficiency measurement of model (4) and managerial ability can be seen in Fig. 3.

Applying linear regression method, the impact of the contextual variables mentioned before on efficiency and following that its management ability is measured and given in Table 7. Accordingly, contextual variables co-efficient of a number of doctors -3.1×10^{-8} means that percentage of efficiency increase (5) is related to one unit reduction of that variable (number of people) equals $100 \times (e^{-3.1\times10^{-8}} - 1) = -3.1 \times 10^{-6}$. The impact of this variable on efficiency is reverse and its one-unit increase will result in management ability reduction. To put it simply, the increase in number of doctors may lead to compression and later cause system inefficiency and reduction of management ability. The second effective variable is density. Alike number of doctors, density has a reverse impact on management ability and one-unit increase results in -1.5×10^{-5} reduction of management ability. However, unlike

Table 6 Efficiency resulting from model (4), managerial ability and ranking

Observation	Efficiency	Residuals	Pure efficiency
1	1	0.025525	0.97448 (21)
2	0.96	−0.00025	0.95605 (26)
3	1	0.012773	0.98723 (6)
4	0.88	−0.04045	0.91545 (27)
5	1	0.017267	0.982733 (12)
6	1	0.013062	0.98694 (7)
7	0.72	−0.11633	0.83743 (30)
8	1	0.023776	0.97622 (16)
9	0.75	−0.11253	0.85903 (29)
10	1	0.015376	0.98462 (10)
11	0.71	−0.12332	0.83422 (31)
12	1	0.010172	0.98983 (3)
13	1	0.024482	0.97552 (18)
14	1	0.016756	0.98324 (11)
15	1	0.026248	0.97375 (22)
16	1	0.03472	0.96853 (25)
17	1	0.024888	0.97511 (20)
18	1	0.018839	0.98116 (14)
19	1	0.02254	0.97746 (15)
20	1	0.017444	0.98256 (13)
21	1	0.024717	0.97528 (19)
22	1	0.015161	0.98484 (9)
23	1	0.011769	0.98823 (4)
24	1	0.030704	0.96930 (24)
25	1	0.012072	0.98793 (5)
26	1	0.014637	0.98536 (8)
27	1	0.006323	0.99368 (1)
28	0.79	−0.08119	0.86969 (28)
29	1	0.026243	0.97376 (23)
30	1	0.023903	0.97610 (17)
31	1	0.00793	0.99207 (2)

two previous variables, as it is expected, one-unit increase of a set of assets can increase management and efficiency of the system (Fig. 4).

The value of R-squared is 0.021245and it means that regression has covered %2 of the whole observation.

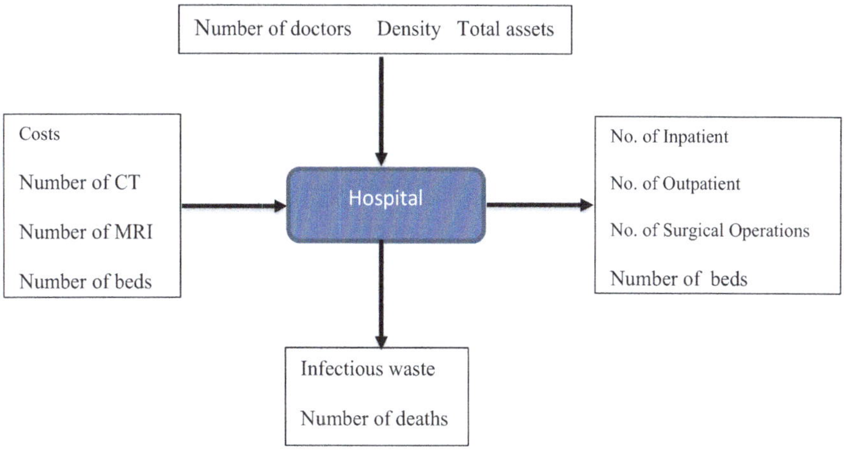

Fig. 3 A view of indicators

Table 7 The results of logarithm regression in base 10 efficiency on contextual variables

Particulars	Coefficient	Standard Error	t Stat	P-value
Intercept	0.063436	0.138905	0.456685	0.65155
Total assets	−3.1E-08	5.87E-08	−0.53325	0.59822
Density	−1.5E-07	3.28E-07	−0.46145	0.648175
Number of physicians	6.56E-06	4.3E-05	0.152692	0.879777
R-squared		0.021245		
Adjusted R-squared		−0.08751		
Sum squared residual		3.361579		
Multiple R		0.145758		
Observations		31		

5 Findings and Results

Hospitals in a country are the building blocks of its healthcare system. The hospitals taken into consideration are in different provinces in Iran. In previous efficiency measurement studies, the pre-supposition was that a decision- making unit has its own specific inputs and outputs while in this study, it is stated that despite specific inputs and outputs of a decision-making unit, other variables such as contextual variables can leave impact on a decision-making unit. In this study, efficiency analysis and managerial ability of some selected hospitals in Iran with contextual variables and undesirable outputs are considered. To do so, throughout a two-stage procedure, first

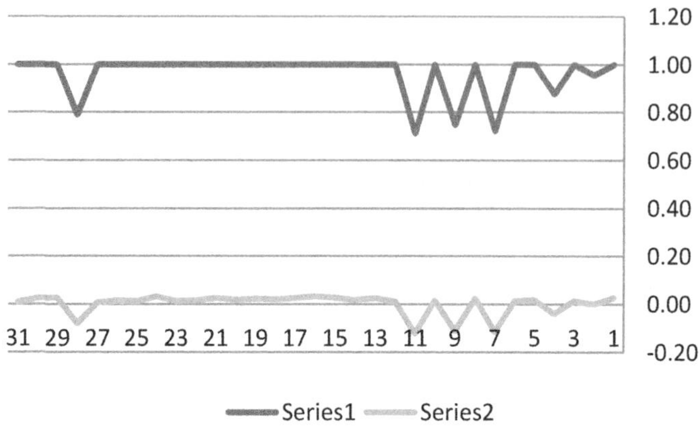

Fig. 4 Diagrams of efficiency and managerial ability of 31 hospital units

using basic models and undesirable units, the efficiency of units is calculated and in the next step, the article suggests a two-stage procedure where in the first place, an efficiency measurement model with undesirable outputs are given and in the next step, technical efficiency logarithm of the first stage has been regressed on a set of contextual variables of hospital performance.

Then, a criterion for ranking units based on managerial ability is given. Furthermore, the impact of contextual variables including a set of assets, density and a number of doctors on efficiency of units are measured. Some of limitations of the research are that all input and output data are considered as deterministic system. Since the data of different time period were not available and hospitals do not record their dataset, finding input and output datasets were difficult. To get precise information, one should attend these hospitals one by one and it was not possible for the researcher so it is limited to library data which are not verified yet. For further research, such theoretical model can be applied to uncertainty situation. Additionally, due to different functions, the way of measuring efficiency can be different. Applying meta-frontier on different social and economic approaches can be mentioned.

References

1. Farell, M.J.: The measurement of productive efficiency. J. R. Stat. Soc. Ser. A (General), **120**(3), 253–290 (1957)
2. Charnes, A., Cooper, W.W., Rhodes, E.: Measuring the efficiency of decision-making units. Eur. J. Oper. Res. **2**(6), 429–444 (1978)
3. Banker, R.D., Charnes, A., Cooper, W.W.: Some models for estimating technical and scale inefficiencies in data envelopment analysis. Manage. Sci. **30**(9), 1078–1092 (1984)
4. Charnes, A., Cooper, W.W., Golany, B., Seiford, L., Stutz, J.: Foundations of data envelopment analysis for Pareto-Koopmans efficient empirical production functions. J. Econometr. **30**(1–2), 91–107 (1985)
5. Russell, R.R.: Measures of technical efficiency. J. Econ. Theory **35**, 109–126 (1988)

6. Sueyoshi, T.: A special algorithm for an additive model in data envelopment analysis. J. Oper. Res. Soc. **41**(3), 249–257 (1990)
7. Green, R.H., Cook, W., Doyle, J.: A note on the additive data envelopment analysis model. J. Oper. Res. Soc. **48**(4), 446–448 (1997)
8. Tone, K.: A slacks-based measure of efficiency in data envelopment analysis. Eur. J. Oper. Res. **130**(3), 498–509 (2001)
9. Dyson, R.G., Allen, R., Camanho, A.S., Podinovski, V.V., Sarrico, C.S., Shale, E.A.: Pitfalls and protocols in DEA. Eur. J. Oper. Res. **132**(2), 245–259 (2001)
10. Coelli, T. J., Rao, D.S.P., O'Donnell, C.J., Battese, G.E.: An Introduction to Efficiency and Productivity Analysis. Springer Science & Business Media (2005)
11. Zhu, J., Cook, W.D.: Modeling Data Irregularities and Structural Complexities in Data Envelopment Analysis. Springer Science & Business Media (2007)
12. Cooper, W., Seiford, L.M., Tone, K.: Data Envelopment Analysis: A Comprehensive Text with Models, Applications, References and DEA-Solver Software. Kluwer Academic Publishers, Boston (2007)
13. Emrouznejad, A., Tavares, G., Parker, B.: Evaluation of research in efficiency and productivity: a survey and analysis of the first 30 years of scholarly literature in DEA. Soc. Econ. Plann. Sci. **42**(3), 151–157 (2008)
14. Zhu, J.: Quantitative models for performance evaluation and benchmarking: data envelopment analysis with spreadsheets. Int. Ser. Oper. Res. Manage. Sci. **126**, 14–40 (2009)
15. Wu, J., Zhu, Q., Chu, J., Liang, L.: Two-stage network structures with undesirable intermediate outputs reused: a DEA Based approach. Comput. Econ. **46**(3), 455–477 (2015)
16. Chu, J., Wu, J., Zhu, Q., An, Q., Xiong, B.: Analysis of China's regional eco-efficiency: A DEA two-stage network approach with equitable efficiency decomposition. Comput. Econ. (2016). https://doi.org/10.1007/s10614-015-9558-8
17. Castanias, R.P., Helfat, C.E.: Managerial resources and rents. J. Manag. **17**(1), 155–171 (1991)
18. Barr, R., Siems, T.: Bank failure prediction using DEA to measure management quality (1997)
19. Adner, R., Helfat, C.: Corporate effects and dynamic managerial capabilities. Strateg. Manag. J. **24**(10), 1011–1025 (2003)
20. Helfat, C., Peteraf, M.: Managerial cognitive capabilities and the micro foundations of dynamic capabilities. Strateg. Manag. J. **36**(6), 831–850 (2015)
21. Demerjian, P., Lev, B., McVay, S.: Quantifying managerial ability: a new measure and validity tests. Manage. Sci. **58**(7), 1229–1248 (2012)
22. Demerijian, P., Lewis-Western, M., McVay, S.: How does intentional earnings smoothing vary with managerial ability? J. Acc. Audit. Financ. **35**(2), 1–32 (2020)
23. Murthi, B., Srinivasan, K., Kalyanaram, G.: Controlling for observed and unobserved managerial skills in determining first-mover market share advantage. J. Mark. Res. **33**(3), 329–336 (1996)
24. Leverty, J.T., Grace, M.F.: Dupes or incompetents? An examination of management's impact on firm distress. J. Risk Insur. **79**(3), 751–783 (2012)
25. Kweh, Q.L., Chan, Y.C., Ting, I.W.K.: Measuring intellectual capital efficiency in the Malaysian software sector. J. Intellect. Cap. **14**(2), 310–324 (2013)
26. Banker, R.D., Park, H.: A Statistical Foundation for the Measurement of Managerial Ability. Working Paper, Temple University, Philadelphia, PA (2020)
27. Banker, R.D., Luo, J., Oh, H.: Measuring managerial ability in the insurance industry. Data Envelop. Analysis J. **5**(1), 115–143 (2021)
28. Cvetkoska, V., Eftimov, L., Ivanovsky, I., Kamenjarska, T.: Measuring the managerial ability in the insurance companies in the Republic of North Macedonia, Croatia, Serbia and Slovenia and identifying its determinants. Int. J. Banking Risk Insur. 10(1), (2022)
29. Shephard, R.W.: Theory of Cost and Production Functions. Princeton University Press, Princeton (1970)
30. Fare, R., Grosskopf, S.: Nonparametric productivity analysis with undesirable outputs: comment. Am. J. Agr. Econ. **85**, 1070–1074 (2003)

31. Kuosmanen, T.: Weak disposability in nonparametric productivity analysis with undesirable outputs. Am. J. Agr. Econ. **87**, 1077–1082 (2005)
32. Zhu, J.: Quantitative Models for Performance Evaluation and Benchmarking: Data Envelopment Analysis with Spreadsheets and DEA Excel Solver. Kluwer Academic Publishers, Boston (2002)
33. Rivera, B.: The effects of public health spending on self-assessed health status: an ordered probit model. Appl. Econ. **33**(10), 1313–1319 (2010)
34. Shwartz, M., BurgessJr, J.F., Zhu, J.: A DEA based composite measure of quality and its associated data uncertainty interval for health care provider profiling and pay-for-performance. Eur. J. Oper. Res., 489–502 (2016)
35. Darabi, N., Ebrahimvandi, A., Hosseinichimeh, N., Triantis K.: A DEA evaluation of U.S. States' healthcare systems in terms of their birth outcomes. Expert Syst. Appl. 182 (2021)
36. Ortega-Díaz, M.I., Martín J.C.: How to detect hospitals where quality would not be jeopardized by health cost savings? A methodological approach using DEA with SBM analysis. Health Policy **126**(10), 1069–1074 (2022)
37. Liu, H., Wu, W., Yao, P.: A study on the efficiency of pediatric healthcare services and its influencing factors in China—estimation of a three-stage DEA model based on provincial-level data. Soc. Econ. Plann. Sci. 84 (2022)
38. Banker, R.D., Natarajan, R.: Evaluating contextual variables affecting productivity using data envelopment analysis. Oper. Res. **56**(1), 48–58 (2008)
39. Banker, R.D., Natarajan, R., Zhang, D.: Two-stage estimation of the impact of contextual variables in stochastic frontier production function models using data envelopment analysis: second stage OLS versus bootstrap approaches. Eur. J. Oper. Res. **278**(2), 368–384 (2019)
40. Caballer-Tarazona, M., Moya-Clemente, I., Vivas-Consuelo, D., Barrachina-Martínez, I.: A model to measure the efficiency of hospital performance. Math. Comput. Model. **52**, 1095–1102 (2010)
41. Al-Shayea, A.M.: Measuring hospital's units efficiency: a data envelopment analysis approach. Int. J. Eng. Technol. IJET-IJENS **11**(06) (2011)
42. Asanduluia, L., Romanb, M., Fatulescua, P.: The efficiency of healthcare systems in Europe: a data envelopment analysis approach. Proc. Econ. Financ. **10**, 261–268 (2014)
43. Yeşilaydin, G.: Health efficiency measurment in turkey by using data envelopment analysis: a systematic review. Ankara Sağlık Bilimleri Dergisi (1–2–3), 49–69 (2017)
44. Stefko, R., Gavurova, B., Kocisova, K.: Healthcare efficiency assessment using DEA analysis in the Slovak Republic. Heal. Econ. Rev. **8**(6) (2018)
45. Ibrahim, M.D., Daneshvar, S.: Efficiency analysis of healthcare system in lebanon using modified data envelopment analysis. J. Healthc. Eng. 6
46. Kocisova, K., Hass-Symotiuk, M., Kludacz-Alessandr, M.: Use of the DEA method to verify the performance model for hospitals. Ekonomika Manage. **21**(4), 125–140 (2018)

Mental Health on Twitter in Turkey: Sentiment Analysis with Transformers

Qamar Alshammari and Süreyya Akyüz

Abstract Social media are regarded as excellent mediums for capturing individuals' everyday routines, interests, and ideologies. Also, these platforms are now used to exchange health-related information. By collecting and analyzing data from social media, hidden patterns of peopleâŁ™s activities, status, etc., can be gathered. The goal of this study is to employ machine learning to conduct sentiment analysis and assess the mental health of Turkish Twitter users. Using terms relating to common mental health issues such as anxiety, stress, depression, suicide, and eating disorders, we collected over 25,000 tweets. The data was then analyzed, and automated sentiment scoring for the Turkish language was applied using a transformer-based machine learning model. By utilizing BERT, our final deep-learning classifier showed 82.6% accuracy in predicting sentiment from tweets. This study shows how effective deep learning models and transformers are for Turkish natural language processing tasks. The findings may help to improve mental health services by providing a better understanding of the sentiment expressed in Turkish tweets about mental health.

1 Introduction

1.1 Background

Mental health has become a growing concern globally, with rates of depression, anxiety, and other mental health disorders increasing in recent years [1, 2]. There is a considerable prevalence of mental health disorders in Turkey, with a significant portion of the population reporting symptoms of depression, anxiety, and other related

Q. Alshammari
Department of Computer Engineering, Bahcesehir University, Istanbul, Turkey
e-mail: qamar.alshammari@bahcesehir.edu.tr

S. Akyüz (✉)
Department of Mathematics, Faculty of Engineering and Natural Sciences, Bahcesehir University, Istanbul, Turkey
e-mail: sureyya.akyuz@bau.edu.tr

T. Allahviranloo et al. (eds.), *Decision Making in Healthcare Systems*,
Studies in Systems, Decision and Control 513,
https://doi.org/10.1007/978-3-031-46735-6_17

disorders. As per the statistics provided by the Ministry of Health of Turkey (MoH), approximately 17% of the populace in Turkey encounters mental health problems, and a total of 3.2 million individuals experience depression.[1] Understanding the attitudes and perceptions of individuals towards mental health is important in efforts to improve mental health services and support. Twitter has become an increasingly popular platform for individuals to share their experiences and discuss mental health-related issues [3–6]. Twitter provides a valuable resource for understanding public perceptions of mental health, as it allows for real-time analysis of large volumes of data and allows for the capture of individual experiences and perspectives [7, 8]. Several other studies [9–11] also report that Twitter is used as a platform to share symptoms [10], seek help, and exchange advice [11]. Mental health-related tweets can provide a rich source of information on the attitudes, beliefs, and experiences of individuals, including their experiences with mental health services, their perceptions of the stigma associated with mental health, and their beliefs about the causes of mental health disorders. This information can be valuable in informing efforts to improve mental health services, reduce stigma, and increase awareness of mental health issues. Several studies have been conducted to predict mental health issues such as anxiety, depression, and insomnia by analyzing Twitter data [12–14].

Twitter sentiment analysis, or the process of automatically classifying the sentiment expressed in tweets, has become a popular area of research in the field of mental health. This method allows researchers to gain a better understanding of public perceptions and attitudes toward mental health. The use of machine learning (ML) and deep learning techniques has been shown to be effective in sentiment analysis of mental health-related tweets [15].

1.2 Turkish Twitter and Sentiment Analysis

The literature on sentiment analysis of Turkish tweets using ML approaches is quite extensive, with studies covering a range of topics, from analyzing emojis to detecting depression and anxiety symptoms. One of the earliest studies of using vector representations in sentiment analysis in Turkish tweets was done by Riza et al. [16], which applied bag-of-words and fastText to predict Turkish tweets over emojis. They achieved a high F1-score for binary and a moderate score for multi-class classification. Abhilash et al. [17] proposed a system that uses tweets and SentiStrength sentiment analysis to detect depression in social media posts. The authors collected 61,400 tweets with keywords like anxiety, suicide, and depression and achieved approximately 80% accuracy with a Back Propagation Neural Network (BPNN) model for all keywords. Yasin et al. [18] completed a study on sentiment analysis of Turkish tweets about global warming and climate change and trained ML models on thirty thousand randomly selected Turkish tweets. The authors used KNN, SVM,

[1] https://www.who.int/about/accountability/results/who-results-report-2020-mtr/country-story/2020/supporting-turkish-mental-health-policy-and-service-delivery.

and naive bayes ML classifier models, achieving high precision, recall, and F-score with KNN and SVM. Zekeriya et al. [19] compared the performance of BERT (Bidirectional Encoder Representations from Transformers) models and ML methods for sentiment analysis on Turkish tweets. The authors found that logistic regression outperformed other methods. Another study by Ayşe et al. [20] performed multi-class sentiment analysis from Turkish tweets with RNN (Recurrent Neural Network) architecture. The authors divided the dataset into 5 different emotion categories and used LSTM (Long Short-Term Memory), Bi-LSTM (Bidirectional LSTM), and GRU (Gated recurrent unit) based on RNN architecture to perform sentiment analysis. The BiLSTM model achieved the highest accuracy. Yavuz et al. [21] aimed to identify Twitter users who may suffer from depression and anxiety after Covid-19 and create a suitable predictive model using ML technology. The authors collected 184,000 tweets and used SVM to analyze a total of 7 words that are seen as symptoms of depression and anxiety. Gülengül et al. [22] conducted a study of Twitter sentiment analysis on COVID-19 in Turkey. They used TextBlob[2] for sentiment scoring and found that XGBoost[3] had better scores than other models in different feature engineering techniques.

In previous studies on sentiment analysis of Turkish tweets, the majority of the work has focused on annotated sentiment datasets rather than applying sentiment scoring using machine learning. This paper aims to address this gap in the literature by applying an automated sentiment scoring technique using a BERT model. In addition, several ML algorithms were applied with different preprocessing techniques, and their performance scores were compared.

2 Methods

2.1 Background Materials

2.1.1 Machine Learning Algorithms

Random Forest

Random Forest [23] is a type of ensemble ML algorithm used for classification and regression problems. It combines multiple decision trees (hence the name "forest") to make predictions, each tree providing a "vote" for the final output. In training, Random Forest builds each decision tree on a random sample of the data with replacement (i.e., bootstrapping), and each tree splits on a random subset of the features. This creates diversity among the trees and helps reduce overfitting, which can be a problem in single-decision trees. This ML algorithm provides an effective way to

[2] https://github.com/sloria/TextBlob.

[3] https://github.com/dmlc/xgboost.

reduce the variance of the model and improve the accuracy of predictions compared to single decision trees.

Gradient Boost

Gradient Boosted Decision Trees (GBDT) [24] is a ML technique used for regression and classification tasks. It is an ensemble learning method that combines multiple simple decision trees to create a more robust model. GBDT uses an iterative process to train decision trees, where each new tree is fit to the residual errors of the previous trees. The final prediction is made by taking the weighted sum of predictions from all the trees in the ensemble. GBDT has been shown to be effective for many real-world applications due to its ability to handle non-linear relationships and complex feature interactions. In this study, a histogram-based GBDT estimator [25] was used. This implementation can be orders of magnitude faster than traditional GBDT. It simplifies the input samples by dividing them into integer bins (usually 256 bins). This significantly reduces the number of points that need to be considered for splitting and enables the use of integer-based data structures, such as histograms, instead of sorting continuous values when constructing the trees.

Long Short Term Memory

LSTM is a type of Recurrent Neural Network (RNN) used for modeling sequential data such as time-series data, speech signals, and text. It is specifically designed to handle the problem of vanishing gradients in traditional RNNs by introducing memory cells that can maintain information for a long period of time. A standard LSTM network consists of multiple LSTM cells, with each cell receiving inputs from the previous time step and producing outputs that are used as inputs for the next time step. The internal structure of an LSTM cell is composed of three gates: the input gate, forget gate, and output gate, each of which regulates the flow of information in and out of the cell state. LSTMs are trained using backpropagation through time, where the gradients are propagated from the final time step back to the initial time step. This allows the LSTM to learn long-term dependencies in the input data.

Bidirectional Long Short Term Memory

Bidirectional Long-Short Term Memory (Bi-LSTM) is a type of Recurrent Neural Network (RNN) that processes input sequences in both forward and backward directions. It is used for modeling sequences with context from both past and future information. A Bi-LSTM network consists of two separate LSTM networks, one processing the input sequence in the forward direction and the other processing the same sequence in the backward direction. The outputs from the two LSTMs are then concatenated and used as input for the next layer or for making the final prediction.

Convolutional Neural Network

Convolutional Neural Networks (CNNs) are a type of neural network commonly used for image and video recognition tasks. They are designed to automatically and adaptively learn spatial hierarchies of features from input data through a process called convolution. A typical CNN architecture consists of multiple layers, including convolutional layers, activation layers, pooling layers, and fully connected layers. In this study, CNN combined with LSTM was used. The CNN is used to extract high-level representations of word sequences, which are then fed into an LSTM network to produce sentence representations. This enables the model to capture both the local features of the text and the temporal semantics of the sentence, resulting in improved performance in tasks such as our text classification.

2.2 *Data Collection*

We collected a total of 26,170 tweets based on different phrases and hashtags that represent an individual's mental health. For this study, we considered four themes for mental health tweets and considered including both English and Turkish similar keywords for data collection. The themes are - self-hate, anxiety, depression, and an eating disorder. The phrases and hashtags are as follows—"hatemyself", "suicidal", "anxiety", "depresyon", "kaygı", "yeme bozukluğu" etc. The tweets were collected until October, 2022. The majority of the tweets falls between 2014 to 2022 with 6,429 tweets as the highest in 2022.

We used SNSscrape[4] to scrape only Turkish tweets containing the above-mentioned keywords and phrases. SNSscrape is a popular tool used in research for collecting data from social media platforms, such as Twitter and Facebook. It has been widely used to collect large amounts of data, including posts, comments, and images, from social media platforms [26–28] to conduct various data mining tasks, such as sentiment analysis [29–31] or other text mining tasks.

For raw data processing, the first step is to clean the data to remove any irrelevant or redundant information. We removed the usernames and mentions from the tweets. Then we normalized the tweets using BeautifulSoup4[5] HTML parser to convert the character to their proper Unicode form. We discarded the URLs and other web links because these data can not be analyzed by lexical methods. We also removed hashtags and cashtags from the tweets because they are irrelevant to the context of a meaningful sentence. We kept the preposition and punctuation because they are essential for the context of the sentence while using transformer-based word embedding techniques such as BERT. We also converted the emojis to their meaningful words by using demoji.[6] Table 1 displays the statistics describing the tweets of the data set.

[4] https://github.com/JustAnotherArchivist/snscrape.

[5] https://www.crummy.com/software/BeautifulSoup.

[6] https://github.com/bsolomon1124/demoji.

Table 1 Tweets statistics

Tweets	N	
Total number of tweets	25,667	
Number of unique tweets	24,923	
Total number of retweets	29,602	
Total number of likes	267,247	
Total number of users	12,867	
Number of unique hashtags	13,099	
Tweets	Mean	Standard deviation
Number of tweets per day	5.38	34.15
Number of likes for daily tweets	56.08	1228.89
Number of retweets per day	6.21	86

2.3 Sentiment Scoring

To conduct sentiment analysis on the dataset, it is required to determine the sentiment level of the tweets. This can be achieved through the process of sentiment scoring, which aims to determine the emotional tone of the tweets. This information can be used to analyze public opinion or to gain insights into people's attitudes and emotions about a particular topic. The sentiment scores generated from this process can then be used as input for the sentiment analysis algorithms and models, allowing for the identification of patterns and trends in the emotional content of the tweets.

There are several methods for sentiment scoring, including manual scoring and automated scoring. Manual scoring involves having human annotators rate the sentiment of the text. Automated scoring uses algorithms and models to determine the sentiment of the text. Automated sentiment scoring can be performed using ML models, such as sentiment analysis algorithms and deep learning models. These models are trained on large datasets of text and sentiment labels and then used to predict the sentiment of new text. The sentiment scores generated by the models can be numerical values, such as positive and negative scores, or binary values, such as positive, negative, or neutral. The scores are generated based on the algorithms and models used and the training data used to train the models.

In this study, we used an automated sentiment scoring method using Transformers [32] model *bert-base-turkish-sentiment-cased*.[7] This model is based on the BERTurk[8] for the Turkish Language that employs BERT as its underlying architecture, which is a widely used deep-learning model for Natural Language Processing (NLP) tasks. This model was specifically trained for sentiment scoring on Turkish text. The training data for this model consisted of Turkish tweets and movie and

[7] https://huggingface.co/savasy/bert-base-turkish-sentiment-cased.

[8] https://github.com/stefan-it/turkish-bert.

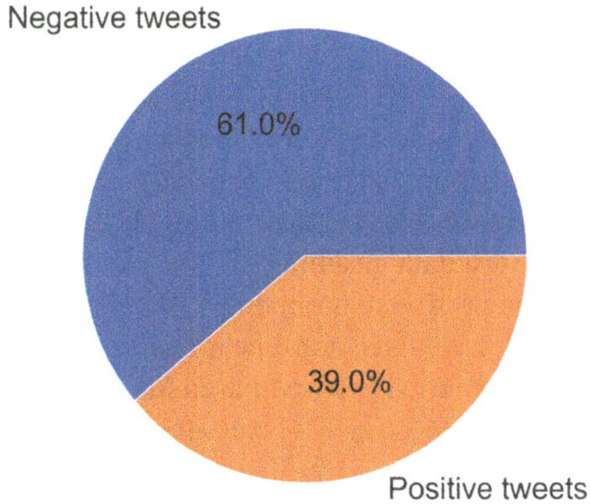

Fig. 1 Sentiment distribution of mental health-related Turkish tweets

product reviews [33–35] that were annotated with sentiment labels. We used the auto tokenizer tool for that model, which automatically tokenizes and preprocess text data for model input. After conducting the automated sentiment scoring of the tweets, we discovered that approximately 39% of the tweets were positive, which means that the majority of the tweets expressed negative sentiments. Figure 1 displays the sentiment distribution of the tweets.

2.4 Model Building

The ML models were developed in two steps. In the first step, a pretrained word embedding model was used to convert the tweets to embeddings. After that, some ML algorithms and deep learning models were used to develop the final model.

To create embeddings from tweets, we used Sentence-Transformers [36] model *emrecan/bert-base-turkish-cased-mean-nli-stsb-tr*[9] which is a pre-trained ML model developed NLP tasks like clustering or semantic search of Turkish text. The model was trained on Turkish machine-translated versions of the NLI (Natural Language Inference) [37] and STS-b (Semantic Textual Similarity Benchmark[10] datasets. The NLI dataset contains pairs of sentences and labels indicating whether the second sentence is entailed, contradicted, or neutral with respect to the first sentence. The STS-b dataset contains pairs of sentences and similarity scores, indicating how similar the two sentences are in meaning. This model maps the input sentences to a dense vector space of 768 dimensions, allowing for the calculation of semantic similarity between sentences. The model's auto tokenizer was used to convert the tweets as input for embeddings.

After creating the word embedding using Sentence-Transformers pretrained model, the next step in the process of building our classifiers. The prepared embed-

[9] https://huggingface.co/emrecan/bert-base-turkish-cased-mean-nli-stsb-tr.

[10] https://github.com/emrecncelik/sts-benchmark-tr.

ding dataset has 768 independent variables and one dependent variable, which is the target class (either positive or negative). The dataset was split into train and test sets with an 80:20 ratio. Since the classes are imbalanced, the stratified sampling technique was applied that ensures that the proportion of the target class is maintained in both the training and test sets. This is important because if the target class is underrepresented in the training data, the model may not be able to generalize well to the test data, resulting in poor accuracy. Also, before applying the ML algorithms, the features were normalized, and the labels were encoded.

Since we have non-linear features, the linear models will not be able to perform better. We tried two tree-based ML algorithms—Random Forest [38] and Histogram Gradient Boosting [24] classifiers using *sklearn* python library [25]. While training, the train data was shuffled, and five-fold cross-validation was applied. We also conducted hyperparameter optimization for these models. The evaluation metrics used include Area Under the Curve (AUC), accuracy, loss, and F1-score. Apart from tree-based classification algorithms, we also developed several Neural Network (NN) models using *keras*[11] and *tensorflow*[12] library.

Apart from the classic ML algorithms, several NN architectures - dense NN, CNN, LSTM, and CNN-LSTM were used for classification tasks. For training the neural networks, 10% of the train data was used for validation. The deep learning model type, batch size, number of neurons, epochs, and layers were varied with different architectures to optimize the performance. The relu [39] activation function was used in hidden layers, and for the output layer *sigmoid* activation function was used. The loss metric for all deep learning models was *binary cross-entropy*, and *Adam* [40] optimizer was used. We also implemented a learning rate scheduler that monitored the validation loss. To prevent overfitting, we applied the early stopping mechanism.

3 Results

Tables 2 and 3 display the performance of tree-based ML algorithms and deep learning, respectively, with the superior performances being emphasized in bold font. The results show that the dense NN model performed the best, with an AUC score of 0.901 and an F1-score of 0.775 on the test data. The next best model is Bi-LSTM with a single layer which performed better than the dense NN on the training data but slightly worse on the test data. The deep learning models performed comparatively better than the classic ML algorithms. The receiver operating characteristic curves for the training and test data sets on the best classification model (dense NN) are displayed in Fig. 2.

[11] https://keras.io.

[12] https://www.tensorflow.org.

Table 2 Comparison of the ML algorithm performance

ML algorithms	Train (80%)				Test (20%)			
	AUC	Accuracy	Loss	F1-score	AUC	Accuracy	Loss	F1-score
Random forest	0.999	0.981	0.701	0.980	0.881	0.803	7.083	0.801
Histogram gradient boost[a]	0.974	0.921	2.854	0.920	**0.888**	**0.813**	**6.725**	**0.812**

[a] Histogram-based Gradient Boosting Classification Tree

Table 3 Comparison of the deep learning model performance

Deep learning models	Train 80%, (validation 10%)				Test (20%)			
	AUC	Accuracy	Loss	F1-score	AUC	Accuracy	Loss	F1-score
Dense neural network	0.961	0.901	0.269	0.871	**0.901**	**0.826**	**0.393**	**0.775**
LSTM[a]	0.906	0.831	0.377	0.782	0.892	0.813	0.404	0.761
Bi-LSTM[b]	0.976	0.927	0.192	0.906	0.897	0.824	0.452	0.771
CNN-LSTM[d]	0.962	0.898	0.245	0.867	0.887	0.816	0.482	0.755

[a] Long short-term memory with three layers
[b] Bidirectional Long short-term memory with a single layer
[d] 1D Convolutional neural network with LSTM

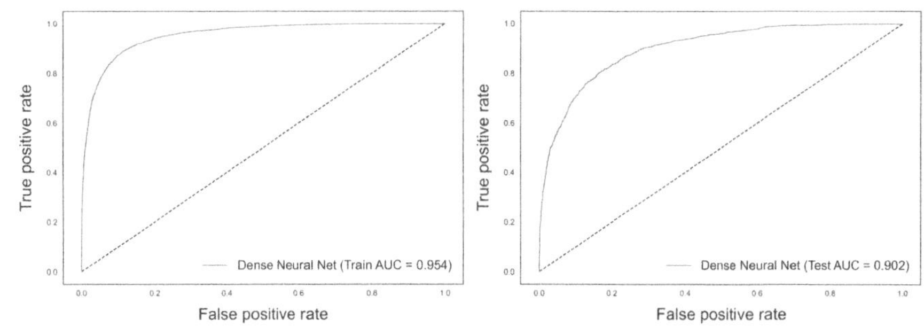

Fig. 2 Receiver operating characteristic curves for sentiment classification for the training set and test set

4 Conclusion

This study used ML techniques to analyze the sentiment of mental health-related tweets in Turkey. In this research, only the automatic sentiment scoring technique was applied for the analysis and classification model development. Future efforts could focus on improving the accuracy and nuance of sentiment analysis through the use of a combination of ML and deep learning techniques with human annotation and on understanding the attitudes and perceptions of Turkish individuals towards mental health.

In conclusion, social media and health data mining are important tools for gaining insights into public perceptions and attitudes toward health and healthcare. By analyzing social media data, researchers can gain valuable insights into public perceptions and attitudes towards health and healthcare, which can inform health policy and practice. The potential of social media and health data mining to revolutionize the field of health and healthcare is vast, and it is an area that is likely to continue to grow in importance in the coming years.

References

1. Kunzler, A.M., et al.: Mental health impact of early stages of the COVID- 19 pandemic on individuals with pre-existing mental disorders: a systematic review of longitudinal research. Int. J. Environ. Res. Public Health **20**(2), 948 (2023)
2. Charlson, F., et al.: New WHO prevalence estimates of mental disorders in conflict settings: a systematic review and meta-analysis. The Lancet **394**(10194), 240–248 (2019)
3. Berry, N., et al.: Why we tweet MH: understanding why people use Twitter to discuss mental health problems. J. Med. Internet Res. **19**(4), e107 (2017)
4. Bucci, S., Schwannauer, M., Berry, N.: The digital revolution and its impact on mental health care. Psychol. Psychother. Theory Res. Pract. **92**(2), 277–297 (2019)
5. Wilson, M.L., Ali, S., Valstar, M.F.: Finding information about mental health in microblogging platforms: a case study of depression. In: Proceedings of the 5th Information Interaction in Context Symposium, pp. 8–17 (2014)
6. Robinson, J., et al.: Social media and suicide prevention: a systematic review. Early Interv. Psychiatry **10**(2), 103–121 (2016)
7. Rabbi, M.F., et al.: Predicting fans' FIFA world cup team preference from tweets. In: Cyber Security and Computer Science: Second EAI International Conference, ICONCS 2020, Dhaka, Bangladesh, 15–16 Feb 2020, Vol. 2, pp. 280–292. Springer (2020)
8. Kuppusamy, S., Thangavel, R.: Deep non-linear and unbiased deep decisive pooling learning-based opinion mining of customer review. Cogn. Comput., 1–13 (2023)
9. Paul, M., Dredze, M.: You are what you tweet: analyzing twitter for public health. In: Proceedings of the International AAAI Conference on Web and Social Media, Vol. 5(1), pp. 265–272 (2011)
10. Sullivan, S.J., et al.: 'What's happening?'A content analysis of concussion related traffic on Twitter. Br. J. Sports Med. **46**(4), 258–263 (2012)
11. Scanfeld, D., Scanfeld, V., Larson, E.L.: Dissemination of health information through social networks: twitter and antibiotics. Am. J. Infect. Control **38**(3), 182–188 (2010)
12. Sakib, A.S., et al.: Identifying insomnia from social media posts: psycholinguistic analyses of user tweets. J. Med. Internet Res. **23**(12), e27613 (2021)
13. Ziwei, B.Y., Chua, H.N.: An application for classifying depression in tweets. In: Proceedings of the 2nd International Conference on Computing and Big Data, pp. 37–41 (2019)
14. Kumar, A., Sharma, A., Arora, A.: Anxious depression prediction in real-time social data. Preprint at arXiv:1903.10222 (2019)
15. Eker, A.G., Eker, K., Duru, N.: Multi-class sentiment analysis from Turkish tweets with RNN. In: 2021 6th International Conference on Computer Science and Engineering (UBMK), pp. 560–564 (2021). https://doi.org/10.1109/UBMK52708.2021.9558958
16. Velioğlu, R., Yıldız, T., Yıldırım, S.: Sentiment analysis using learning approaches over emojis for Turkish tweets. In: 2018 3rd International Conference on Computer Science and Engineering (UBMK), pp. 303–307 (2018). https://doi.org/10.1109/UBMK.2018.8566260

17. Biradar, A., Totad, S.G.: Detecting depression in social media posts using machine learning. In: Recent Trends in Image Processing and Pattern Recognition: Second International Conference, RTIP2R 2018, Solapur, India, 21–22 Dec 2018, Revised Selected Papers, Part III 2, pp. 716–725. Springer (2019)
18. Kirelli, Y., Arslankaya, S.: Sentiment analysis of shared tweets on global warming on twitter with data mining methods: a case study on Turkish language. Comput. Intell. Neurosci. (2020)
19. Guven, Z.A.: Comparison of BERT models and machine learning methods for sentiment analysis on Turkish tweets. In: 2021 6th International Conference on Computer Science and Engineering (UBMK), pp. 98–101. IEEE (2021)
20. Eker, A.G., Eker, K., Duru, N.: Multi-class sentiment analysis from Turkish tweets with RNN. In: 2021 6th International Conference on Computer Science and Engineering (UBMK), pp. 560–564. IEEE (2021)
21. Balcıoûlu, Y.S.: Detection of depression and anxiety symptoms via twitter after COVID-19 with machine learning. In: Baskent International Conference on Multidisciplinary Studies, Ankara, Turkey, 24–25 Feb 2022
22. Mermer, G., Özsezer, G.: Discussions about COVID-19 vaccination on Twitter in Turkey: sentiment analysis. Disaster Med. Public Health Prepared. **17**, e266 (2023)
23. Breiman, L.: Random forests. Mach. Learn. **45**, 5–32 (2001)
24. Friedman, J.H.: Greedy function approximation: a gradient boosting machine. Annals Stat., 1189–1232 (2001)
25. Pedregosa, F., et al.: Scikit-learn: machine learning in Python. J. Mach. Learn. Res. **12**, 2825–2830 (2011)
26. Sarkar, T., Rajadhyaksha, N.: TLA: twitter linguistic analysis. Preprint at arXiv:2107.09710 (2021)
27. Alp, E., et al.: Covid-19 and vaccine tweet analysis. In: Social Media Analysis for Event Detection, pp. 213–229. Springer (2022)
28. Algefes, A., et al.: A text-mining approach for crime tweets in Saudi Arabia: from analysis to prediction. In: 2022 7th International Conference on Data Science and Machine Learning Applications (CDMA), pp. 109–114. IEEE (2022)
29. Abednego, L., Nugraheni, C.E., Fedora, A.: Forex sentiment analysis with Python. Int. J. Adv. Res. Econ. Financ. **4**(1), 46–55 (2022)
30. Blair, J., et al.: Using tweets to assess mental well-being of essential workers during the covid-19 pandemic. In: Extended Abstracts of the 2021 CHI Conference on Human Factors in Computing Systems, pp. 1–6 (2021)
31. Ridhwan, K.M., Hargreaves, C.A.: Leveraging Twitter data to understand public sentiment for the COVID-19 outbreak in Singapore. Int. J. Inf. Manage. Data Insights **1**(2), 100021 (2021)
32. Wolf, T., et al.: Transformers: state-of-the-art natural language processing, pp. 38–45. Association for Computational Linguistics (2020). https://www.aclweb.org/anthology/2020.emnlp-demos.6
33. Yildirim, S.: Comparing deep neural networks to traditional models for sentiment analysis in Turkish language. In: Deep Learning-Based Approaches for Sentiment Analysis, pp. 311–319 (2020)
34. Demirtas, E., Pechenizkiy, M.: Cross-lingual polarity detection with machine translation. In: Proceedings of the Second International Workshop on Issues of Sentiment Discovery and Opinion Mining, pp. 1–8 (2013)
35. Hayran, A., Sert, M.: Sentiment analysis on microblog data based on word embedding and fusion techniques. In: 25th Signal Processing and Communications Applications Conference (SIU), pp. 1–4. IEEE (2017)
36. Reimers, N., Gurevych, I.: Sentence-bert: sentence embeddings using siamese bert-networks. In: Proceedings of the 2019 Conference on Empirical Methods in Natural Language Processing. Association for Computational Linguistics. arXiv:1908.10084 (2019)
37. Budur, E., et al.: Data and representation for turkish natural language inference. Preprint at arXiv:2004.14963 (2020)

38. Ho, T.H.: Random decision forests. In: Proceedings of 3rd International Conference on Document Analysis and Recognition, Vol. 1, pp. 278–282. IEEE (1995)
39. Agarap, A.F.: Deep learning using rectified linear units (relu). Preprint at arXiv:1803.08375 (2018)
40. Kingma, D.P., Ba, J.: Adam: a method for stochastic optimization. Preprint at arXiv:1412.6980 (2014)

Roe v Wade in Twitter: Sentiment Analysis with Machine Learning

Hiba Ayad Allami and Süreyya Akyüz

Abstract Abortion policy has long been a contentious issue in the United States, and the recent overturning of the Roe v Wade ruling has reignited the national debate on this topic. With the widespread use of social media, it is now easier than ever to gather data on public perceptions and attitudes towards healthcare policies such as abortion. The objective of this study is to conduct sentiment analysis on US abortion policy tweets using machine learning techniques. To achieve this goal, a random selection of tweets available to the public was gathered from January 2021 to October 2022. The tweets were filtered based on relevant hashtags related to abortion and the Roe v Wade ruling. The collected dataset comprised over 450,000 tweets, which were then analyzed using an automated sentiment scoring technique based on a lexicon-based approach. A 78.6% accuracy in predicting the sentiment of tweets was achieved through the use of BERT and deep learning. The insights gained from this study can be useful for policymakers and stakeholders in the healthcare industry to understand public sentiment towards abortion policy and formulate effective communication strategies.

1 Introduction

1.1 Background

Abortion policy in the United States has been a topic of heated debate for decades. Since the landmark Supreme Court case Roe v. Wade[1] in 1973, which legalized abor-

[1] https://supreme.justia.com/cases/federal/us/410/113/.

H. A. Allami (✉)
Department of Computer Engineering, Bahcesehir University, Istanbul, Turkey
e-mail: hiba.allami@bahcesehir.edu.tr

S. Akyüz
Department of Mathematics, Faculty of Engineering and Natural Sciences, Bahcesehir University, Istanbul, Turkey
e-mail: sureyya.akyuz@bau.edu.tr

T. Allahviranloo et al. (eds.), *Decision Making in Healthcare Systems*,
Studies in Systems, Decision and Control 513,
https://doi.org/10.1007/978-3-031-46735-6_18

tion across the country, there have been ongoing efforts to restrict access to abortion through various legislative and judicial means. The issue has divided Americans along political and ideological lines, with those in favor of abortion rights arguing for women's autonomy over their own bodies and those opposed to abortion arguing for the protection of fetal life.

In recent years, the political landscape surrounding abortion has shifted. In Jun 2022, the Supreme Court overturned[2] Roe v. Wade, returning the decision on abortion regulation to the states. This has reinvigorated the national debate on abortion, with activists on both sides of the issue fighting for their respective positions. Abortion policy is not just a political issue; it also has significant implications for public health [1]. Access to safe and legal abortion services is essential for ensuring that women can make informed choices about their reproductive health [2]. However, restrictive abortion policies can have negative consequences, including increased rates of maternal mortality, unsafe abortions, and restricted access to other essential reproductive health services [3–5]. Given the ongoing debate surrounding abortion policy in the United States and its potential impact on public health, it is important to understand public attitudes and opinions on the issue. Social media provides a valuable platform for analyzing these attitudes and opinions. Twitter, in particular, has become a popular platform for individuals and organizations to express their opinions on a wide range of issues, including public policy. Twitter enables the analysis of vast amounts of data in real-time and provides an opportunity to capture personal experiences and viewpoints [6, 7]. Several other studies also report that Twitter is used as a platform to analyze public health [8, 9] or mental health issues [10, 11].

Sentiment analysis is a valuable technique used to analyze the emotional tone of a text or a collection of texts. It can provide insights into the attitudes and opinions of individuals and groups towards specific topics, including public policy. By analyzing Twitter data, sentiment analysis can offer a valuable window into public attitudes towards policy issues such as healthcare, immigration, and gun control. In the context of public policy, sentiment analysis has the potential to inform policymakers and other stakeholders about the views of the public on various policy issues. It can also help to identify areas where communication and messaging efforts may be needed to shape public opinion and build support for specific policies. In this regard, sentiment analysis of Twitter data on US abortion policy can be particularly valuable. Machine learning (ML) and deep learning techniques have demonstrated their efficacy in analyzing the sentiment of tweets related to public policy [12].

1.2 Public Policy and Sentiment Analysis

The analysis of public sentiment through social media has become increasingly popular in recent years, with various studies using ML techniques to analyze the sentiment towards different policy issues such as same-sex marriage, hybrid work

[2] https://supreme.justia.com/cases/federal/us/597/19-1392/.

models, nuclear energy, and vaccination. One study [13] focused on the impact of the Supreme Court's decision to legalize same-sex marriage on public sentiment toward gay rights in the United States using Twitter data and a difference-in-difference estimator. The study collected 5,996,741 tweets, mapped 1,028,151 messages to a specific state, and performed sentiment scoring on the most retweeted tweets to represent a larger portion of the data. Another study [14] analyzed public sentiment toward hybrid work models using the RoBERTa approach and Twitter API. The study found that 62.5% of tweets related to hybrid work were classified as positive. Additionally, the study compared public sentiment toward hybrid work with that of remote work. Xu et al. [15] examined public sentiment regarding nuclear energy in German-speaking countries based on public comments on social media. The study used decision tree, random forest, and long short-term memory networks (LSTM) for sentiment analysis and found that LSTM had the highest accuracy at approximately 85.6%. Siegel et al. [16] assesses media coverage of the Tobacco 21 policy using supervised and unsupervised ML methods. The study developed an ML classifier to identify tobacco-related media texts that contained mentions of the policy and used LDA for topic modeling. Valdez et al. [17] employed sentiment analysis to examine the semantic structures of restrictive and protective abortion bills enacted in 2019. The study identified 19 bills using the Legiscan tool and categorized each as restrictive or protective. Chen et al. [18] analyzed public perception towards vaccination in the US by using social media data and ML techniques. The study identifies three vaccine sentiments (Pro-vaccine, Anti-vaccine, Neutral) by using word embedding and ML techniques.

Most of the previous research on sentiment analysis has concentrated on manual sentiment annotation technique or annotated sentiment datasets. In contrast, this paper utilizes an automated sentiment scoring approach through the use of a lexicon method. Furthermore, multiple ML algorithms and deep learning models were employed to develop sentiment classification model.

2 Methods

2.1 Background Materials

2.1.1 Machine Learning Algorithms

Logistic Regression

Logistic regression is a statistical method used to analyze the relationship between a categorical dependent variable and one or more independent variables. It is commonly used for binary classification problems where the dependent variable has only two possible outcomes.

$$p = \frac{1}{1 + e^{-z}}, \tag{1}$$

where p is the probability of the dependent variable taking the value 1, e is the base of the natural logarithm, and z is a linear combination of the independent variables and their coefficients:

$$z = b_0 + b_1x_1 + b_2x_2 + ... + b_nx_n, \tag{2}$$

where b_0 is the intercept term and $b_1, b_2, ..., b_n$ are the coefficients for the independent variables $x_1, x_2, ..., x_n$. In logistic regression, the coefficients are estimated using maximum likelihood estimation, which finds the values of the coefficients that maximize the likelihood of observing the dependent variable given the independent variables. Once the coefficients are estimated, the logistic regression model can be used to predict the probability of the dependent variable taking the value 1 for new observations based on the values of the independent variables. If the predicted probability is greater than a threshold value (usually 0.5), the dependent variable is predicted to take the value 1; otherwise, it is predicted to take the value 0.

Random Forest

Random Forest [19, 20] is a type of ensemble ML algorithm used for classification and regression problems. It combines multiple decision trees (hence the name "forest") to make predictions, each tree providing a "vote" for the final output. For a given input x and number of trees N, the prediction y of Random Forest is obtained as the average of the predictions from each of the N decision trees, i.e.,

$$y = 1 \div N \times (y^1 + y^2 + ... + y^N), \tag{3}$$

where y^i is the prediction from the i-th decision tree. In training, Random Forest builds each decision tree on a random sample of the data with replacement (i.e., bootstrapping), and each tree splits on a random subset of the features. This creates diversity among the trees and helps reduce overfitting, which can be a problem in single-decision trees. This ML algorithm provides an effective way to reduce the variance of the model and improve the accuracy of predictions compared to single decision trees. For this study, we used *sklearn* [21] library to implement random forest.

Gradient Boost

Gradient Boosted Decision Trees (GBDT) [22] is a ML technique used for regression and classification tasks. It is an ensemble learning method that combines multiple simple decision trees to create a more robust model. GBDT uses an iterative process to train decision trees, where each new tree is fit to the residual errors of the previous trees. The final prediction is made by taking the weighted sum of predictions from all the trees in the ensemble. GBDT has been shown to be effective for many real-world applications due to its ability to handle non-linear relationships and complex feature interactions. In this study, a histogram-based GBDT estimator [21] was used. This implementation can be orders of magnitude faster than traditional GBDT. It simplifies the input samples by dividing them into integer bins (usually 256 bins). This significantly reduces the number of points that need to be considered for splitting and enables the use of integer-based data structures, such as histograms, instead of sorting continuous values when constructing the trees.

XGBoost

XGBoost [23] is a machine learning algorithm that is designed to optimize gradient boosting, a technique that iteratively adds weak learners to an ensemble to improve the model's predictive power. It is particularly useful for solving supervised learning problems with large, complex datasets. The formula for the XGBoost model is:

$$\hat{y}_i = \sum k = 1^K f_k(x_i), \tag{4}$$

where $\hat{y}_i$ is the predicted value for the i-th observation, K is the number of weak learners, and $f_k(x_i)$ is the prediction of the k-th weak learner for the i-th observation. XGBoost uses gradient boosting to iteratively add weak learners to the model. At each iteration, the algorithm calculates the negative gradient of the loss function concerning the current model's prediction and trains a new weak learner to predict the negative gradient. The weak learner is then added to the ensemble by multiplying its prediction by a learning rate parameter, which determines the contribution of the weak learner to the final prediction. The formula for updating the model at each iteration is:

$$\hat{y}_{i,new} = \hat{y}_{i,old} + \eta \sum_{k=1}^{K} f_k(x_i), \tag{5}$$

where $\hat{y}_{i,new}$ is the updated prediction for the i-th observation, $\hat{y}_{i,old}$ is the previous prediction, η is the learning rate parameter, and $f_k(x_i)$ is the prediction of the k-th weak learner for the i-th observation. XGBoost also incorporates regularization techniques such as L1 and L2 regularization to prevent overfitting and improve the generalization performance of the model.

LightGBM

LightGBM [24] is a gradient boosting framework that is designed to be efficient and scalable for handling large, high-dimensional datasets. It uses histogram-based algorithms [25–27] to bin continuous features into discrete values, reducing the algorithm's memory usage and computation time. Unlike XGBoost, LightGBM uses a different splitting criterion called the leaf-wise approach, which grows the tree by splitting on the leaf with the largest potential gain in the objective function. This can result in a deeper and more unbalanced tree than traditional depth-wise approaches, but it can also improve the model's performance by exploring more complex feature interactions. It also includes several other optimizations such as data parallelism, feature parallelism, and histogram-based gradient computation, which allow it to handle large, high-dimensional datasets with high accuracy and efficiency.

Long Short Term Memory

Long Short Term Memory (LSTM) [28] is a type of Recurrent Neural Network (RNN) used for modeling sequential data such as time-series data, speech signals, and text. It is specifically designed to handle the problem of vanishing gradients in traditional RNNs by introducing memory cells that can maintain information for a long period of time. A standard LSTM network consists of multiple LSTM cells, with each cell receiving inputs from the previous time step and producing outputs that are used as inputs for the next time step. The internal structure of an LSTM cell is composed of three gates: the input gate, forget gate, and output gate, each of which regulates the flow of information in and out of the cell state. LSTMs are trained using backpropagation through time, where the gradients are propagated from the final time step back to the initial time step. This allows the LSTM to learn long-term dependencies in the input data.

Bidirectional Long Short Term Memory

The Bidirectional Long-Short Term Memory (Bi-LSTM) [29] is a form of Recurrent Neural Network (RNN) that can analyze input sequences in both forward and backward directions. It is useful in modeling sequences with context from both past and future data. A Bi-LSTM network comprises two independent LSTM networks, where one processes the input sequence in a forward direction and the other processes the same sequence in a backward direction. The outputs from both LSTMs are combined and utilized as input for the subsequent layer or for generating the final prediction.

Table 1 Tweets count by hashtags

Hashtags	N
RoeVWade OR RoeVsWade	357,055
AbortionIsHealthcare	165,795
AbortionIsAWomansRight	9,453
WomensReproductiveRights	1,212

2.2 Data Collection

We initially collected 533,515 tweets based on different phrases and hashtags that represent the USA abortion rights policy using SNSscrape[3]. The phrases and hashtags are as follows—"RoeVWade" or "RoeVsWade", "AbortionIsHealthcare", "AbortionIsAWomansRight", and "WomensReproductiveRights". The dataset was composed of tweets that different users posted. It included metadata fields such as the date and time the tweet was posted, the tweet's ID, the tweet's content, the username of the person who posted the tweet, the number of likes, the number of retweets, and hashtags used in the tweet. The tweets were collected from January 2021 to October 2022. Table 1 summarizes the distribution of the tweets based on different hashtags.

Figure 1 displays the data gathered from January to October 2022, indicating a noticeable surge in the number of tweets related to abortion policy during May, June, July, and August. The highest count of tweets collected based on the hashtags exceeded 300,000 in total during May and June 2022. Of significance, the US Supreme Court overturned Roe v. Wade, which was a significant piece of legislation guaranteeing access to abortion as a federal right in the United States, on June 24, 2022. This event might have influenced the increased tweets about abortion policy during the summer of 2022.

For raw data processing, the first step is to clean the data to remove any irrelevant or redundant information. After eliminating tweets that had the same tweet id, we ended up with a total of 457,368 tweets. We removed the usernames and mentions from the tweets. Then we normalized the tweets using BeautifulSoup4[4] HTML parser to convert the character to their proper Unicode form. We discarded the URLs and other web links because these data can not be analyzed by lexical methods. We also removed hashtags and cashtags from the tweets because they are irrelevant to the context of a meaningful sentence. We kept the preposition and punctuation because they are essential for the context of the sentence while using a transformer-based word embedding techniques such as BERT. We also converted the emojis to their meaningful words by using demoji[5]. Table 2 displays the statistics describing the tweets of the data set (Fig. 2).

[3] https://github.com/JustAnotherArchivist/snscrape/.

[4] https://www.crummy.com/software/BeautifulSoup/.

[5] https://github.com/bsolomon1124/demoji/.

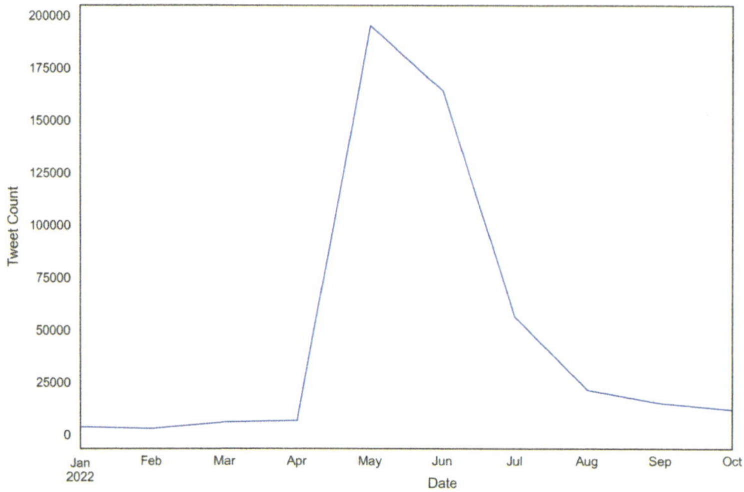

Fig. 1 Number of tweets realted to USA abortion rights from 1 Jan-30 Oct 2022

Table 2 Tweets statistics

Tweets	N	
Total number of tweets	457,368	
Number of unique tweets	450,529	
Total number of retweets	1,265,469	
Total number of likes	5,009,442	
Total number of users	180,499	
Number of unique hashtags	193,720	
Tweets	Mean	Standard deviation
Number of tweets per day	684.68	3174.35
Number of likes for daily tweets	7499.16	48156.24
Number of retweets per day	1894.41	10674.64

The wordcloud analysis revealed the most frequently occurring terms in the dataset, providing insight into the key themes and topics present in the text. The analysis was performed using a custom script with a Python library[6], which generated a wordcloud image based on the frequency of each word in the corpus. The results showed that certain words were more prevalent than others, with some terms appearing particularly salient. The word "abortion" stands out as the most prominent term in the word cloud, which is not surprising given that the theme of the analysis is abortion policy tweets. This finding is significant because it indicates that abortion is a central and highly debated issue on Twitter. Other common terms included "women",

[6] https://github.com/amueller/word_cloud/.

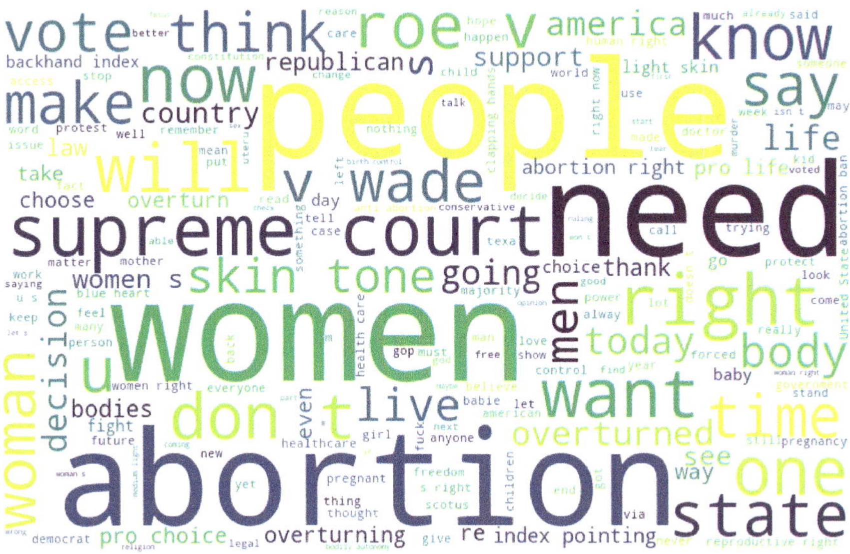

Fig. 2 Word cloud of the USA abortion rights related tweets

"people", "need", "supreme court", "overturned", etc. The significant occurrence of the term "women" in the tweets emphasizes the attention given to the impact of abortion policies on women's reproductive healthcare and their rights. The significance of the term "people" could imply that the conversation is centered around the opinions and experiences of individuals affected by the issue rather than just the policies and regulations surrounding it. Additionally, It could also indicate that the issue being discussed has a widespread impact on society as a whole. In the context of abortion policy, the term "need" highlights the importance of access to safe and legal abortion for those who require it. The term "Supreme Court" reflects the ongoing debate and political attention given to abortion policies, particularly regarding the potential overturning of Roe v. Wade. The word "overturned" highlights the fear and concern expressed in the tweets regarding the potential loss of abortion rights. The repeated use of the term "live" may suggest a focus on the real-life consequences of abortion policies and their impact on individuals. Figure 1 displays the word cloud of the USA abortion rights related tweets.

2.3 Sentiment Scoring

To perform sentiment analysis on the dataset, it is necessary to ascertain the sentiment level of the tweets. This can be accomplished through sentiment scoring, which is the process of determining the emotional tone of the tweets. The sentiment scores derived from this process can be utilized to examine public opinion and understand people's attitudes and emotions toward a particular subject. These sentiment scores can also be input into sentiment analysis algorithms and models to detect emotional patterns and trends within the tweets. In this study, we used an automatic sentiment scoring technique using VADER (Valence Aware Dictionary and sEntiment Reasoner) [30], a rule-based sentiment analysis tool that works well with social media texts. By applying the VADER sentiment library to the tweets, sentiment scores were obtained, which were then filtered to exclude neutral tweets. The resulting tweets consisted of positive and negative tweets only. The resulting dataset was found to have a balanced distribution of positive and negative (51:49 ratio) tweets totaling 371,057 observations. Using VADER allowed for a more nuanced understanding of the sentiment expressed in the tweets and provided valuable insights into the public's perception of the issue.

2.4 Model Building

A two-step process was followed to develop the ML models. Initially, a pretrained word embedding model was utilized to transform the tweets into embeddings. Following this, several ML algorithms and deep learning models were employed.

To generate embeddings from tweets, we used Sentence-Transformers [31] model *all-MiniLM-L6-v2*[7], a pre-trained language model that is intended to serve as an encoder for sentences and short paragraphs. When an input text is provided, the model produces a vector that encapsulates semantic information. The resulting vector for the sentence can then be utilized for various tasks such as information retrieval, clustering, or determining the similarity between sentences. This model was trained using a massive dataset of over 1 billion sentence pairs. Given that the maximum length of a tweet is 280 characters and the model can only process up to 256-word pieces, it is a fitting choice for encoding tweets.

We started building our classifiers by preparing the embedding dataset after generating the word embedding. The dataset consisted of 384 independent variables and one dependent variable, the target class—either positive or negative. We divided the dataset into 80:20 train and test sets. Before applying the ML algorithms, the features were normalized, and the labels were encoded. We initially applied logistic regression as our baseline. We also tried four tree-based ML algorithms—Random Forest, Histogram Gradient Boosting, XGBoost, and LightGBM. Five-fold cross-validation was applied during training, and hyperparameter optimization was conducted for these models. These models' performance was evaluated using metrics such as Area Under the Curve (AUC), accuracy, loss, and F1-score. Since we have non-linear features, we also developed several Neural Network (NN) models—dense NN, LSTM, and Bi-LSTM using *keras*[8] and *tensorflow*[9] library. The deep learning model type,

[7] https://huggingface.co/sentence-transformers/all-MiniLM-L6-v2/.

[8] https://keras.io/.

[9] https://www.tensorflow.org/.

batch size, number of neurons, epochs, and layers were varied with different architectures to optimize the performance. We used 10% of the train data for validation during the training of neural networks. The hyperparameters, such as—the number of neurons, layers, and batch size, were varied to optimize the performance. The *ReLU* [32] activation function was used in hidden layers, and the *sigmoid* activation function was used in the output layer. The loss metric for all deep learning models was *binary cross-entropy*, and *Adam* [33] optimizer was used. To prevent overfitting, early stopping, and a learning rate scheduler were implemented.

3 Results

Tables 3 and 4 display the performance of tree-based ML algorithms and deep learning, respectively. The results show that XGBoost and LightGBM outperformed the other ML algorithms in both the train and test sets in terms of AUC, accuracy, and F1-Score. Logistic Regression had the lowest performance among the ML algorithms. Overall, the dense NN model performed the best, with an AUC score of 0.915 and 0.870 on the train and test data, respectively. The next best deep learning model is the Bi-LSTM which performed slightly worse on the test data. The deep learning models performed comparatively better than the ML algorithms. It's worth noting that the

Table 3 Comparison of the ML algorithm performance

ML algorithms	Train (80%)				Test (20%)			
	AUC	Accuracy	Loss	F1-score	AUC	Accuracy	Loss	F1-score
Logistic regression	0.836	0.756	0.498	0.760	0.837	0.757	8.749	0.757
Random forest	0.825	0.741	8.946	0.744	0.828	0.742	9.291	0.744
Histogram gradient boost	0.820	0.738	0.524	0.741	0.820	0.738	9.433	0.738
XGBoost	0.866	0.778	0.520	0.781	**0.867**	**0.782**	**7.534**	**0.784**
LightGBM	0.856	0.771	0.470	0.774	0.858	0.772	8.203	0.772

Table 4 Comparison of the deep learning model performance

Deep learning models	Train 80%, (validation 10%)				Test (20%)			
	AUC	Accuracy	Loss	F1-score	AUC	Accuracy	Loss	F1-score
Dense neural network	0.915	0.827	0.369	0.829	**0.870**	**0.786**	**0.456**	**0.788**
LSTM	0.869	0.782	0.449	0.789	0.863	0.776	0.459	0.782
Bi-LSTM	0.914	0.829	0.371	0.830	0.866	0.780	0.468	0.780

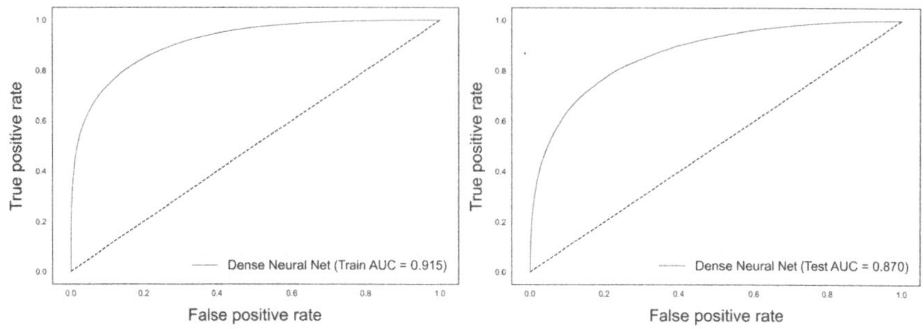

Fig. 3 Receiver operating characteristic curves for sentiment classification for the training set and test set

deep learning models had a smaller difference in performance between the training and test sets compared to the XGBoost model, indicating that they may generalize better to new data. Additionally, the deep learning models had lower losses on both the training and test sets, indicating better optimization compared to the XGBoost model. The receiver operating characteristic curves for the training and test data sets on the best classification model (dense NN) are displayed in Fig. 3.

4 Conclusion

In conclusion, this study highlights the potential of social media and health data mining to provide valuable insights into public perceptions and attitudes toward healthcare policies such as abortion. By applying machine learning techniques for sentiment analysis of social media data, this research sheds light on the public opinion on abortion policy in the United States. However, future studies can further improve the accuracy and nuance of sentiment analysis through the use of a combination of ML and deep learning techniques with human annotation. Additionally, it would be interesting to investigate the factors that influence the sentiment of tweets related to abortion policy, such as political affiliation, gender, and geographic location.

Overall, the findings of this research can be useful for policymakers and other stakeholders in understanding public sentiment toward abortion policy and formulating effective communication strategies. As the potential of social media and health data mining to revolutionize the field of policymaking is vast, it is an area that is likely to grow in importance in the coming years. Further studies can be conducted to explore the impact of sentiment on abortion policy decisions and public opinion.

References

1. Crawford, B.L., et al.: Examining the relationship between Roe v.Wade knowledge and sentiment across political party and abortion identity. Sex. Res. Soc. Policy **19**(3), 837–848 (2022)
2. Lewandowska, M.: The fall of Roe v Wade: the fight for abortion rights is universal (2022)
3. Berg, J.A., Woods, N.F.: Overturning Roe v. Wade: consequences for midlife women's health and well-being. Women's Midlife Health 9(1), 1–6 (2023)
4. Feinberg, E.C., Kawwass, J.F., Cedars, M.I.: Roe v Wade and the threat to fertility care. Obstet. Gynecol. **140**(4), 557–559 (2022)
5. Bermas, B.L.: The unintended consequence of the overturn of Roe v Wade: restrictions on methotrexate use. J. Rheumatol. **49**(11), 1284–1285 (2022)
6. Rabbi, M.F., et al.: Predicting Fans' FIFA world cup team preference from tweets. In: Cyber Security and Computer Science: Second EAI International Conference, ICONCS 2020, Dhaka, Bangladesh, 15–16 Feb 2020, vol. 2, pp. 280–292. Springer (2020)
7. Kuppusamy, S., Thangavel, R.: Deep non-linear and unbiased deep decisive pooling learning-based opinion mining of customer review. Cogn. Comput., 1–13 (2023)
8. Paul, M., Dredze, M.: You are what you tweet: analyzing twitter for public health. In: Proceedings of the International AAAI Conference on Web and Social Media, Vol. 5(1), pp. 265–272 (2011)
9. Li, C., et al.: Public health policy monitoring through public perceptions: a case of covid-19 tweet analysis. Information **13**(11), 543 (2022)
10. Sakib, A.S., et al.: Identifying insomnia from social media posts: psycholinguistic analyses of user tweets. J. Med. Internet Res. **23**(12), e27613 (2021)
11. Marshall, C., et al.: Using natural language processing to explore mental health insights from UK tweets during the COVID-19 pandemic: infodemiology study. Jmir Infodemiol. **2**(1), e32449 (2022)
12. Verma, S.: Sentiment analysis of public services for smart society: literature review and future research directions. Govern. Inf. Q. **39**(3), 101708 (2022)
13. Adams-Cohen, N.J.: Policy change and public opinion: measuring shifting political sentiment with social media data. Am. Polit. Res. **48**(5), 612–621 (2020)
14. Trivedi, S., Patel, N.: Mining public opinion about hybrid working with RoBERTa. Empir. Quests Manage. Essences **2**(1), 31–44 (2022)
15. Xu, H., et al.: Automatic sentiment analysis of public opinion on nuclear energy. Kerntechnik **87**(2), 167–175 (2022)
16. Siegel, L.N., et al.: Do longitudinal trends in Tobacco 21-related media coverage correlate with policy support? An exploratory analysis using supervised and unsupervised machine learning methods. Health Commun. **37**(1), 29–38 (2022)
17. Valdez, D., Goodson, P.: Neutral or framed? A sentiment analysis of 2019 abortion laws. Sex. Res. Soc. Policy **19**(3), 936–945 (2022)
18. Chen, Q., Crooks, A.: Analyzing the vaccination debate in social media data Pre-and Post-COVID-19 pandemic. Int. J. Appl. Earth Observ. Geoinf. **110**, 102783 (2022)
19. Breiman, L.: Random forests. Mach. Learn. **45**, 5–32 (2001)
20. Ho, T.K.: Random decision forests. In: Proceedings of 3rd International Conference on Document Analysis and Recognition, Vol. 1, pp. 278–282. IEEE (1995)
21. Pedregosa, F., et al.: Scikit-learn: machine learning in Python. J. Mach. Learn. Res. **12**, 2825–2830 (2011)
22. Friedman, J.H.: Greedy function approximation: a gradient boosting machine. Annals Stat., 1189–1232 (2001)
23. Chen, T., Guestrin, C.: Xgboost: A scalable tree boosting system. In: Proceedings of the 22nd ACM SIGKDD International Conference on Knowledge Discovery and Data Mining, pp. 785–794 (2016)
24. Ke, G., et al.: Lightgbm: a highly efficient gradient boosting decision tree. Adv. Neural Inf. Process. Syst. **30** (2017)

25. Ranka, S., Singh, V.: CLOUDS: a decision tree classifier for large datasets. In: Proceedings of the 4th Knowledge Discovery and Data Mining Conference, Vol. 2(8) (1998)
26. Jin, R., Agrawal, G.: Communication and memory efficient parallel decision tree construction. In: Proceedings of the 2003 SIAM International Conference on Data Mining (SIAM 2003), pp. 119–129
27. Li, P., Wu, Q., Burges, C.: Mcrank: learning to rank using multiple classification and gradient boosting. Adv. Neural Inf. Process. Syst. **20** (2007)
28. Hochreiter, S., Schmidhuber, J.: Long short-term memory. Neural Comput. **9**(8), 1735–1780 (1997)
29. Graves, A., Schmidhuber J.: Framewise phoneme classification with bidirectional LSTM and other neural network architectures. Neural Netw. **18**(5–6), 602–610 (2005)
30. Hutto, C., Gilbert, E.: Vader: a parsimonious rule-based model for sentiment analysis of social media text. In: Proceedings of the International AAAI Conference on Web and Social Media, Vol. 8(1), pp. 216–225 (2014)
31. Reimers, N., Gurevych, I.: Sentence-bert: sentence embeddings using siamese bert-networks. In: Proceedings of the 2019 Conference on Empirical Methods in Natural Language Processing. Association for Computational Linguistics. arXiv:1908.10084 (2019)
32. Agarap, A.F.: Deep learning using rectified linear units (relu). Preprint at arXiv:1803.08375 (2018)
33. Kingma, D.P., Ba, J.: Adam: a method for stochastic optimization. Preprint at arXiv:1412.6980 (2014)

Time Scheduling for Staff in Hospitals and Health Care Centres

Nursaç Kurt, Ramazan Bakır, and Amir Seyyedabbasi

Abstract As different departments have different scheduling needs, this chapter provides a comprehensive overview of scheduling physicians, nurses, service workers, and office staff. This chapter also outlines procedures for managing employee absences, vacation requests, and shift changes. It provides guidance for creating a shift schedule that meets the needs of the organization and its employees. Finally, it offers advice for dealing with scheduling conflicts and resolving disputes between staff members. The chapter also outlines the process for disciplining employees who fail to adhere to the organization's scheduling policies. It also provides guidance on how to respond to requests for flexible working arrangements. Finally, it provides advice on how to handle sudden changes in staffing levels due to illness or other unforeseen circumstances. There are a number of problems with the existing review papers that have been addressed in this chapter. This chapter provides detailed information on how to manage flexible working arrangements and how to respond to requests for such arrangements. It also provides an overview of the legal requirements and implications of flexible working. Finally, it outlines the potential benefits of flexible working for employers and employees.

Keywords Time scheduling · Decision-making · Healthcare · Machine learning · Hospital staff

1 Introduction and Motivation

Today, staff employment and planning are seen as an important issue in many institutions. There are important studies on this issue, especially in hospitals and health institutions. A lot of work has been done because different departments have different

N. Kurt · A. Seyyedabbasi (✉)
Istinye University, Software Engineering, Istanbul, Turkey
e-mail: amir.seyyedabbasi@istinye.edu.tr

R. Bakır
Sıtkı Koçman University, Muğla, Turkey

T. Allahviranloo et al. (eds.), *Decision Making in Healthcare Systems*,
Studies in Systems, Decision and Control 513,
https://doi.org/10.1007/978-3-031-46735-6_19

planning needs. One of the points to be considered when conducting these studies is to conduct comprehensive research on doctors, nurses, service workers and staff. As a result of the research, it should be determined how much hours the employees can work, how they can adapt to the shift system and how the working performance can be.

Working time choices of staff working in organizations should be made well. In these elections, it is necessary to consider the absenteeism of the staff, holiday requests and shift changes. Staff and runtime choices must be made correctly to provide patients with timely and good care. While making these choices, it is necessary to comply with the obligation of hospitals and other health institutions to have 24-h staff in nursing and emergency services [8]. With planning procedures, we can solve the staff problem of doctors and nurses with flexible working hours. With flexible working hours, employees will be able to work more comfortably. Thus, both happiness and convenience will be provided for working personnel.

Another important issue in health institutions is cost. There is considerable pressure to reduce the cost of healthcare. A factor that affects cost is staff. It is necessary to minimize the total number of personnel to reduce the cost or to keep it under control. The low number of staff affects shift hours and employee motivations. Considering these factors, planning is of great importance. In this section, we will talk about staff problems in health institutions and work on staff planning.

2 Literature Review

Studies on personnel employment and planning in hospitals and other health institutions are still among the important studies today. Provide timely and good quality care to sick individuals. When making these choices, it is important to note that most hospitals are obliged to have 24-h staff in their nursing and emergency units. There are also many pressures to reduce the costs of health care. Health care providers should control the cost. An element that has a significant impact on cost is the staff [8].

Today, only patients who need highly skilled nursing care remain in hospitals. This situation causes personnel planning and time arrangements to be made in hospitals. Many studies have been conducted on this subject. In this article, we aim to give information about the studies carried out.

In a study, a strategic model was developed to solve the staffing problem of doctors in hospitals with flexible working hours [4]. The purpose of the work is to minimize the total number of personnel working on the employment contract. While conducting this study, various legal restrictions and institution-specific personnel policies are also taken into consideration. The model developed in the study simply decides on the number of personnel for two levels of experience. When it comes to two experience levels, low experience and high experience come to mind. It is determined how many assistants and how many specialists work in the institution. Runtimes are created by the model based on different start times and duration lengths. In this study, the problem was first formulated and then a column-building based method was created [5].

To make short-term planning, Brunner and colleagues present a mixed integer programming (MIP) model [5]. MIP refers to an optimal situation in which all doctors have the highest level of experience and are able to perform any task in the hospital [4]. However, the reality in university hospitals does not reflect this situation. Because the story of the patients is very complex, it does not allow generalization. University hospitals are instructed to train doctors with low experience. As a result, university hospitals have to deal with different levels of experience of their staff [4]. To carry out long-term planning, the optimal number of doctors with different levels of experience is tried to be determined. Thus, the aim is to minimize personnel costs.

The model created by using the mixed integer program is divided into weeks. In this separation, the total number of personnel for each week is determined separately in the 1-year planning. The results obtained by solving any one of the weeks have no effect. To solve these weekly problems, a method based on creating columns was used in the study [9]. Normally, column generation is used to solve linear program relaxations in a search tree to find the optimum for a linear program [4]. According to research, a well-known consequence of creating columns is that it provides a lower bound that is as good as the lower boundary that comes from the relaxation of the linear program. This method adds new columns to the main problem. The search for new columns occurs through sub-problems. It acts as a different optimization, guided by the binary solution of the main problem. As a result, the method of creating columns takes into account only a subset of the columns that are suitable at a time, since the number of schedules is very large. Sub-problems have a special structure that allows to efficiently find the column with the most promising and reduced cost [4]. The flow diagram of the column-building method is shown in Fig. 1.

With this model, the problem of creating flexible work schedules of doctors with different levels of experience has been solved. The model indirectly addresses working hours while flexibly creating a task list in a flexible way on the schedule. It also guarantees appropriate staffing ratios and staffing according to hospital rules [4]. When assistants and specialists are taken into account in the examination of the study, it is seen that the proposed algorithm produces results close to the optimum. Additionally, time scheduling is one of the Np-hard problems (nondeterministic polynomial time), which can be solved using metaheuristic algorithms [19–21].

When we look at the literature, the models used in the studies for personnel planning in health institutions are mostly on a linear program. In their study, Martha and her colleagues developed a tool that combines an integer linear program (ILP) with a simulation. The simulation determines the personnel needs required for each period. The integer linear program produces the most appropriate work schedule for the staff, and how many personnel will work in each shift [8]. These two models are integrated into each other. Staff scheduling problems have been studied for many years. In these studies, different approaches were adopted, including mathematical models as well as computational models [8]. A few of these models are built into scheduling systems. The scheduling system has two purposes;

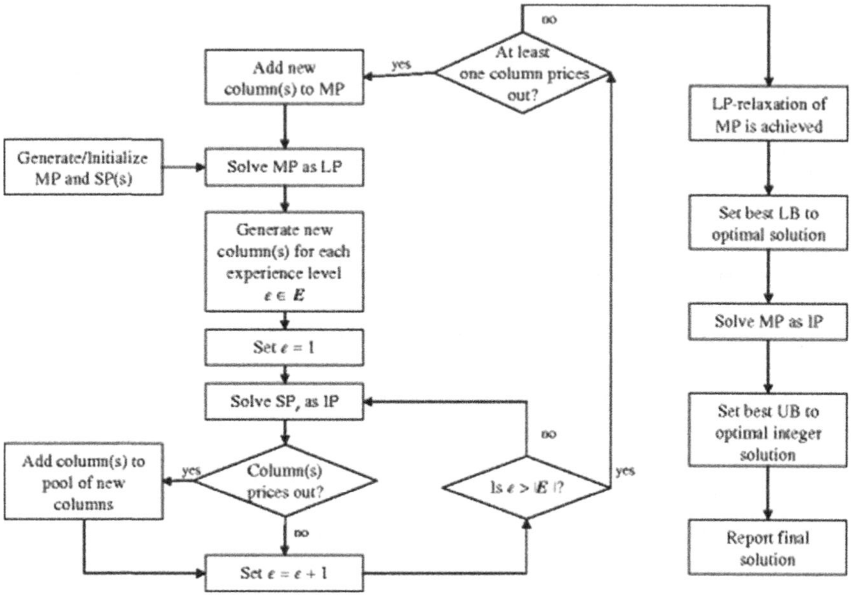

Fig. 1 Flow diagram of a method based on creating columns [4]

(1) To determine the minimum number of personnel to meet the service level requirement.
(2) To create a chart that states when a person should start their shift, the staff level requirement for each period is met and labor law rules are maintained.

More than 60% of the cost of running a hospital comes from hiring staff [13]. Scientific management tools and better timing systems are needed to reduce staff levels. In hospitals, especially in the emergency room, patients may have to wait a long time to get the care they need [8]. Patients are not satisfied with the long wait. Another problem is that the number of employees is reduced for arbitrary purposes. When the number of staff is reduced, both sick individuals and low-staffed personnel are not happy with the situation.

Recently, executives have turned to scientific methods to reduce costs in healthcare and improve their practices. In addition, managers in the healthcare sector are clinicians, not analysts. So they need easy and flexible tools [8]. For this reason, they use a model that integrates simulation and mathematical programming. With this model, it takes into account demand and service times and achieves the optimum number of nurses required per shift. The model was written in AMPL and solved using the CPLEX optimization package. The result of the solution is obtained as a text file that lists all scheduled rounds. However, mathematical models provide few complete answers, but real problems offer partial solutions to better understand the problem [8]. Examining studies in the literature, Khan presented a model proposal in 1991 to minimize resource flow through the network [15]. The resource mentioned in this model is the nurse staff, who must be assigned to departments in hospitals. In his study, Khan proved that using the minimum flow algorithm to solve problems would give the same results as the simplex method. This study may provide some information about the personnel scheduling issue [15]. The problem of staff planning, which is a major problem in health centers, was addressed by Hancock and Chan in a study. With the increasing workload day by day, staff planning by managers has become difficult [13, 14]. While the study was carried out, some aspects such as average levels of personnel, fixed level personnel, permissible overtime and labor capacity were taken into account. For each of these considerations, managers calculated labor cost and productivity for staff [1.7]. Another scientist, Tine, and Ramayana, suggested that the timing problem consists of five stages, or sub-problems. These five stages consist of determining the needs of manpower, recreation blocks, work schedules, and shift schedules. They proposed a different algorithm for each stage and compared each algorithm and solution. They used existing algorithms to analyze each of the stages of the timing problem [23].

The basis of personnel and time planning work is mathematical models. In Baker's work, he solved problems such as shift planning and day planning using mathematics. Provided the service level policy for staff needs on shift timing. In the planning system, he created a model that provides equal assignments of individuals during the daily leave cycle [1].

3 Simulation Usage in Planning

Simulation is used to model and analyze real problems that cannot be solved by analytical techniques. In recent years, the use of simulation as a planning tool has been rapidly increasing in the field of health. According to research, many simulation projects have been carried out for hospitals around the world, especially in Emergency departments [11]. Pitt's work, i.e. resource planning tool simulation, is reported. The overall framework of the project is a model for testing different scenarios in resource and strategic planning in hospitals [18]. The different scenarios cover the comparison of staff levels and patients. In addition, the simulation creates a schedule for the required personnel based on patient waiting time, patient time in the system, and the number of patients treated during the total day.

Simulation models can be an accurate and insightful tool for analyzing and predicting the performance of a system, such as a hospital emergency room, a complex system created by a large number of units. Integer linear programming is an optimization technique used to find the best possible answer to a problem. At the time of an emergency room, the program must meet certain conditions to protect personnel and patients, including maximum shift length or maximum overtime hours [8]. To make simulation and linear programming model useful for emergency department management, these two methods are integrated under a VBA for ARENA implementation. This application is shown in Fig. 2.

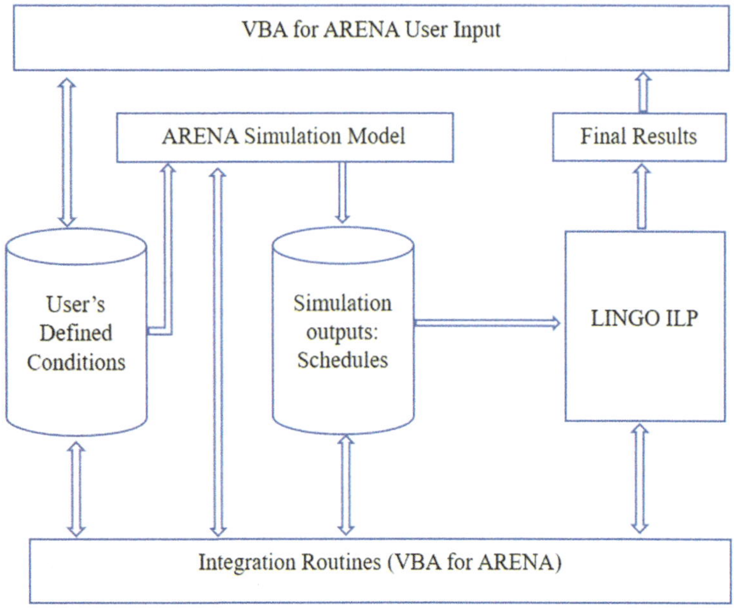

Fig. 2 System integration

The simulation model determines personnel requirements in each of the predetermined periods in a day, given the current demand and service conditions. Member nurses in each of these periods are then automatically fed into the ILP model to create a shift-based 24-h schedule [8]. The analyst patient's arrival model provides the conditions of the current system, such as the service patterns of the servers in the ER system and the target performance level, thanks to user-defined conditions. There are two options to import data into the simulation model. The first option allows the user to manually enter the data into the simulation model. The second option is to allow the user to create text files that contain data for each category. In this study, the second option was chosen for no other reason than to reduce the amount of programming required for this prototype. The user creates text files with a predefined format [8].

The ARENA simulation model calculates the minimum number of personnel required for each of the defined periods. In addition to data exchange from simulation model to ILP model and back to user, a VBA integration routine is embedded in the simulation model to support data retrieval from user [8]. This work provides a tool that combines two tools, such as simulation and integer linear programming, to help the ER and to properly manage departments without overspending.

4 ILP MODEL (Integer Linear Programming Model)

The integer linear programming model deals with the solution of mathematical programming problems that assume that some or all of the variables will receive positive integer values. The difference between linear programming model and integer programming is that in linear programming, the decision variables must be zero and greater than zero, while integer linear programming is expected to receive positive values equal to or greater than zero [3].

The ILP problem is formulated as follows:

$$\text{Minimum } Z = \sum_{j=1}^{n} c_j x_j$$

$$\sum_{j=1}^{n} a_{ij} x_{ij} \leq b_i \; i = 1, 2, \ldots m$$

$$x_j = 0, 1, 2, \ldots tamsayı \; (J = 1, 2, \ldots n)$$

The integer linear programming model is examined in two categories [10]. These are,

1. Mixed integer programming model; there is an integer condition for k of n decision variables, and a positive condition for n-k.
2. Pure integer programming is the integer value of all decision variables.

ILP, an optimization model that is very often used in planning problems, is used to find the optimal number of personnel needed to work each shift. The first step to build the model is to determine the shifts used by the hospital [8]. In addition, the ILP model is used in traveling salesman problems, material use, problems assigning workers to machines, critical road problems and planning problems.

The hospital's emergency services are a complex system of probabilities in which discrete event simulation can be implemented. Discrete event simulation treats time as a continuous variable. Changes in the system occur at different points in time. Continuous simulation is the name given to the continuous occurrence of changes made in the model as time changes. Discrete event simulation has been implemented for production Control, material handling and inventory systems. Simulation analysis has been used in service sector operations. It was used specifically to model queues for a transportation system, bank or hospital admissions Department [16].

Another study presents simulation analysis using a unique approach to programming nursing staff of the emergency room at Georgetown University Hospital (GUH) [16]. This analysis was carried out in three phases.

(a) Patient classification system: Patient sharpness levels are a system designed to determine the degrees of resource needs by objectively specifying nursing tasks at each level of sharpness.

(b) Data collection: A computer-based database is specifically designed to collect ER workload information.
(c) Modeling and simulation: The model is designed according to hourly levels of patient sharpness mix. The simulation was carried out over a period of 1000 h using the computer-based bird.

The first 120 h of the simulation were ignored to allow the system to reach steady state. Upon arrival, patients were given a sharpness, directed to the triage, and sent to the treatment site according to sharpness. In the field of treatment, the patient is examined by the nurse every hour until the period of stay the nurse is completed. The number of nurses provided to a patient depended on the level of nursing care and the level of sharpness [16]. The model was later incorporated into assisted patient care. The auxiliary maintenance parameters were based on the probabilities generated from the database. The current program was first simulated to validate the model by comparing the simulation output with real-time data. To study the impact of these programs on the emergency room patient workload, different types of programs are simulated that may work with fewer shifts or fewer staff. Outputs of CURRENT simulation reports are patient waiting time before being seen to the nurse in the treatment area, patient queues in the waiting area, and personnel use by hours [16]. As a result of this study, a cost-effective program consisting of 12-h shifts is implemented based on simulation experiments.

The model was initially validated by comparing the output of the simulation with the actual data collected in the database using the current personnel program. As a result of this verification, patient waiting time and tail lengths were found to be the same. A cost and benefit analysis comparison of the three options used in this study with the current program revealed that it was the most suitable program for ER in GUH [16].

In modern hospital management, programming people and resources is an important issue. Good planning practices require a variety of financial and social benefits. However, timing is a difficult and time-consuming task due to increased pressure and regulation on missing resources. Fortunately, the ever-increasing computational power of computers and advances in the database has provided an opportunity to improve today's planning applications. In one of his studies, Belien identifies scheduling problems in hospitals and formulates them mathematically. He then develops algorithms to solve them efficiently [2].

Health care is becoming very expensive. The importance of this increase is even more apparent when compared to the growth of GDP. During the same period, GDP growth percentages fluctuated between 2.5% and 5.2% annually [2]. As a result, the increase in health spending outpaces the growth of GDP. The proportion of GDP spent on health services has increased by 1.3% [17].

Planning is an important topic for successful health management. Planning in hospitals is done to specify which resources and time samples will serve what purposes. This research suggests an intuitive algorithm that offers practical solutions to scheduling problems encountered in hospitals [2]. First, it may be preferable to do the work in hospitals, as algorithms help in creating programs. Second, programs created by well-thought-out algorithms should be better than programs created manually. Third, better planning practices can lead to social benefits such as shorter waiting [6]. In addition, studies in psychology have shown that better staff programs have an impact on nurses' well-being and job satisfaction, leading to safer work environments [12, 24].

5 Precise and Heuristic Algorithms

The difference between precise and intuitive algorithms is that they guarantee optimization. Precise algorithms can guarantee the optimization of a system. In contrast, intuitive algorithms are designed to find the best solution with small calculations. Often, intuitive methods lack an optimization proving mechanism. Therefore, it does not give any information about the quality of the solution except that it is the best solution found [2]. In everyday life, intuitive methods are the best choice to be able to solve problems practically. If the problem area is too large, intuitive methods are the only option. Because precise algorithms require infinite computational times. In everyday life, the only thing that matters is to arrive at a solution that is as quick and convenient as possible [2]. In other words, precise algorithms are better suited to developing basic knowledge about the mathematical complexity of the problem. An exact algorithm can be used to integrate the nurse and surgical planning process.

Programming is an important topic for successful health management. The quality of the programs produced and the efficiency with which the programs are developed contribute greatly to the overall hospital performance. Good timing practices lead to more efficient use of resources and reduced costs. Almost all problems are specified using integer programming formulation. Various mathematical techniques are taken into account when developing algorithms. Frequently used techniques are column production, branch and deterministic dynamic programming [2]. When we examine the literature, most of the timing problems encountered are short-term shift scheduling problems involving some type of set or set segmentation formulation [7].

Column generation is used to analyze simple algorithms. The output created by the model made with column production is shown in Fig. 3.

In the study, the problem was first solved by formulating a mathematical formula and then by creating a precise algorithm. Using precise algorithms as well as heuristic algorithms, the results are further strengthened.

When we look at the literature, we see that in planning and scheduling problems, integer programming, column production, and intuitive algorithms are often used. Another nurse shift planning study used exact numbered programming [22]. In this article, the impact of nurse recruitment and planning on both hospital management and health services is also mentioned. In addition, the importance of personnel and timing choices to provide timely and high-quality care to patients is emphasized [22].

As a result of the literature research, many studies have been conducted to solve the complex problem of scheduling and personnel planning. The majority of the methods used in this study are mathematical techniques. These techniques are also known to

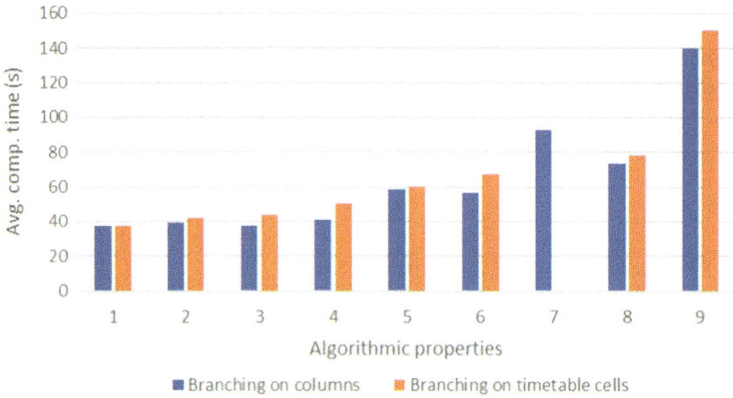

Fig. 3 Contributions of algorithmic improvements

be very effective in algorithm development. Models such as integer programming, integer linear programming, column production and deterministic algorithms have been used to solve the problem.

References

1. Baker, K.B.: Workforce allocation in cyclical scheduling problems: a survey. J. Oper. Res. Soc. **27**(1), 155–167 (1976). https://doi.org/10.1057/jors.1976.30
2. Belien, J.: Exact and heuristic methodologies for scheduling in hospitals: problems, formulations and algorithms. 4OR, **5**(2), 157–160 (2007). https://doi.org/10.1007/s10288-006-0006-4
3. Bronson, R., Naadimuthu, G.: Schaum's Outline of Operations Research. McGraw Hill Professional (1997)
4. Brunner, J.O., Edenharter, G.M.: Long term staff scheduling of physicians with different experience levels in hospitals using column generation. Health Care Manag. Sci. **14**(2), 189–202 (2011). https://doi.org/10.1007/s10729-011-9155-x
5. Brunner, J.O., Bard, J.F., Kolisch, R.: Flexible shift scheduling of physicians. Health Care Manag. Sci. **12**(3), 285–305 (2009). https://doi.org/10.1007/s10729-008-9095-2
6. Buhaug, H.: Long waiting lists in hospitals-Operational research needs to be used more often and may provide answers. BMJ **324**, 252–253 (2002)
7. Caprara, A., Monaci, M., Toth, P.: Models and algorithms for a staff scheduling problem. Math. Program. **98**(1–3), 445–476 (2003a). https://doi.org/10.1007/s10107-003-0413-7
8. Centeno, M.A., Giachetti, R.E., Linn, R.J., Ismail, A.M.: Emergency departments II: a simulation-ilp based tool for scheduling ER staff. In: Winter Simulation Conference, pp. 1930–1938 (2003b). https://doi.org/10.5555/1030818.1031086
9. Desaulniers, G., Desrosiers, J., Solomon, M.M.: Column Generation. Springer Science & Business Media (2006)
10. Doğan, İ.: Yöneylem araştırması teknikleri ve işletme uygulamaları (1995)
11. Fitzpatrick, K.E., Baker, J.R., Dave, D.S.: An application of computer simulation to improve scheduling of hospital operating room facilities in the United States. J. Comp. Appl. Technol. (2014). https://doi.org/10.1504/IJCAT.1993.062626

12. Folkard, S.: Shift work, safety and productivity. Occup. Med. **53**(2), 95–101 (2003). https://doi.org/10.1093/occmed/kqg047
13. Hancock, W.M., Chan, T.Y.K.: Productivity and staffing of hospital units with uncertainty in the demand for service. IIE Trans. **20**(4), 346–353 (1988a). https://doi.org/10.1080/07408178808966190
14. Hancock, W.M., Chan, T.Y.K.: Productivity and staffing of hospital units with uncertainty in the demand for service. IIE Trans. **20**(4), 346–353 (1988b). https://doi.org/10.1080/07408178808966190
15. Khan, Z.A.: A note on a network model for nursing staff scheduling problems. Inf. Decis. Technol. **17**(1991), 63–69 (1991)
16. Kumar, A., Kapur, R.: Discrete simulation application-scheduling staff for the emergency room (1989). https://doi.org/10.1145/76738.76880
17. OECD (2005). OECD health data 2005: Statistics and indicators for 30 countries. www.oecd.org
18. Pitt, M.: A generalised simulation system to support strategic resource planning in healthcare (1997). https://doi.org/10.1145/268437.268753
19. Seyyedabbasi, A.: WOASCALF: a new hybrid whale optimization algorithm based on sine cosine algorithm and levy flight to solve global optimization problems. Adv. Eng. Softw.Softw. **173**, 103272 (2022). https://doi.org/10.1016/j.advengsoft.2022.103272
20. Seyyedabbasi, A.: A reinforcement learning-based metaheuristic algorithm for solving global optimization problems. Adv. Eng. Softw.Softw. **178**, 103411 (2023). https://doi.org/10.1016/j.advengsoft.2023.10341
21. Seyyedabbasi, A.: Binary sand cat swarm optimization algorithm for wrapper feature selection on biological data. Biomimetics **8**(3), 310 (2023)
22. Siferd, S.P., Benton, W.C.: Workforce staffing and scheduling: Hospital nursing specific models. Eur. J. Oper. Res. **60**(3), 233–246 (1992). https://doi.org/10.1016/0377-2217(92)90075-k
23. Tien, J.M., Kamiyama, A.: On manpower scheduling algorithms. Siam Rev. **24**(3), 275–287 (1982). https://doi.org/10.1137/1024063
24. Wilkinson, R.J., Allison, S., Feeney, M., Kaminska, Z.: Alertness of night nurses: two shift systems compared. Ergonomics **32**(3), 281–292 (1989). https://doi.org/10.1080/00140138908966088

Transportation Models in Health Systems

Nursaç Kurt, Ramazan Bakır, and Amir Seyyedabbasi

Abstract Providing transport systems for objects and people that meet the needs of medical centers can be one of the most challenging topics in health care. These models can include single and multi-goods depending on their type and costs. This is because the transport system must be designed to accommodate the specific requirements of the medical center, such as the types of goods that need to be transported, the distances that need to be covered, the speed of transport, and the costs associated with transporting the goods. For example, single-good models are suitable for scenarios where the medical center only needs to transport one type of good, such as blood samples, over a short distance. Multi-good models, on the other hand, are suitable for scenarios where the medical center needs to transport several types of goods, such as medical supplies, over a long distance. The purpose of this chapter is to provide a general overview of the transportation systems and the needs of medical centers within the healthcare system.

Keywords Transportation · Decision-making · Healthcare · Medical transportation

1 Introduction and Motivation

Recently, difficulties in health care have increased. Providing transportation systems in health institutions is one of the most difficult issues in health services. It is necessary to provide transportation systems for objects and people that meet the needs of health institutions. These systems can be costly based on the uniqueness and multiplicity of goods. The transport system needs to be designed to meet the special needs of health institutions, such as the types of goods to be transported. Therefore, the cost

N. Kurt · A. Seyyedabbasi (✉)
Istinye University, Software Engineering, Istanbul, Turkey
e-mail: amir.seyyedabbasi@istinye.edu.tr

R. Bakır
Sıtkı Koçman University, Muğla, Turkey

T. Allahviranloo et al. (eds.), *Decision Making in Healthcare Systems*,
Studies in Systems, Decision and Control 513,
https://doi.org/10.1007/978-3-031-46735-6_20

is too high. The reason for the high cost is the distance to be transported, the speed of transportation, and the costs associated with the transportation of goods.

Health costs in the field of health services have increased greatly in recent years. The transport system is also one of the factors that cause increased costs. One of the factors that are important in-patient care is that patients move from one section to another. It is important to transport patients safely and on time. This transport is critical to meeting certain standards, health status, work, and financial goals. Any other situation may cause a delay in moving. In most health centers, queues are formed almost immediately caused by waiting. These queues and discomforts are experienced by everyone in polyclinics [8]. Doctors, nurses, administrative staff, and patients may be adversely affected. Such situations should also be taken into account when arranging the transport system.

It is known that the transportation system is proportional to cost. The transport system should be well organized in medical centers, hospitals, and other health institutions. Various models have been developed to create these transport systems. In this section, we will provide general information about the needs of health institutions and transport systems from the developed models.

2 Literature Review

In recent years, health care costs have increased significantly. The transportation of patients from one department to another within the hospital is an important part of patient care. The transportation department provides the transportation of thousands of patients. The efficient, safe and timely transportation of patients is critical to meet certain standards, health status, work and financial goals. Delays that may occur can also cause delays in interventions. Queues and discomfort caused by waiting in queues are experienced by everyone in outpatient clinics. This phenomenon is specific to dense, urbanized, "high-tech" societies. We also wait in line in many places in our lives, for example; we wait in line at booths, traffic jams, supermarkets, hospitals, etc. Today, society demands not only high-efficiency and comfortable systems, but also systems that work with minimal cost, without pollution, with little or no delay. Transportation service can also be classified as an intermediate service. A typical intermediate service consists of designing vehicle routes and schedules for 'x' number of users with a pickup and drop-off location.

Transportation is provided by a fleet of 'n' vehicles or a group of employees in a hospital setting [8]. The most common example is door-to-door transportation service for elderly/disabled people or the transportation of patients within the hospital to various test/laboratory centers or various outpatient clinics and then back to their rooms. Many authorities are setting up or restructuring intermediate services in response to the increasing demand for this service. While some existing systems cannot meet the demand, others face increasing operating costs [24]. By 2020, national health expenditures are expected to reach $4.3 trillion and account for about one-fifth (18.4 percent) of Gross Domestic Product (GDP) (Fig. 1).

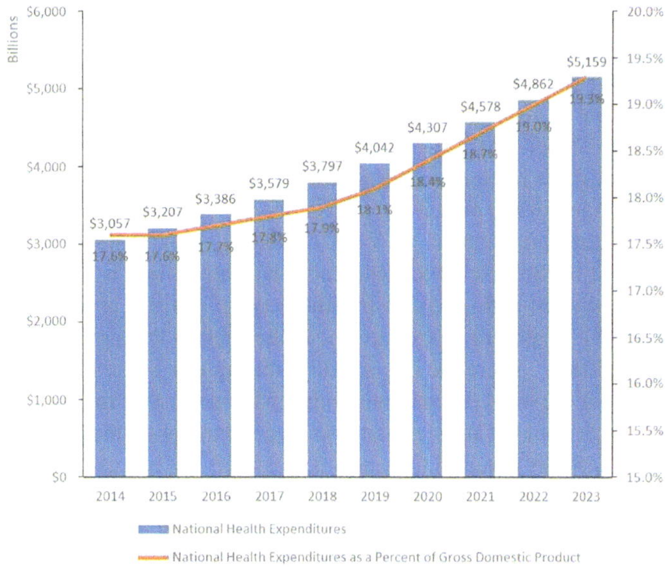

Fig. 1 CMS projected healthcare spending [24]

There is a real need for reliable and cost-effective systems and operations research can help achieve this goal. The transportation of patients within the hospital and the sequencing of outpatient clinics, laboratories and test centers, the design of the practicality of their locations within the hospital must be determined by hospital management. This design can be positioned depending on hundreds of parameters such as the most visited points and points of congestion in the hospital [8]. Patients are usually transported by stretcher, bed or wheelchair. Failure to transport the patient to the unit or department on time causes delays in the services provided to patients, which increases hospital costs, lowers patient satisfaction scores and affects the use of valuable resources. This causes staff to work longer hours in valuable areas such as operating rooms, thus increasing costs to the hospital. In the worst case scenario, a 'domino effect' or 'wave effect' can be seen in these departments. The effect occurs because the patient is delivered late from the appointment time and often delays subsequent appointments, this increases waiting time and patient discomfort [8]. It also increases waiting times for other future patients. In a study conducted at a community general hospital in the US, a software called Tele-Tracking is used for transporting patients within the hospital. Tele-Tracking is a software that nurses enter requests to transport patients from one place to another [8]. This software then assigns tasks according to porters, similar to a central dispatch office. The nurse can also enter special requirements for transporting the patient, such as requiring a wheelchair to transport the patient or other requirements such as an IV pole or other medical equipment [8]. Nurses enter requests to transport patients from one place to another in a software called Tele-Tracking. The software also assigns a priority level to each transport request. For example, a patient transfer request from the emergency department or intensive care unit has a higher priority level than a patient transfer request from one of the medical surgical units. If a higher priority is required for the transportation of a patient, the nurse must call the central dispatch and assign a higher priority depending on the reasons given [8]. When the porter is idle, he calls the system from his current location and the system assigns him a job. The system assigns a job to the porter from the job list according to his current location to minimize his time and distance traveled. If there is only one job in the system, the system assigns it to the first porter who calls. Dispatch Time is the time when the porter calls the system and accepts a transfer request job and is dispatched to pick up the patient [8]. When the porter arrives at the pickup location, the job changes to "In Progress Time". There are major delays during this time. The reasons for the delay may be that the nurse is busy with other patients or that the patient has to go to the bathroom or wait for another porter to come to transport the patient [8]. When more than one porter is required to transport a patient, In Progress Time starts when the first porter arrives at the pickup location. The job changes to "Completion Time" when the patient is dropped off at the drop-off location and the equipment is moved to appropriate storage locations. Sometimes wheelchairs and beds need to be moved to storage areas after a transfer request [8].

The basic problem can be seen as a dynamic intermediate service problem (DARP) with complications due to hospital environment settings. These settings may result from special equipment needs that can significantly increase the time required for patient transportation, such as patient isolation to prevent infection spread [8]. Patient transportation is very dynamic, as most transportation requests are reserved within a short time and it is difficult to plan porters in advance and meet the department's goal of transferring the patient within 27 min from the time the request is reserved until completion [8]. Queue theory is based on A. K. Erlang's work and he initiated the field with his article titled 'Probability Theory and Telephone Conversations [3]. Its applications were initially limited mainly to the functioning of telephone systems. Erlang assumed a spreading distribution for the arrival traffic pattern in the telephone network [6]. Based on the M/D/1 model, he initiated the process of characterizing delay in queue models and completed it in the 1930s as expressed in the formula for average delay [14]. Welch and Bailey pioneered its use in health care by evaluating appointment systems for outpatient departments and scheduling systems and waiting times continued to be the main application in health care until Haussmann took a different perspective to create an index of care quality based on waiting times [25, 36]. Since then, it has been extended and applied to a wide range of applications such as production, inventory management, supermarkets, call centers, computer and communication systems, hospitals, etc. [8]. A queue system can be defined as a system where customers come for service, wait for service if service is not immediately available, and leave the system after receiving service (Figs. 2 and 3).

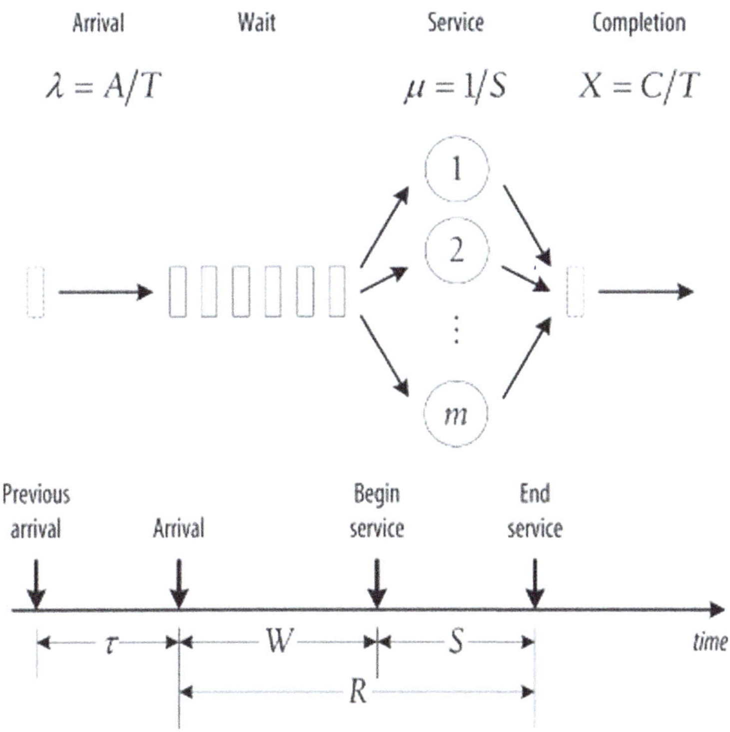

Fig. 2 Fundamental Relationship among queuing theory parameters [8]

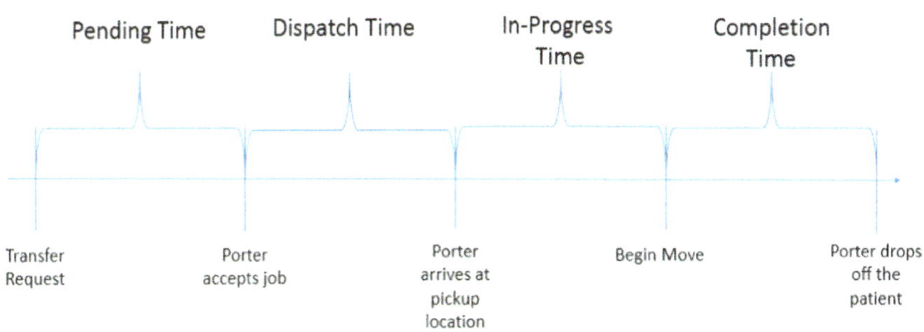

Fig. 3 Time line for transporter movement [8]

The text explains the six basic characteristics of queuing theory, which are [8]:

- Arrival pattern of customers
  - How often customers arrive for service.
- Service pattern of servers
  - How long it takes for servers to serve customers.
- Queue discipline
  - How customers are chosen for service when there is a line.
- System capacity
  - How much space is available for waiting customers.
- Number of service channels
  - How many servers can serve customers at the same time.
- Number of servers
  - How many servers are working to serve customers.

Kendall proposed three factors written as A/S/c to classify a queue model. Here, 'A' indicates the inter-arrival time of the customers to the queue, 'S' indicates the service model described by the probability distribution of the service time and 'c' indicates the number of servers available. The model can also be defined as A/S/c/K/N/D. Here, 'k' indicates the capacity of the queue, 'N' indicates the population size of the jobs to be served and 'D' indicates the queue discipline [13].

A lot of research has been done to show that queuing theory can be used in healthcare situations. A queuing system can be explained by the arrival rate, service rate, and queue mechanism. Siddharthan et al. reported a priority queuing model to reduce patient waiting times in an emergency department as non-emergent patients tend to increase length of stay and delays in the ER [33]. The priority queuing model helped to decrease the overall patient waiting time by 10%, which translated to savings of more than 8000 h of patient waiting time over a year. Tucker et al. used queuing theory to determine the staffing needs for operating room. The study was done to determine the need to activate a backup OR team during the night shift at a designated, verified Level II trauma center [35]. Using data analysis and queuing theory, they concluded that they did not need to activate the second OR team as the probability of two or more cases occurring simultaneously on the night shift is less than 0.1%. Green et al. [9] discuss how to adapt stationary queuing models for use in non-stationary environments so that time dependent performance is captured and staffing requirements can be determined. Dershin et al. used queuing theory to determine the porter staffing level based on a set service level to meet the demand [5]. They also talk about quality improvement project, a centralized communication system between a scheduler and porter using radio and using queuing theory to determine staffing levels. Their analysis also led to relocate an x-ray machine next to the emergency room. This resulted in almost 8000 plus transports per year being eliminated. A redesign of the transport system proved to be a success for the hospital. Singer et al. [34] used queuing theory to improve operations of an ambulance service in Chile. They calculated the key performance indicators [KPI] that concerned the manager and the patient. Episodes of low demand might be interpreted as evidence of excessive idleness. A temporarily high demand might lead to over-investing on resources. In the case of private ambulance services, being mistaken either way can be literally a matter of life and death [34]. An inadequate timely response can be fatal for the patient, while an inefficient operation can drive the organization bankrupt. After identifying when performance was unsatisfactory, for example during shift changes, a tighter supervision was enforced. Instead of over-investing in new vehicles, they concentrated on reducing cycle times. Cochran et al. [4] used queuing theory and simulation to determine the number of beds required in each department (L&D, OB, PACU, NICU, and Triage) for a 200 + bed hospital. The aim is to balance bed unit utilizations in an entire hospital and minimize the blocking of beds from upstream units within given constraints on bed reallocation, which can be applied in any hospital, regardless of busyness level. Balancing the demand for beds can allow highly utilized hospitals to increase throughput [4]. Gupta et al. used queuing theory to optimize staffing levels for the messenger services Department [10]. Queuing theory helped them choose the optimum staffing level based on the waiting time and service level or gives the manager the option of providing more messengers while balancing the operating cost of the Department. A natural way to model porter services is to model it as a multiple server, closed, and priority queuing system. Hillier and Lieberman [11] modeled this to determine the optimum number of porters required for the transportation department in order to meet certain department time targets. Dershin and Schaik used queuing theory to evaluate the effect of porter services on patient waiting times [5]. The model helps in providing insights into service level, centralized- decentralized hybrid systems and setting quality metrics for the department.

McManus et al. [17] used queuing theory to accurately model the need for critical care resources. First, it clearly demonstrates that the realistic capacity of an ICU is significantly overestimated by measures that fail to account for the variability of demand. Since patient arrivals are random, occupancy rates are more appropriately discussed in terms of probabilities. Common measures of utilization, such as daily census and average occupancy, fail to capture flow related stresses in the system and mask the reality that patients may frequently be denied access even if the unit seems less than "full." Also when utilization is maintained at high levels, there is increasing probability that patients will be rejected from the system [17]. The findings were consistent with this because utilization above 85% was associated with rapidly increasing rejection rates. The queuing model shows the exquisite sensitivity of "bed crises" to sudden staffing shortfalls or the presence of patients with extremely long durations of stay. Because both conditions effectively lower the number of available "servers," they rapidly degrade the performance of the system [8]. For this reason, analyses that depend on basic duration of stay averages but do not suitably adjust the number of available servers may tend to overvalue the performance of the system. However, as demonstrated here, if server number is accurately accounted for, queuing theory may be useful in making decisions regarding staffing costs and construction of step-down units. However, queuing theory can only generate the number of transporters required per hour based on service level and patient waiting time. In order to obtain the optimum shift schedule based on the number of transporters required per hour, integer programming needs to be exploited. Integer programming would give us the optimum shift schedule based on 8 h, 6 h, 5 h and 4 h shifts [8]. In the healthcare industry, Zhang et al. [37] utilized mixed integer programming approach for allocating operating room capacity. The mixed integer programming was utilized to develop a model which determines a weekly operating room allocation template that minimizes inpatients' cost measured as their length of stay. MIP model was developed to determine optimal operating room allocation to each specialty. A simulation analysis was utilized to assess the performance of the operating room template [37]. The templates generated by the optimization model could perform poorly in practice when there are high variances associated with surgery length and volatile patient arrival patterns since the optimization model does not account for uncertainty in the problem parameter. Blake et al. [2] utilized linear programming for strategic resource allocation for cases in acute care hospitals. One model sets case mix and volume for physicians, while holding service costs fixed,the other translates case mix decisions into a commensurate set of practice changes for physicians. Conventional models allow decision makers to set case mix and case costs in such a way that the institution is able to break even, while preserving physician income and minimizing disturbance to various practices. The model also helps in finding trade-offs between case mix and physician practice parameters. These models were utilized to investigate the impact of growth and decline within particular segments of the Perioperative Planning Council. The model results suggested growth in the dental/eye/ENT group and decline in the thoracic and oncology services. Ronnberg and Larsson [26] utilized integer programming to improve nurse scheduling in hospital wards as previous scheduling involved self-scheduling by the nurses and final schedules is determined through informal negotiations. Mulholland et al. [19] used linear programming to determine the procedure mix for the surgical department and to evaluate the impact of constrained resources such as operating room time, ICU availability to help determine the procedure mix. Lin, C.K [15] describes using a microcomputer based algorithm to help schedule a monthly roster for porters in a community based hospital. The algorithm helps in generating a schedule in which the hours are fixed but there are other constraints such as if the worker works 2 straight night shift then he/she gets the next day off. Melachrinoudis et al. [18] proposed a model that used mixed integer programming and tabu search heuristics to address a static, dial a ride problem with soft time windows. Beaumont [1] used integer programming for staff scheduling for the police department and taxis service. The problem was a particularly difficult one, as the optimal solution was to weigh in over the customer waiting time for the taxi service or the response based on the severity of the call for the police department. They used the model to invalidate certain assumption amongst people such as it would be better to have no employees and rely entirely on contractors. The model also helped them to ascertain a benchmark for its operating cost. They could compare the actual operating cost to the theoretical minimum from the model [18]. The analyst must decide how to represent the historical data as random variables for each object in the simulation model. The model depends on the input data in order to mimic the real life situation. If the variables are independent, there are three ways to determine the type of input data. One way is to assume that the data is deterministic based on historical data. However, if there is variation in the historical data then the data can invalidate the simulation results. The second method is to fit the historical data in a probability distribution. There are many software available in order to obtain the probability distribution. SPSS can be used for probability distribution. If no probability distribution fits the data, then the last option is to feed the actual historical data itself into the model. The data can be fed as a flat file format or CSV file format. Odegaard et al. focused on the study of porter operations at Vancouver General Hospital [22, 23]. The study focused on the importance of good communications between the departments for efficient porter services. In part 2 of the paper, they used linear programming to optimize the shift schedules and used simulation to assess "what if" scenarios. One of the key findings of the study is that even small and insignificant changes can have dramatic effects. An improved staff schedule not only leads to improved overall performance but helps to meet increased demand and shorter response-time targets. The simulation also helped them to assess and maintain a hybrid centralized-decentralized transporter system. Hillier and Lierberman [11] focused on the effect of porter shift schedule changes using discrete event simulation. The simulation helped in obtaining the effect of change in shift schedule, time varying demand, and increasing the number of prescheduled jobs. The main advantage of simulation was to explore the impact of proposed system changes before implementation. Segev et al. [28] used simulation to study the effects of porter services in a hospital during a construction. Simulation helped them decide on the number of dedicated elevators and transporters required to transport patients to the operating room on time in order for first case starts to start on time. Simulation also helped in understanding the relationship between key parameters such as dedicated elevators, staff, transportation means, magnitude of patient lateness and delayed surgical operations. Nickel and colleagues [21] used simulation to evaluate the use of radiological devices such as MRI machines. They evaluated two different scenarios using simulation. The first scenario suggests preparing the patient immediately after arrival instead of delaying the preparation until an MRI device is available. The second improvement strategy suggests combining the patient queues of three MRI devices into a single queue. The scenario provided high time savings compared to the current situation in the clinic and increased machine utilization by an average of 6.56%. Schoenmeyr and colleagues [27] focused on understanding the delicate relationship between surgical load and the number of recovery beds in PACU and the magnitude of recovery congestion using queue theory and simulation. Small changes in PACU capacity, such as adding three beds, reduced the waiting time for recovery beds by about 60%. A similar simulation study by Ferreira and colleagues [7] observed that flexible surgical planning or increasing the number of post-anesthetic beds significantly increased the efficiency of the surgical center. Flexible planning was better than rigid planning because any surgical team could use the operating room when it was available. In some studies, simulation was used for a specific application. McAleer and colleagues [16] used simulation to find the result of increasing a specific resource for the surgical unit. Since building and improving new space for post-anesthesia care was expensive, they used simulation to determine whether increasing recovery beds would help them and also increase the efficiency of the surgical center.

The text describes how the hospital uses Tele-Tracking software for transport requests and how the historical data is updated every month. It also explains how the number of transporters required to transport a patient depends on the acuity of the case and how it affects the scheduling. The text also mentions some examples of simulation studies that evaluated different improvement strategies for the transport system (Table 1).

Pareto analysis is used to identify the locations with high transfer requests within the hospital. The G/G/c model is used to calculate the minimum number of transporters required at half-hour intervals. The model takes inputs from the user such as service rate and waiting time and gives results using an excel add-in called Queuing Toolpak 4.0 [12].

It has understood the steps involved in patient transport with the porter timeline activity shown in Fig. 4. This activity also helped it to understand the data obtained from the software and the requirement to calculate other metrics based on that. The data also helped it to obtain the distributions for the waiting time and service time. These distributions were used in the excel model and the simulation model. Various departments depend on the transportation department to deliver their patients to their units. The transportation department handles thousands of intra-hospital patient transports. This makes it difficult for the transporters to transport the patients to various locations within the hospital in a timely manner. Any delays in transporting patients can lead to a delay in performing certain procedures, which in turn affects factors such as cost, customer satisfaction. The thesis addresses the manual scheduling of transporters by the manager as a problem [8]. To create a better and feasible schedule for the transporters, the thesis looks into the implementation of a computerized scheduling system that uses queueing theory, integer programming and simulation. The excel model uses queueing theory to determine the number of

Table 1 Attribute explanation [8]

Attribute	Definition
Pending time	Time when the RN/tech keys in the request to transfer a patient
Dispatch time	Time when the transporter who is free accepts the transport job
In-progress time	Time when the transporter picks up the patient
Completion time	Time when the transporter drops off the patient at the destination
Waiting time	Difference in time between dispatch time and pending time
Service time	Difference in time between completion time and dispatch time

transporters required based on user input parameters and constraints that are set by department rules and standards. The generated results are optimized using linear integer programming. The shift schedules for the transporters are completely generated using macros programmed in excel. The main relation that exists between the excel model and simulation model is the validation that is provided by the simulation model for the results obtained in the excel model. The excel model generates the shift schedules based on demand for patient transport, utilizes queuing theory to determine the approximate number of transporters required to meet the demand and also based on departmental metrics. Integer programming was used to optimize the previously determined number of transporters required. Simulation was used to validate the shift schedules obtained from the excel model. This way, one can be certain that the shift schedules that were generated from the excel model were correct and if utilized the department would be able to meet the patient transfer time of 27 min from start to finish [8]. The aim of this research is to improve the staff schedule and the system performance of the transportation department in a hospital. The research combines forecasting, queuing theory, integer programming, and simulation to generate and validate the optimal shift schedules for the transporters. The research also shows how the improved staff schedule can increase patient satisfaction and reimbursement rates for the hospital.

Metaheuristic algorithms can be used to develop transportation models in health care. To ensure access to healthcare services, these models can be used to identify the best routes and schedules for transportation. Additionally, they can be used to estimate the costs associated with providing transportation services. Furthermore, they can be used to estimate the health benefits of improving access to healthcare services [29–32].

When another study is examined, the development of smart cities and big data presents unprecedented challenges and opportunities for operations managers: they need to develop new tools and techniques for network planning and control, and the increased transparency and convenience that can be derived from smart city infrastructure and services call for the development of new operations models [18]. The study aims to make a contribution to theory by presenting the potential of big data to facilitate a city-network perspective to capacity sharing decision making, which is more efficient than individual health care transport schemes taking independent decisions, which often leads to duplication and inefficiency with ambulance capacity failing to meet volatile and rapidly changing demand with resulting unacceptable levels of performance variance, in particular in dealing with emergencies [18]. Our primary purpose was to build a framework and to provide initial Markovian results investigating the interplay of big data and smart cities with transport sharing and to assess how this could improve performance. To advance the framework and preliminary Markovian model we intend to extend our research investigation through intensive case studies of health care transport operations in the UK, US, France, and the Middle East. We emphasize the importance of "big data" orientations and related management and operations issues to be analyzed with Markovian theoretical framing as an area in which further research is urgently needed. Future operational performance is linked with these sharing orientations which can ensure

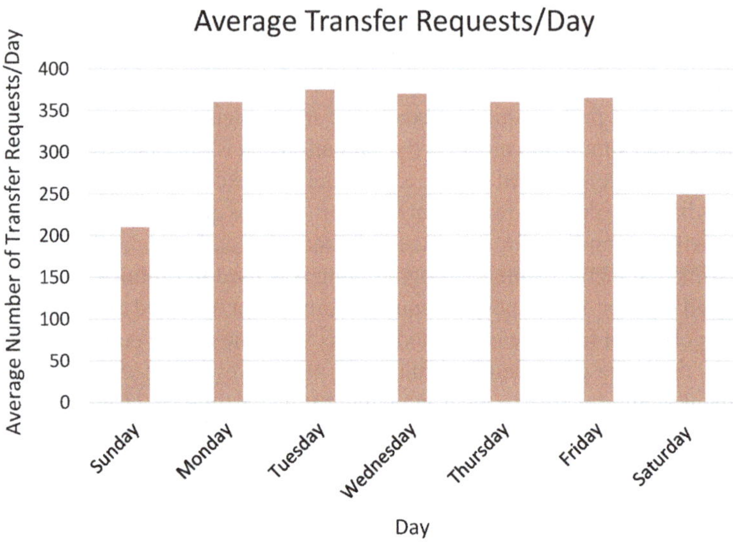

Fig. 4 Average number of transfer request/day [8]

unique service delivery competitive advantage and urban performance. Further case studies are therefore needed.

References

1. Beaumont, N.B.: Scheduling staff using mixed integer programming. Eur. J. Oper. Res. **98**(3), 473–484 (1997). https://doi.org/10.1016/s0377-2217(97)00055-6
2. Blake, J.G., Carter, M.R.: A goal programming approach to strategic resource allocation in acute care hospitals. Eur. J. Oper. Res. **140**(3), 541–561 (2002). https://doi.org/10.1016/s0377-2217(01)00219-3
3. Brockmayer, E.: Table of Erlang's loss formula, the life and works of AK Erlang. Trans. Danish Acad. Tech. Sci. **1**, 268–275 (1948)
4. Cochran, J.K., Bharti, A.: Stochastic bed balancing of an obstetrics hospital. Health Care Manag. Sci. **9**(1), 31–45 (2006). https://doi.org/10.1007/s10729-006-6278-6
5. Dershin, H., Schaik, M.S.: Quality improvement for a hospital patient transportation system. PubMed **38**(1), 111–119 (1993). https://pubmed.ncbi.nlm.nih.gov/10127289
6. Erlang, A.K., Brockmeyer, E., M, Halstr, H.L., Jensen, A.: The Life and Works of AK Erlang. Danish Academy of Technical Sciences (1948)
7. Ferreira, R.L., Coelli, F.C., De Albuquerque Pereira, W.C., De Almeida, R.M.V.R.: Optimizing patient flow in a large hospital surgical centre by means of discrete-event computer simulation models. J. Eval. Clin. Pract. **14**(6), 1031–1037 (2008). https://doi.org/10.1111/j.1365-2753.2007.00939.x
8. Gopal, K.: Modeling and Optimization of Hospital Transportation System (2016)
9. Green, L.K.: Queueing Analysis in Healthcare. In: International series in management science/operations research, pp. 281–307. Springer Science+Business Media (2006). https://doi.org/10.1007/978-0-387-33636-7_10

10. Gupta, I.D., Zoreda, J., Kramer, N.: Hospital manpower planning by use of queueing theory. PubMed **6**(1), 76–82 (1971). https://pubmed.ncbi.nlm.nih.gov/5569229
11. Hillier, F.S., Lieberman, G.J.: Introduction to Operations Research. Technometrics **10**(2), 410 (1968). https://doi.org/10.2307/1267061
12. Ingolfsson, A.: Queueing ToolPak. http://queueingtoolpak.org/. Accessed 1 Jan 2015
13. Kendall, D.A.: Stochastic processes occurring in the theory of queues and their analysis by the method of the imbedded Markov Chain. Ann. Math. Stat. **24**(3), 338–354 (1953). https://doi.org/10.1214/aoms/1177728975
14. Kleinrock, L.: Queueing Systems, Vol. 1: Theory (1975). https://www.bookdepository.com/Queueing-Systems---Theory-Volume-1-Leonard-Kleinrock/9788126546039
15. Lin, C.K.Y.: Microcomputer-based workforce scheduling for hospital porters. J. Manag. Med. **13**(4), 251–262 (1999). https://doi.org/10.1108/02689239910290992
16. McAleer, W., Turner, J.J., Lismor, D., Naqvi, I.: Simulation of a hospital's theatre suite. J. Manag. Med. **9**(5), 14–26 (1995). https://doi.org/10.1108/02689239510096785
17. McManus, M.L., Long, M.C., Cooper, A., Litvak, E.: Queuing theory accurately models the need for critical care resources. J. Am. Soc. Anesthesiol. **100**(5), 1271–1276 (2004)
18. Mehmood, R., Graham, G.: Big data logistics: A health-care transport capacity sharing model. Proc. Comput. Sci. **64**, 1107–1114 (2015). https://doi.org/10.1016/j.procs.2015.08.566
19. Melachrinoudis, E., Ilhan, A.B., Min, H.: A dial-a-ride problem for client transportation in a health-care organization. Comput. Oper. Res. **34**(3), 742–759 (2007). https://doi.org/10.1016/j.cor.2005.03.024
20. Mulholland, M.W., Abrahamse, P., Bahl, V.: Linear programming to optimize performance in a department of surgery. J. Am. Coll. Surg. **200**(6), 861–868 (2005). https://doi.org/10.1016/j.jamcollsurg.2005.01.001
21. Nickel, S., Schmidt, U.A.: Process improvement in hospitals: a case study in a radiology department. Quality Manag. Healthc. **18**(4), 326–338 (2009)
22. Ødegaard, F., Chen, L., Quee, R., Puterman, M.L.: Improving the efficiency of hospital porter services, part 1: study objectives and results. J. Healthc. Qual. **29**(1), 4–11 (2007a). https://doi.org/10.1111/j.1945-1474.2007.tb00169.x
23. Ødegaard, F., Chen, L., Quee, R., Puterman, M.L.: Improving the efficiency of hospital porter services, part 2: schedule optimization and simulation model. J. Healthc. Qual. **29**(1), 12–18 (2007b). https://doi.org/10.1111/j.1945-1474.2007.tb00170.x
24. Projected|CMS. (n.d.). https://www.cms.gov/Research-Statistics-Data-and-Systems/Statistics-Trends-and-Reports/NationalHealthExpendData/NationalHealthAccountsProjected
25. Rk, H.: Waiting time as an index of quality of nursing care. PubMed **5**(2), 92–105 (1970). https://pubmed.ncbi.nlm.nih.gov/5482376
26. Rönnberg, E., Larsson, T.: Automating the self-scheduling process of nurses in Swedish health-care: a pilot study. Health Care Manag. Sci. **13**(1), 35–53 (2010). https://doi.org/10.1007/s10729-009-9107-x
27. Schoenmeyr, T., Dunn, P.O., Tsitsiklis, J.N., Levi, R., Berger, D.H., Daily, B., Levine, W.C., Sandberg, W.S.: A model for understanding the impacts of demand and capacity on waiting time to enter a congested recovery room. Anesthesiology **110**(6), 1293–1304 (2009). https://doi.org/10.1097/aln.0b013e3181a16983
28. Segev, D., Levi, R., Dunn, P.O., Sandberg, W.S.: Modeling the impact of changing patient transportation systems on peri-operative process performance in a large hospital: insights from a computer simulation study. Health Care Manag. Sci. **15**(2), 155–169 (2012). https://doi.org/10.1007/s10729-012-9191-1
29. Seyyedabbasi, A.: WOASCALF: a new hybrid whale optimization algorithm based on sine cosine algorithm and levy flight to solve global optimization problems. Adv. Eng. Softw. **173**, 103272 (2022). https://doi.org/10.1016/j.advengsoft.2022.103272
30. Seyyedabbasi, A.: A reinforcement learning-based metaheuristic algorithm for solving global optimization problems. Adv. Eng. Softw. **178**, 103411 (2023). https://doi.org/10.1016/j.advengsoft.2023.10341

31. Seyyedabbasi, A.: Binary sand cat swarm optimization algorithm for wrapper feature selection on biological data. Biomimetics **8**(3), 310 (2023)
32. Seyyedabbasi, A., Kiani, F., Allahviranloo, T., Fernandez-Gamiz, U., Noeiaghdam, S.: Optimal data transmission and pathfinding for WSN and decentralized IoT systems using I-GWO and Ex-GWO algorithms. Alex. Eng. J. **63**, 339–357 (2023)
33. Siddharthan, K., Jones, W.W., Johnson, J.R.: A priority queuing model to reduce waiting times in emergency care. Int. J. Health Care Qual. Assur. **9**(5), 10–16 (1996). https://doi.org/10.1108/09526869610124993
34. Singer, M., Donoso, P.: Assessing an ambulance service with queuing theory. Comput. Oper. Res. **35**(8), 2549–2560 (2008). https://doi.org/10.1016/j.cor.2006.12.005
35. Tucker, J.D., Barone, J.E., Cecere, J., Blabey, R.G., Rha, C.: Using queueing theory to determine operating room staffing needs. J. Trauma-Inj. Infect. Crit. Care **46**(1), 71–79 (1998). https://doi.org/10.1097/00005373-199901000-00012
36. Welch, J.D., Bailey, N.: Appointment systems in hospital outpatient departments. The Lancet **259**(6718), 1105–1108 (1952). https://doi.org/10.1016/s0140-6736(52)90763-0
37. Zhang, B., Murali, P., Dessouky, M., Belson, D.: A mixed integer programming approach for allocating operating room capacity. J. Oper. Res. Soc. **60**(5), 663–673 (2009). https://doi.org/10.1057/palgrave.jors.2602596

Correction to: Boosting Facial Action Unit Detection with CGAN-Based Data Augmentation

Duygu Cakir, Gorkem Yilmaz, and Nafiz Arica

Correction to:
Chapter "Boosting Facial Action Unit Detection with CGAN-Based Data Augmentation" in: T. Allahviranloo et al. (eds.), *Decision Making in Healthcare Systems, Studies in Systems*, Decision and Control 513, https://doi.org/10.1007/978-3-031-46735-6_13

In the original version of the book was inadvertently published without including the second author name (Gorkem Yilmaz) in chapter 13. The Author has been now updated as "Duygu CAKIR, Gorkem YILMAZ, Nafiz ARICA". The correction chapter and the book have been updated with the changes.

The updated version of this chapter can be found at
https://doi.org/10.1007/978-3-031-46735-6_13

T. Allahviranloo et al. (eds.), *Decision Making in Healthcare Systems*,
Studies in Systems, Decision and Control 513,
https://doi.org/10.1007/978-3-031-46735-6_21

The manufacturer's authorised representative in the EU is Springer Nature Customer Service Centre GmbH, Europaplatz 3, 69115 Heidelberg, Germany. If you have any concerns regarding our products, please contact ProductSafety@springernature.com

Printed and bound by CPI Group (UK) Ltd, Croydon, CR0 4YY
28/09/2026
02224056-0008